Ethics: Working with Ethical and Moral Dilemmas in Psychotherapy

Ethics: Working with Ethical and Moral Dilemmas in Psychotherapy

PETRŪSKA CLARKSON FBPsS, FBAC

Professor of Counselling and Psychotherapy,
University of Surrey

W

WHURR PUBLISHERS

LONDON AND PHILADELPHIA

© 2000 Whurr Publishers
First published 2000 by
Whurr Publishers Ltd
19b Compton Terrace, London N1 2UN, England and
325 Chestnut Street, Philadelphia PA 1906, USA

British Library Cataloguing in Publication Data
A catalogue record for this book is available from the
British Library.

ISBN: 1 86156 112 1

Printed and bound by CPI Antony Rowe Ltd, Eastbourne

Contents

Contributors   viii

Dedication   x

Marianne Fry Resigns   xi

Preface   Ethics, the Heart of the Matter   xiii

Acknowledgements   xxix

Chapter 1   1

Ethical Dilemmas of Psychotherapists (with Geoff Lindsay)

Item 1   17

The Psychotherapy and Counselling Oath (with Mark Aveline)

Chapter 2   20

Ethical Relationships

Item 2   41

A Decision-making Hierarchy Regarding Ethical Issues

Chapter 3   48

Values in Counselling and Psychotherapy

Item 3   59

Discovering Your Own Values

Chapter 4   61

Bystanding in Counselling and Psychotherapy

Item 4   73

Bystanding and Responsible Involvement in Psychotherapy, Organisations and Society

Chapter 5   **75**
In Recognition of Dual Relationship

Item 5   89
Information for Prospective Clients

Chapter 6   **96**
Vengeance of the Victim

Item 6   107
'Asking the Client's Permission' to do a Case Study

Chapter 7   **113**
When Rules are not Enough: The Spirit of the Law in Ethical Codes
(with Lesley Murdin)

Item 7   122
Professional Practices and Ethical Guidelines for Administrative/
Ancillary Staff at Counselling and Psychotherapy Practices, Institutes
and Colleges

Chapter 8   **126**
Collegial Working Relationships – Ethics, Research and Good
Practice (with Geoff Lindsay)

Item 8   150
Libel, Slander and Defamation and their Derivatives in Professional
Codes of Ethics (with Vincent Keter)

Chapter 9   **154**
The Ethical Dimensions of Supervision (with Lesley Murdin)

Item 9   168
What Happens if a Psychotherapist Dies? (with Barbara Traynor)

Chapter 10   **173**
Ethical Dilemmas in Supervision, Training and Organisational Contexts
(with Geoff Lindsay)

Item 10   191
Seven Domains of Discourse in Exploring Ethical and Moral Dilemmas

Chapter 11   **199**
Whose Idea is it Anyway? (and Writing for Publication)

Item 11 219
A Code of Ethics for Counselling and Psychotherapy Publications

Chapter 12 222
Psychotherapy Ethics in the Context of 'Schoolism'

Item 12 237
Physis – or 'a Pleasing Illusion'

Chapter 13 242
Judicial Review of Psychotherapy Self-regulation (with Vincent Keter)

Item 13 250
Thought Experiments and Imaginary Dilemmas for People Involved in Complaints Procedures

Chapter 14 253
Integrative Relational Research: An Approach to Ethics

Item 14 288
Extract from *Letters to a Young Poet* by Rainer Maria Rilke

Appendix 1 289
A Traveller's Guide to Psychotherapy: a Companion for Clients and Patients

Appendix 2 305
Dysfunction in Training Organisations (by Chris Robertson)

Contributors

Mark Aveline has been a consultant medical psychotherapist in Nottingham since 1974. His chief interests are in the development of a range of effective psychotherapies suitable for NHS practice, and teaching the necessary skills at undergraduate, post-qualification and specialist levels. He has a special interest in group and focal therapy and programming in 4th Dimension, a relational database. Administrative responsibilities include: member of the Governing Board of the United Kingdom Council for Psychotherapy (1992–98), President of the British Association for Counselling (1994), Chair of the Psychotherapy Training Specialist Advisory Committee of the Royal College of Psychiatrists (1995–98) and UK President of the Society of Psychotherapy Research (1996–99).

Petrūska Clarkson is a consultant philosopher, chartered clinical, counselling and chartered occupational psychologist, registered child, individual and group psychotherapist, accredited supervisor and management consultant with almost 30 years' international experience and more than 150 publications (22 languages) in these fields. She works at the Centre for Qualitative Research in Psychotherapy Training and Supervision at PHYSIS, London, is Professor of Counselling and Psychotherapy at Surrey University, Roehampton and is visiting professor at Westminster University as well as at other training institutions and universities in the UK and abroad. She was Honorary Secretary of the Universities Psychotherapy Association and has served on many ethics boards including being the chair of the PS section of the UKCP.

Vincent Keter is an artist who has trained as a barrister in order to assist his wife and others to obtain justice and fair process. He then fell in love with the law as well. He is the author of several papers and is currently researching for a book on psychotherapy and the law while doing a Ph.D. at Birkbeck College, University of London on psychoanalysis and the law.

Geoff Lindsay is Director of the Psychology and Special Needs Research Unit and of the Centre for Educational Development Appraisal and Research in the Institute of Education, University of Warwick, and is a Chartered Psychologist. He is a former President of the British Psychological Society, a former Chair of its Investigatory Committee, and now a member of the Society's Disciplinary Board. He is also convenor of the European Federation of Professional Psychologists Associations Standing Committee on Ethics.

Lesley Murdin is a psychoanalytic psychotherapist with a private practice in Cambridge. She organises training for the Westminster Pastoral Foundation in Psychodynamic Counselling and Psychotherapy where she teaches and supervises. She is the Chair of the Psychoanalytic Section of the United Kingdom Council for Psychotherapy, a member of the Governing Board and is past Chair of its Ethics Committee.

Chris Robertson is a registered psychotherapist and has been a supervisor and a trainer since 1978. As well as psychosynthesis, he has studied meditation, child psychotherapy and family therapy. He is a co-founder and director of Re·Vision and acts as a consultant to other training organisations.

Barbara Traynor is a registered psychotherapist and has been a supervisor and a trainer for many years. She is a Provisional Teaching and Supervising Transactional Analyst (with Clinical Speciality), a past editor of the *ITA News*, and runs training courses for organisations and groups. She has a private psychotherapy and supervision practice in London.

Dedication

In memoriam
MARIANNE FRY
A good friend and spiritual person,
and co-founder of
the Gestalt Psychotherapy Training Institute (UK)

Marianne Fry was heard and sanctioned by junior colleagues with apparent bias on a code of ethics which did not even exist at the time. Whatever the rights and wrongs of her actions, this kind of *process* is considered a violation of natural justice. Her letter of resignation and the announcement of her death in the GPTI Newsletter are reprinted here as profound food for thought and reflection on the theory and practice of ethics and complaints processes in our profession.

Reprinted from the Gestalt Psychotherapy Training Institute (UK) Newsletter

Marianne Fry Resigns

Marianne has sent us her resignation letter that she sent to The Executive and has asked us to print it. We include it below in full.

Dear GPTI Executive,

Peter has just spoken to me on the telephone, and I understand that some decision in this long drawn-out process is essential for your survival as an accredited institution. I have therefore decided to tender my resignation as a registered member of GPTI.

My feelings are a mixture of sadness and relief. The event which led to the complaint against me happened four years ago. I can only describe my own process over that time. My first reaction was disbelief and angry pride which led to my refusal to take action, or defend myself adequately. I saw myself unjustly victimised and found it hard to believe that my own colleagues and friends could take actions against me. Surely everyone knew that I have always been a respected and ethical practitioner.

During the last year I have started looking inwards. Life events have significantly contributed to this. My husband Peter's death, my accident, my long illness. When Peter died last October, I said to a friend, 'this is the end of my apprenticeship'. My friend replied 'then now you must be a master'. I think that the events in my professional life echo this. I have stopped seeing myself as a victim and now regard the complaint as a last clearing out of the shadows of the old persecution I experienced in my youth.

As you know, what hasn't been dealt with keeps re-emerging. The other important factor for me is my difficulty in letting go – of the past, of people, of work, of old connections. The Buddhists have taught me much about constant change, and the illusion of regarding any structures as permanent. I am learning that resistance never really succeeds, and that controlling the flow of life is impossible. I have become aware that in this situation nobody truly acted out of love (without fear) and that includes me. Arriving at a place of mutual love was the furthest thing on my mind.

I now see my resignation as a surrender rather than defeat – leaving the level of ego where only one side can win. Surrender is faith in the power of love. Struggle is always against myself and I am committed to end struggle and to come from love. I frequently fail in that direction, but I have set a spiritual goal for myself which can act as a constant reminder to substitute awareness for reactions. I want my future – the years I have left – to be open and free; to cease holding on to anger, pride and mistrust. I want to part from you with love, appreciation and gratitude for our past connection and the transforming work that flowed between us. I leave you feeling happy in the knowledge that our contact will be unchanged in spirit – free from the ballast of the imprisoning past.

Yours as ever

Marianne Fry

Since this newsletter went to press, we received the sad news that Marianne had died.

Preface

Ethics, the Heart of the Matter

> What the postmodern mind is aware of is that there are problems in human and social life with no good solutions, twisted trajectories than cannot be straightened up, ambivalences that are more than linguistic blunders yelling to be corrected, doubts which cannot be legislated out of existence, moral agonies which no reason-dictated recipes can soothe, let alone cure.
> (Bauman 1993, p. 245)

The word ethics is essentially derived from the Greek *ethos* which means the prevalent tone of sentiment of a people or community; the genius of an institution or system.

Introduction

Moral and ethical dilemmas are the mainsprings of most human dramas and arguably the most challenging dimension of working as a mental health professional in any sphere. Most such dilemmas involve us as persons *and* as professionals in a social–legal cultural context which require increasing demands on our abilities to deal with conceptual complexity and practical skills in generating, considering and implementing possibilities.

This book has a very modest aim – to contribute an invitation to *stimulate your own thinking* and feeling, imagination and valuing about ethics and morality in the helping professions – particularly in psychoanalysis, psychology, psychotherapy and counselling. (These terms, as well as client or patient, are used interchangeably throughout the book.)

It is possible to see the primary task of psychotherapy as the restoration of relationship with oneself, with others, with the world. The work of the psychotherapist is, in one way or another, conducted through relationship. Like all other relationships, therefore, it is vulnerable to all the ills which we already know. Because of its particular intimacy, the therapeutic relationship is perhaps more vulnerable than most.

A good way to start reading this book is to think of the most difficult professional ethical problem you yourself ever had to face, and to keep that problem in mind until the end of the book – or of whichever chapter you choose to read first – when you may want to discuss it further with others.

The definition of ethics in all its senses which I am using in this book comes from the *Concise Oxford Dictionary:* (a) relating to morals, (b) a treatise on the science of morals, (c) the rules of conduct recognised in certain limited departments of human life such as psychotherapy, and (d) the science of human duty in its widest extent, including besides ethics proper, the science of law whether civil, political or international.

Personal introduction

My own interest in ethics came as birthright – I was born a white South African. I was thus catapulted from the very beginning into ethical and moral and legal dilemmas by my very existence. I have since been active in the development and enactment and researching of ethics and ethics codes conducting new research and replicating studies done in North America and elsewhere. From disciplinary and theoretical points of view, I have worked as a chartered clinical, counselling and accredited research psychologist, management consultant, supervisor, trainer and professional founder, chair and leader of several professional organisations. In this process, I have acquired extensive training and experience to supervisor or teaching member level in psychoanalytic, Jungian, integrative, existential and humanistic approaches over a period of almost 30 years and several continents.

Much as I value and love the craft and the poetry of each of these unique 'psycho-languages', I also try to heed Jung's (1928) advice to: 'Learn your theories as well as you can, but put them aside when you touch the miracle of the living soul' (p. 361). During this last quarter-century, I have also been privileged to work formally with ethics complaints; for example, I was Chair of the Ethics Committee of the HIPS section of the UKCP and on the Ethics Committee of the British Association for Psychoanalytic and Psychodynamic Supervision. Often I think: 'now I've heard it all'. Equally often I realise that my learning has only just begun.

I have been influenced by my education as a philosopher with a particular interest in epistemology, ethics and aesthetics. Particular authors whom my students and I have also found particularly helpful are Holmes and Lindley (1989) on values, Bond (1997) on standards and ethics, Thompson (1990) and his distinctions between ethical and unethical in terms of whether they are also alegal, illegal and legal; Jenkins (1997) on law, Palmer Barnes' (1998) work on ethics and complaints procedures as well as our own researches and concerns. Textbooks on ethics generally such as Hare (1989), Singer (1994) and the politics of postmodernism (Anderson, 1990; Bauman, 1993) have deeply influenced me, as do my daily encounters with the news of the world in and around me and the vicissitudes of my own personal and professional life and those of my colleagues and supervisees. *Ethics for Beginners* (Robinson and Garratt, 1996) is a good place to start or revise.

Frequently I have had to remind myself of the words of Smuts (1987), the last South African prime minister before apartheid, who was one of the founders of what is today the United Nations:

> It has been my lot to have passed many of the years of life amid the conflicts of men, in their wars and their Council Chambers. Everywhere I have seen men search and struggle for the Good with grim determinations and earnestness, and with a sincerity of purpose which added to the poignancy of the fratricidal strife. But everywhere too I have seen that it was at bottom a struggle for the Good, a wild striving towards human betterment; that blindly, and through blinding mists of passions and illusions, men are yet sincerely, earnestly groping towards the light, towards the ideal of a better, more secure life for themselves and for their fellows. . . . The real defeat for men as for other grades of the universe would be to ease the pain by a cessation of effort, to cease from striving towards the Good. (pp. 344–5)

Caveats

In keeping with our theme, caveats are of the first priority. The field of ethics – human, professional, national – is infinitely complex. It is therefore extremely rare that a simple clear answer will suffice. My purposes are to research, deepen and problematise these issues, not particularly to 'solve' them. (See for example my research book Clarkson 1998a.) Human beings are as interested in good and evil as we know we are by the popularity of movies, tales and energies around the themes of sex (Libido) and aggression (Mortido), often closely entwined with those of secrets and money. Of course, the creative physis is the teller of these stories (see Clarkson, 1995, pp. 105–7).

Further complications arise when we consider that there are differences, contrasts and conflicts between what could be considered ethical, moral, professional or legal. For example, South African psychiatrists and psychologists wrote official documents certifying that certain white young men were too mentally ill to go to war on black people in Angola – knowing full well that this was untrue. Many of these young men were healthy people of principle who did not want to kill others in the name of the apartheid state. Thus these psychotherapists were breaking the law of their country – and as we know psychotherapists are ethically required to keep the laws of the countries in which they practice. Yet some people made this *moral* choice, knowing that they might have to take responsibility for their actions and choosing to risk that perhaps they might even have to spend time in jail.

Current concerns

Having written some, researched many and participated in the implementation of codes of ethics over some decades, I find certain concerns
seem particularly vivid at this time. One is the fervent human hope that
we can legislate our problems away – that if we can just get all possible
situations anticipated in 'the code', we will have solved our problems. Of
course, it does not happen like this. As any family or community knows
who has ever made 'written down rules', as soon as they are written
down, new problems emerge. The writing down of ethics codes is
merely always a beginning. A code of any kind only begins to live when it
is 'taken to heart' as part of the ongoing warp and woof of the human
existential dilemma.

When that does not happen, one finds the simplistic introjection of
ethical code items, without any genuine understanding of the issues
involved in our profession. For example, in an assessment situation for
becoming a training analyst or equivalent in a particular approach,
someone asked the prospective teaching member what they would do if
one of their trainees had sexual relations with a client. The trainer/super-
visor was adamant: 'They should not do this.' Then the examiner asked:
'Why should psychotherapists not have sexual relations with their client
or trainee?' The candidate answered with all the certainty of a three-year-
old: 'Because it's a no-no!'

So, on the one hand there is the uncritical and ignorant adaptation to
code items and on the other hand there are people who follow the letter
of the law in their declarations, but actually live according
to very different principles. This is the difference between *avowed* values
and *lived* values; between 'talking the talk' and 'walking the walk'; and
between a congruent matching of social and psychological level communication or an incongruent public espousal of certain values (such as
marital fidelity) with private behaviour which makes a lie of it.

There is, as Severin (1965) has shown also an ethical element to every
act or non-action, whether we are conscious of it or not. According to
Taylor's definition of a value as

'... an idea on which people act, or a principle on which they judge how to act
[we cannot ever act in a value free way], since very choice and action must be
based upon explicit or implicit acceptance of a value'. (Taylor, 1954, p. 368)

So, the practitioner's values are always being communicated and
sometimes the more 'neutral' they claim to be, the clearer the communication at the *implicit, psychological or ulterior* level. Someone once
said: 'Who you are speaks so loudly that I cannot hear what you are
saying.'

It is perhaps possible that the perceived increase in ethical
complaints is the result of a greater sense of ethical awareness in the

practitioners of our profession, rather than an increase in unethical behaviour. Ethical guidelines exist as changing and developing articulations of the best moral thinking of a professional group at any particular time. Changing circumstances, special situations and exceptions as well as case law influence, shape and also change practice. Theoretical developments take place. Political and cultural currents and world events affect emergent sensibilities in addition to challenging previous certainties.

According to Pedersen (1995), counsellors should distinguish between fundamental ethical principles and discretionary aspects of ethics. The former are non-negotiable and should not be compromised. They are not modifiable. The ethical guidelines of professional associations are discretionary and unresponsive to culturally diverse populations and the ethics guidelines need to be modified accordingly.

Ethics is also evolving as a complex adaptive system. We certainly need to take into account that ethics, like laws and morality, changes over time and that what was once considered OK, such as having sex with one's clients and trainees (like Jung) or analysing one's friends' children (like Freud) or one's own (like Klein), will no longer be tolerated. Of course, few situations are this clear. Unfortunately, research on both sides of the Atlantic still demonstrates a shocking degree of ignorance – some 25% of psychotherapists believe that they have not had to face serious ethical dilemmas. As one respondent in our research wrote: 'I am fortunate that in thirty years of practice as a psychotherapist, I have never had to face any ethical dilemma.'

With the increase in consumer education and public awareness and the development of counselling and psychotherapy as a growth industry there has been an concomitant explosion of concerns about not making mistakes, insuring against client claims. Unfortunately, what I see, among many practitioners is this rather regrettable attempt to be more and more careful, more and more conscious of third parties listening, interpreting and judging on degrees of reality that can only ever be mediated by the two (or ten) people in the confines of the consulting room. There is increasing preoccupation with being 'error-free', with avoiding spontaneity and intuitive authenticity of the kind from which our forefathers (however clumsily) birthed this profession. (It is almost a cliché to point out that few of them – such as those I mentioned above – would either pass our present-day exams or be considered 'ethical' by today's standards!) There is a growing feeling in some quarters that the joy and excitement of practising counselling and psychotherapy have somewhat abated and that the risks of experimentation and creativity are being minimised to the level of the kind of bland, self-conscious carefulness. (See Kvale, 1992, p. 52.)

It is patently uncomfortable to live up to the House of Lords statement that:

professionals, whether in practice or in employment, must be independent in
thought and outlook, willing to speak their minds without fear or favour, and
not be in the control or dominance of any person or organisation. (Lord
Benson, *Hansard* 618, LD92/93 July 6-11 1207)

Can one speak of psychotherapy as a profession in this sense? Or is it
true what Szasz (1999) said, at the 1997 UPA Conference that
psychotherapy organisations exist to protect the professionals from the
public? Or perhaps the training organisations?

Over the past 25 years, a number of criticisms have been raised by various
progressive or marginalized groups in psychology, as well as by the supposed
beneficiaries of these ethical codes, our students and clients. These critics –
most frequently from feminist psychology, mental patient liberation groups,
and groups of psychologists of color – ask who truly benefits from organized
psychology's formal ethical guidelines. They have inquired repeatedly into
whether the dominant culture's code existed simply to uphold a certain
oppressive status quo within psychology and to protect psychologists from
those over whom they hold power, rather than the reverse . . . [they]
continue to question whether these are genuine attempts to transform the
meaning of ethics codes in psychology, or merely strategies to silence
through cooptation. (Brown, 1997, p. 53)

Brown also mentions the harm done by practitioners behaving
'ethically' and 'scientifically' by offering and then requiring the involun-
tary incarceration – hospitalisation – of suicidal patients since they have
been advised by experts that otherwise they open themselves to lawsuits
for malpractice. In her view

It exposes people at their most vulnerable to the abuses and risks found in
psychiatric institutions, including forced drugging, physical restraint,
[electroconvulsive shock in Britain] and the risks of sexual assault by staff and
patients alike. (p. 55)

So a kind of clinical practice has been developing which I would call
'defensive psychotherapy' This is an appropriation of the term 'defensive medicine' which is used in the US to describe an ethos in which
doctors and paramedics refuse to become involved, for example, with
accident victims on the road. This is reportedly because they are frightened of or protecting themselves against potential lawsuits that may
implicate them in malpractice suits or potential financial or reputation
loss on the basis of an unpremeditated act of merciful intervention. Too
many psychotherapists are now concerned to practice in ways that are
beyond criticism of their supervisors or training organisations and fear
being misunderstood by their patients. They are often worried about
'protecting themselves and their friends' at the cost of protecting their
patients, trainees or members of the public.

It is perhaps essential for each one of us to begin *a relationship to ethics, morality, our profession and the law* which is continuous and ongoing, problematised and questioning rather than adapted or formalistic and rote. Personally I would like to think of ethics processes as educative and ameliorative in the first instance and only in the last instance involving sanctions. The first principle in considering ethical relationships in psychotherapy may be to maintain healthy and effective working relationships. Where there appear to be difficulties, the principle should be to work toward restoring the interrupted or disturbed relationship between therapist and patient in the first place – if at all possible. Many problems could be prevented from the beginning if a client or patient openly discussed the discomforts with the analyst giving him or her the opportunity to change, explain, seek supervision or other help as needed. Supervisors, mediators or independent consultants could perhaps even be involved in some cases to the benefit of all concerned.

I am surprised by the difference between experiences of psychotherapy ethics processes where 'reconciliation' often receives mere lip-service. It may appear in the codes, but it may in fact be absent from practice. The Institute of Management Consultants to which I belong publicises that since, as *management consultants*, our business is *relationships*, if there is a problem, our immediate attention is devoted to the *restoration* of that relationship between the client and practitioner. Facilitators or mediators may be used, but the primary energy is not in creating an adversarial, pseudo-legal climate, but rather a dialogic mutual problem-solving climate.

In my opinion, only when such attempts at reconciliation, problem-solving and mutual understanding have demonstrably failed, should there be recourse to formal complaints procedures. It is my hope that as the primary function of ethical codes in psychotherapy and related professions becomes more educational and nourishing of the therapeutic relationship, the policing and punitive functions may in time become less important. Psychotherapy is after all about love and hate and we cannot avoid entanglement with the most profound and distorted of human emotions. In many cases discussion, working through, insight into the complex dynamics of the analysis can resolve apparently irrevocable breakdowns. There are certain exceptions – as always – particularly in cases which concern sexual behaviour between therapist and client (or supervisor and supervisee).

Most codes of ethics assume that their purpose is primarily to protect clients and members of the public from the wrongdoing of therapists, supervisors and training institutes. That certainly is their major purpose. We might also consider the need of therapists for protection and help. Therapists may sometimes be particularly vulnerable to displaced feelings of vengeance or retaliation for the same complex reasons that doctors who go to help earthquake victims may be attacked.

Transference theory also teaches us that clients (and others) may see us in illusional and at times, delusional ways as the need arises for them. This is also open to misinterpretation and abuse – as well as therapeutic transformation – from both sides.

The heart of the matter is that ethics is concerned with *relationship* – the betweenness of people. This has been true since the beginning of time and is still true even in all countries where psychotherapy or consultancy does not even exist. Even physicists no longer conceive of the world outside of relationship (see for example, *New Perspectives in Supervision*, Clarkson, 1991, 1998b, and the chapter called 'New Perspectives in Counselling and Psychotherapy', Clarkson, 1993). Notions from these universes of discourse may upset (beneficially or otherwise) many of our cherished beliefs about causality, development, productivity, intersubjectivity and the nature of individuality.

> Epistemologically, the things we see (people, objects, etc.) exist only in relationship and, when analysed microscopically, they too are best viewed as relationships. It is no secret in physics (Capra, 1975; 1982) that the closer we analyse some 'thing' the less it appears as a thing and the more it appears as a dynamic process (things in relationship). Consequently, relationships become a primary source of our knowledge of the world. This can be taken to the ontological extreme by stating that things do not exist . . . that, in fact, things ultimately *are* relationships. (Cottone, 1988, p. 360)

In psychology Mesmer said it and so did Freud. It was the first thing I understood about psychotherapy as a teenage suicide counsellor. In recent years I have even defined psychotherapy as *the intentional use of relationship. Relationship is the heart of the matter.*

As psychotherapists we claim expertise in relationship, yet we repeatedly fail most miserably – witness endless schisms, the Jungian 'shadow' of our profession when our skills are used for abuse of our clients, misleading the public or the exploitation or destruction of each other's work and reputation. I do not believe anyone can – or should – give an easy yes-or-no answer to whether they are 'ethical' or not. We are all implicated in the great struggle between good and evil. Usually there is a trend, like the veer on a car in one way or another. Ziegler (1988) in *Morbidezza* characterises the profession of psychotherapy as the city of the morbid in order to capture the sense in which we are fascinated and involved in pathology, dysfunction and our own humanly mixed motivations.

Some of the deepest offences against ethics, against our human relationship, seem to be in fact those where certainty is assumed. I remember as a young child chilling when I heard on the radio the South African prime minister John Voster say with ultimate authority and pride: 'Never in the darkest night have I ever asked myself whether I could be wrong.' With Bauman (1993) I believe that ' the frustration of certainty is morality's gain.' (p. 223) But the very worst is where ignorance is claimed as a badge of honour. I also remember Mary Goulding, an honoured teacher on a Council, getting angry when someone was claiming 'ignorance' about the South African situation in a debate on sanctions. Vehemently she asked the psychotherapist: 'How dare you *not* know enough about it?'

Relationship is indeed where the healing is possible, but it is also (a) where the injury happened first and (b) where violation and abuse and neglect is once again experienced, retraumatising people and damaging whatever healing was made possible through the new relationships. The greatest violence is to a hope for the restoration of faith in human nature.

Organisation of the book, style and terms

I have organised this book according to some major themes per chapter with an 'item' which is somehow connected with the theme to follow each chapter. This is partly to create some rhythm between long and shorter pieces and also between more theoretical and more practical moments. The issues touched on in this book apply as much to education, supervision or training and organisational work.

Although considerable thought has gone into the sequencing of chapters, the book does not have to be read in such order. It will probably be most useful to find a chapter with issues close to your current interests or concerns and to stay with it and your own thoughts and feelings about what it imaginatively *evokes*, rather than taking it too literally or concretely. It is concerned with what Kant called "moral imagination".

> Broadly speaking . . . it is moral imagination that we use when confronted with a pressing, problematic, and especially, conflict-laden situation. Moral imagination is one means by which we apply our imagination to complex social and political issues. *Moral* because a choice may have to be made; *imagination* because that choice may have to be ingenious, less than clear-cut, a compromise or a creatively improved adaptation. (Samuels, 1989, p. 201)

I have included many ethical dilemmas as exercises in moral imagination. If we allow that there are active and passive forms of meditation in most spiritual traditions, I could have called this book *Meditations on Morality*, since that is its truest intent.

There is a variety of styles and tones throughout the book, from scientific research reports to prose poetry; from the deeply personal to the apparently objective. Some are well-researched papers, others less academic or even more personal spiritual exercises in trying to grapple or even understand an ethical or a moral problem. I have tried to show how one can get involved with human ethical and moral dilemmas through a multitude of prisms refracting light in different directions, but hopefully making our experience more profound and more conscious. I hope that this diversity may bring people different options of approaching and immersing ourselves in these ongoing and never-ending challenges. It also makes it easy for people to ignore or avoid chapters which are not to their taste and select those whose style and content are more useful.

The terms counselling, psychotherapy, psychoanalysis, counselling psychology, clinical psychology and psychological counselling are all used interchangeably. The relevant professional bodies have ethics codes and complaints procedures which should be available on request. Please read the appellations as they apply to you. The application of this volume to the individual fields needs to be undertaken as theoreticians and practitioners move from the general to the particular and from the generic to the unique. Often I use the term psychotherapist generically to include all the other professions. I also interchange the terms patient and client. Following Muhlhausler and Harré's (1991) recommendation I have also frequently adopted the vernacular device of the gender-neutral third person singular usage of *they*, *their* and *them*.

Every chapter and every item has been wrought from my own experiences – as a researcher in inextricable subjective relationship with the world of my exploration, as a teacher of professionals accountable for substantial portions of the future and as a human being constantly engaged in the vicissitudes of existence. Each one represents a problem or set of problems I have encountered through my clients, students and colleagues; none of them represents a problem solved or a dilemma finally laid to rest. It is about relationship in terms of keeping each other's secrets, about the forces of sex and death and creativity and about money, not only in a literal sense, but also a symbolic sense as standing for freedom, power, creativity, barter, exchange, professionalism and all their other associated meanings. In psychotherapy and psychoanalysis we work with some of the greatest forces in the world – and the importance of these forces was well-evidenced in the research which forms the backbone of this work. This book is also a work in progress – which is why I finally sub-titled it *'Working with ethical and moral dilemmas in psychotherapy'*. My hope is that others will not necessarily take on its content, but that *demonstrating the process* may perhaps in some moment prove a warning or an inspiration.

- Chapter 1, 'Ethical dilemmas of psychotherapists', with Professor Geoff Lindsay, reports a research study which compares results from similar APA and BPS studies. Many years ago I became interested in collecting 'ethical dilemmas' from colleagues with identifying infor-mation protected. I particularly wanted such information for training purposes so that the richness of real experiences can provide the fertiliser for well-honed ethical reflexes and moral intelligence. I was publicly accused of 'being unethical' to invite such research responses. Some years later I discovered that North American colleagues and the then president of the BPS had conducted just such studies – and gladly we commenced a most fruitful collaboration.

- Item 1, 'The psychotherapy and counselling oath', with Dr Mark Aveline, President of the BAC, came from our long-standing ongoing conversations about professional ethics and our concern that a preoccupation with rules and regulations needs to be balanced against the deepest intentions of the kind which can be formed (or adapted) into an oath.
- Chapter 2, 'Ethical relationships', came from exploring one of my major projects – the discourse analysis of psychoanalysis, counselling psychology and psychotherapy in terms of certain ethical dimensions which focus on the nature, uses and abuses of the different kinds of therapeutic relationship.
- Item 2, 'A decision-making hierarchy regarding ethical issues', is the direct result of having many students and supervisees struggle with prioritising – when there is much to do and little guidance about what to do first. I love complexity as well as simplicity. It is at their recommendation of its usefulness to them, that I include it here along with 21 ethical dilemmas for practice.
- Chapter 3, 'Values in counselling and psychotherapy', is another paper written from the heart engaging with the notions of neutrality and the theoretical, philosophical and practical impossibility of not communicating our values.
- Item 3, 'Discovering your own values' presents a small exercise which has been used and appreciated in many different forums as a starting point for teaching novices or a revision point for veterans.
- Chapter 4, 'Bystanding in counselling and psychotherapy': The denial and retrieval of human relationship, our inevitable reciprocity, our complicity intentional or not, conscious or not is a central theme of my life and my work.
- Item 4, 'Bystanding and responsible involvement in psychotherapy, organisations and society'. The small questionnaire grew from conference and workshop presentations, most recently at the instigation of Earl Hopper, President of the International Group Psychotherapy Association.
- Chapter 5, 'In recognition of dual relationships'. This work grew from constant engagement with the ethical issues and sometimes sheer hypocrisies which can grow like weeds when a profession is at risk of being unquestioned and unquestioning.
- Item 5, 'Information for prospective clients'. These are simple examples – and my choice of examples would probably be different in the course of time and in new circumstances – just to stimulate

discussion and reflection of how practitioners actually deal with similar ethical and professional issues.

- Chapter 6, 'Vengeance of the victim'. Many of my life-long concerns have been about the welfare of clients, supervisees and students, but psychotherapists (and others in helping professions) can also be consciously or even unconsciously abused – sometimes for reasons which are too deep to fathom. This is a meditation on that theme.
- Item 6, 'Asking the client's permission to do a case study'. This was specifically written to counteract certain kinds of bad practice which had grown into 'the norm' by the time I noticed. Clients were being abused and trainees' practice unconscionably compromised by well-meaning but in my opinion ill-thought-through guidance, dealing very superficially with extremely important issues of how trainee therapists may exploit their clients (however unconsciously) for their professional gain – and how clients may be drawn into destructive dynamics. It will probably be of interest only to some people, but I was happy that the BPS Counselling Psychology Board of Examiners supported it and that it is now published in the regulations.
- Chapter 7, 'When rules are not enough: the spirit of the law in ethical codes'. As professionals frequently engaged in ethical hearings, Lesley Murdin and I felt that it is important to remind the profession that the spirit of the law is more important than the letter.
- Item 7, 'Professional practices and ethical guidelines for administrative/ancillary staff at counselling and psychotherapy practices, institutes and colleges'. A secretary who was typing out a transcript of a patient who had been sexually abused became extremely distressed by the material. Sometimes therapists forget to confine their case discussions to closed consulting rooms. Such were the original moments of impetus for working with the ethical needs of those who constantly surround and support us as psychotherapists, overhearing our conversations, mopping our tears, sometimes coping with public complaints and abuse – even violence – and whom we can never appreciate enough.
- Chapter 8, 'Collegial relationships – ethics, research and good practice', with Geoff Lindsay. This is an extrapolation and exploration of the disturbing fact from research and experience that so many ethical dilemmas concern colleagues' misconduct and so few people seem willing to act or even know that our ethical codes require us to act appropriately in such cases. If this is so difficult for reasons of lack of information, fear of retaliation, financial or status loss, psychotherapy can never honestly make a claim to effective self-regulation.
- Item 8, 'Libel, slander and defamation and their derivatives in professional codes of ethics' – guidelines written with my husband Vincent

    Keter from a particularly painful personal experience that other
    professionals may yet find useful.

- Chapter 9, 'The ethical dilemmas of supervision', with Lesley Murdin, also a recognised Supervisor of the British Association for Psychoanalytic and Psychodynamic Supervision (BAPPS). Looking at the ethical dimensions of supervision.

- Item 9, 'What happens if a psychotherapist dies?' Barbara Traynor finally co-wrote this material with me after many years of teaching it and introducing it into ethical codes. It had to be written, because it happened and nobody seemed to know what to do. Our hope is to prevent or ameliorate the distress and damage this kind of event (which is mentioned again in the research studies) can cause to clients and supervisees – but also to the families of psychotherapists.

- Chapter 10, 'Ethical dilemmas in supervision, training and organisational contexts'. More research in process with Geoff Lindsay, exploring qualitatively the kinds of dilemmas faced in supervision.

- Item 10, 'Seven domains of discourse in exploring ethical and moral dilemmas'. Applying the seven-level model to ethical issues. The seven-level model is an epistemological tool which has been effectively used since 1975 (Clarkson, 1975) to unscramble the fact that people live at different levels, talk about different domains and have to learn to tolerate ambiguities, contradictions and paradox while still achieving clarity, compassion and coherence. There are another 21 (or so) ethical dilemmas concerning supervision, training and professional issues.

- Chapter 11, 'Whose idea is it Anyway? (and Writing for publication)'. Many practitioners have said to me that it is only when they write or teach that they discover what they really think and believe. I consider writing as research. I also believe that writing is one of the ways psychotherapists can engage in ethically accountable professional thought and practice. So I include as part 2 'Writing for publication' as an encouragement with lots of practical how-tos which may help aspiring writers and part 1 'Whose idea is it anyway' to explore a potentially confusing part of writing.

- Item 11, 'A code of ethics for counselling and psychotherapy publications'. I was so delighted when Alexandra Chalfont consulted me about ethical matters in the training publication *Dialogue* for which she is the editor, I compiled this code as a starting point for further development.

- Chapter 12, 'Psychotherapy ethics in the context of "schoolism"'. As a management consultant of some 25 years' experience – including the professional leadership in several spheres – it seems to me that psychotherapy is still remarkably unaware of larger systemic social, organisational and cultural influences at work in our practice, our training and our professional organisations. This is a beginning.

- Item 12, *'Physis* – or "a pleasing illusion"'. This elaborates the notion of *physis* as an aspiration ethic for all the human beings involved with psychotherapy and its related disciplines.
- Chapter 13, 'Judicial review of psychotherapy self-regulation' (with Vincent Keter). This chapter is a preliminary report on the judicial review of the UKCP and some of the issues and dilemmas which affect organisations who claim to protect the public but are often found to be protecting the professional members.
- Item 13, 'Thought experiments and imaginary dilemmas for people involved in complaints procedures'. These concern the work of complaints procedures and the issues involved in hearing complaints in psychotherapy, psychology and related professions.
- Chapter 14, 'Integrative relational research: an approach to ethics'. This is a reflection on ethical and moral dilemmas involved in research, particularly those involved in the research which forms both the spine and spirit of this book.
- Item 14, extract from Rainer Maria Rilke, *Letters to a Young Poet*.
- Appendix 1, 'A traveller's guide to psychotherapy: a companion for clients and patients' is an example of the kind of material some people may want to rewrite or give to their clients – or to student psychotherapists who are just beginning to see clients.
- Appendix 2, 'Dysfunction in training organisations'. Chris Robertson kindly gave me permission to reproduce his paper on dysfunction in training organisations. Whether or not one agrees with everything he says, he certainly is among the few who have seriously paid attention to this aspect of our professions.

Compass

As a final orientation to the material which follows I should like to recommend this quotation from Solzhenitsyn (1974):

> If only it were all so simple! If only there were evil people somewhere insidiously committing evil deeds, and it were necessary only to separate them from the rest of us and destroy them. But the line dividing good and evil cuts through the heart of every human being. And who is willing to destroy a piece of his own heart? (p. 168)

References

Anderson, W.T. (1990) Reality Is Not What It Used To Be. San Francisco, CA: Harper and Row.
Ani, M. (1994) Yurugu – an African-centred Critique of European Cultural Thought and Behavior. Trenton, NJ: Africa World Press.
Bauman, Z. (1993) Postmodern Ethics. Oxford: Blackwell.
Bond, T. (1997) Standards and Ethics for Counselling in Action, London: Sage.

Brown, L. S. (1997) Ethics in Psychology: Cui Bono? In D. Fox and I. Prilleltensky (eds) Critical Psychology: An Introduction. London: Sage.

Capra, F. (1975) The Tao of Physics. London: Wildwood House.

Capra, F. (1982) The Turning Point: Science, Society, and the Rising Culture. London: Flamingo.

Clarkson, P. (1975) The seven-level model. Invitational paper delivered at the University of Pretoria, November.

Clarkson, P. (1991) New perspectives in supervision. Paper delivered at conference of British Association for Supervision Research, London.

Clarkson, P. (1993) New perspectives in counselling and psychotherapy, or adrift in a sea of change. In On Psychotherapy, pp. 209–232. London: Whurr.

Clarkson, P. (1995) The Therapeutic Relationship. London: Whurr.

Clarkson, P. (1998a) Counselling Psychology: Integrating Theory, Research and Supervised Practice. London: Routledge.

Clarkson, P. (1998b) Supervised supervision: including the archetopoi of supervision. In P. Clarkson (ed.) Supervision: Psychoanalytic and Jungian Perspectives, pp. 136–146. London: Whurr.

Cottone, R. R. (1988) Epistemological and ontological issues in counselling: Implications of social systems theory. Counselling Psychology Quarterly, 1(4), 357–365.

Hare, R. M. (1989) Essays in Ethical Theory. Oxford: Clarendon Press.

Holmes, J. and Lindley, R. (1989) The Values of Psychotherapy. Oxford: Oxford University Press.

Jenkins, P. (1997) Counselling, Psychotherapy and the Law, London: Sage.

Jung, C.G. (1928). Analytical psychology and education. In Contributions to Analytical Psychology (trans. H.G. Baynes and F.C. Baynes), pp. 313–382. London: Trench Trubner.

Kvale, S. (1992) Postmodern psychology: A contradiction in terms? In S. Kvale (ed.) Psychology and Postmodernism, pp. 31–37. London: Sage.

Muhlhauser, P. and Harré, R. (1991) Pronouns and the People. Oxford: Blackwell.

Palmer-Barnes F. (1998) Complaints and Grievances in Psychotherapy. London: Routledge.

Pedersen, P. B. (1995) Culture-centered ethical guidelines for counselors, in J. G. Ponterotto, J. M. Casas, L. A. Suzuki and C. M. Alexander (eds) Handbook of Multicultural Counseling, pp. 34–49. Thousand Oaks, CA: Sage.

Robinson, D. and Garratt, C. (1996) Ethics for Beginners, Cambridge: Icon Books.

Samuels, A. (1989) The Plural Psyche, London: Routledge.

Severin, F. T. (1965) Humanistic Viewpoints in Psychotherapy. New York: McGraw-Hill.

Singer, P. (ed.) (1994) Ethics. Oxford: Oxford University Press.

Smuts, J. C. (1987) Holism and Evolution. Cape Town: N & S Press.

Solzhenitsyn, A. (1974) The Gulag Archipelago. Glasgow: Fontana Books.

Szasz, T. (1999) Discretion as power: Language and money and status in the situation called psychotherapy. Universities Psychotherapy Association. Review No. 7: 1–14.

Taylor, H. (1954) On Education and Freedom. New York: Abelard-Schuman.

Thompson, A. (1990) Guide to Ethical Practice in Psychotherapy. New York: Wiley.

Ziegler, A. (1988) Morbidezza: The sick society of the healing profession (E. Loewe, trans.), Sphinx 1: 66–81.

Acknowledgements

Grateful thanks to our respondents, research assistants Yuko Nippoda, Mark Donati and other colleagues such as Julie Allen for their assistance; and to the Independent Centre for Qualitative Research in Training and Supervision at PHYSIS in London for financially supporting the research and writing of this book.

Any initial comments on this part of the ongoing research project will be welcomed. We would also like to express our grateful thanks to all respondents who completed our questionnaire, thus helping to further research information and education in this vitally important underpinning of all our work. Without their willingness to share problems, uncertainties and experiences, there would be no progress in this most delicate and painful area of our work. Our grateful thanks also to the University of Surrey and the University of Warwick for financial support for part of this work.

The contributions of my co-authors should not be read as agreement with any of my material in the rest of the book which is solely my responsibility. I extend grateful thanks to them for their enjoyable collaboration on our mutual chapters. I also thank the numerous people who have advised, read and participated in improving the quality of the book and of the quality of ethical theory, practice and research in these professions.

I am grateful to the editors/authors and publishers of the following books and journals for publication of material which forms portions of this book:

Chapter 1: Ethical Dilemmas of Psychotherapists. A version of this chapter was first published in 1999 in *The Psychologist*, 12(4): 182–5.

Item 1: The Psychotherapy and Counselling Oath was first published in 1996 in *The Psychotherapist*, 9(7): 12.

Chapter 3: Values in Counselling and Psychotherapy was first published in 1994 in *Changes*, 13(4): 299–306.

Item 6: 'Asking the Client's Permission' to do a Case Study was published by the British Psychological Society in 1998 as part of the Regulations and Syllabus for the Diploma in Counselling Psychology.

Chapter 5: In Recognition of Dual Relationships was first published in 1994 in the *Transactional Analysis Journal*, 24(1): 32–8.

Chapter 7: When Rules Are Not Enough: The Spirit of the Law in Ethical Codes was first published in 1996 in *Counselling*, 7(1): 31–5.

Item 7: Professional Practices and Ethical Guidelines for Administrative/ Ancillary Staff at Counselling and Psychotherapy Practices, Institutes and Colleges was first published as 'Ethics for the Counselling Office' in *Counselling*, 5(4): 282–3.

Chapter 9: The Ethical Dimensions of Supervision was first published in 1998 in P. Clarkson (ed.) *Supervision: Psychoanalytic and Jungian Perspectives* (pp. 107–20). London: Whurr.

Item 9: What Happens if a Psychotherapist Dies? was first published in 1992 in *Counselling*, 3(1): 23–4.

Item 14 is an excerpt from *Letter to a Young Poet* by Rainer Maria Rilke, translated by M.D. Herter Norton. Translation copyright 1934, 1954 by W.W. Norton & Company, Inc., renewed © 1962, 1982 by M.D. Herter Norton. Reprinted by permission of W.W. Norton & Company, Inc.

Appendix 2: Dysfunction in Training Organisations by Chris Robertson was first published in 1993 in *Self & Society*, 21(4): 31–5.

Excerpt from "East Coker" in *four quarters*, copyright 1940 by T.S. Eliot and renewed 1968 by Esme Valerie Eliot, reprinted by permission of Harcourt, Inc. and Faber and Faber.

Every effort has been made to obtain permission to reproduce copyright material throughout this book. If any proper acknowledgement has not yet been made, the copyright holder should contact the publisher.

CHAPTER 1
Ethical Dilemmas of Psychotherapists

GEOFF LINDSAY AND PETRŪSKA CLARKSON

> Kant defined an entity that has become the centerpiece of modern moral
> theory: the disembodied subject, a subject that knows no culture, history,
> class, race, or gender. This subject qualifies as a moral subject only in the
> sense that he legislates for himself. Furthermore, the laws that this
> autonomous subject legislates and executes (the political terms here are no
> accident) are moral only in that they are universalizable; the deciding factor
> in moral judgments cannot be particular circumstances, concrete empirical
> conditions, but must always be the universalizability of the abstract principle.
> That women are excluded from this realm should be obvious but, just in case
> his readers have missed the point, Kant notes: 'of course, I exclude women,
> children and idiots'. (Hekman, 1995, pp. 35–6)

The ethical basis of psychological practice has received increased atten-
tion in recent years. For example, recent presidential addresses to the
British Psychological Society (Lindsay, 1995), the Irish Psychological
Society (McGee, 1995) and the Canadian Psychological Association
(Pettifor, 1996) have addressed ethics and values. Also, the European
Federation of Professional Psychologists Associations approved a meta-
code of ethics at its General Assembly in 1995 (EFPPA, 1997) whose
requirements all aspiring member associations must meet.

In 1995 Lindsay and Colley argued that there were limitations in the
traditional approach to devising ethical codes, namely an expert
committee working on the basis of principles, devising ethical codes, or
standards of behaviour. They studied ethical dilemmas identified from
their own practice by a sample of BPS members, replicating a study by
Pope and Vetter (1992) of members of the American Psychological
Association (APA). The BPS study identified two kinds of ethical
dilemmas: those that fitted the traditional form of ethical codes for
professionals such as psychologists (e.g. confidentiality) and a second
category which concerned tensions between the psychologist's

preferred practice, and constraints imposed by the organisation within which the psychologist works (e.g. National Health Service).

Further evidence on the usefulness of researching ethical dilemmas empirically to identify important aspects of ethical practice, and the content of ethical codes, has been provided in an international collaboration between researchers in Canada, Colombia, Finland, Norway, Sweden and the UK, and presented to the 1997 European Congress of Psychology in Dublin (see Antikainen, 1997; Colnerud, 1997; Odland, 1997; Sinclair, 1997; Wassenaer and Slack, 1997).

In the present chapter, we report on extension of this approach to psychotherapists. In the UK, the title 'psychotherapist' (as well as 'psychologist') is not protected and there is no single training route. Rather, the UK Standing Conference on Psychotherapy (UKCP) and the British Confederation of Psychotherapists (BCP) recognises a number of training routes. Many recognised psychotherapists are, or are eligible to be, chartered psychologists, but others have alternative professional qualifications. Vetere et al. (1997) have recently described the stage reached in the development towards the accreditation by the Society of psychologists specialising in psychotherapy. We were interested to discover whether this professional group (psychotherapists) would have similar ethical dilemmas to those identified by groups exclusively of psychologists.

The research study

The present study comprised a survey of a random selection of 1000 psychotherapists on the UK Council of Psychotherapy (UKCP) register. The survey form (replicating the USA study) asked respondents to respond to the following question:

> Describe in a few words, or more detail, an incident that you or a colleague
> have faced in the past year or two that was ethically troubling you.

The covering letter asked respondents to state their psychotherapeutic orientation, but not to include any other information which could identify themselves or anybody else. They were asked to reply, even if they had no dilemma to describe, and a reply-paid envelope was enclosed.

Replies were received from 213 psychotherapists, a response rate of 21.3%. This compares with a response rate of 28.4% for the survey of members of the British Psychological Society (Lindsay and Colley, 1995). Of these, 47 (22.1% of respondents) stated that they had no ethical dilemmas to report. This compares with 37% of the BPS sample who reported having had no dilemmas. However, while the psychotherapists are all likely to be in practice, to varying degrees, the BPS sample was drawn from the total membership, not all of whom were practising as psychologists. A further 4.7% reported that they were unable to comment. Reasons for this included retirement, those not in practice and those who had undertaken little practice during the previous 2 years. Consequently, 156 psychotherapists reported having had at least one dilemma (73.2%). Some reported a single dilemma, others more than one. One respondent reported he had dilemmas 'all the time'.

The 156 respondents who reported dilemmas mentioned a total of 254 ethically troubling incidents. These were analysed by the two authors independently and each was allocated to the same 23 categories used in the study of BPS members. This method allowed comparison with surveys of psychologists who were members of the BPS and the APA (Pope and Vetter, 1992).

There were some thought-provoking examples showing the range of people's attitudes towards ethics from:

> to the extent that I drop down into pure awareness as a therapist, I enter a space of just seeing/being – where there are essentially no ethical dilemmas – seeing the light in the client.

to

> Psychotherapy is concerned with ethics in every case all of the time, e.g. how to live a 'good' life – an enjoyable and worthwhile life free from neurotic conflict. So every patient is ethically challenging and dilemmas – if you wish to call ethical decisions such – are everyday.

Another voice:

> I do not wish to describe any incident of ethical dilemma but to point out the dangers inherent in ethical guidelines becoming prescriptive. There are times when, although I may agree in principle with what is defined as proper psychotherapeutic practice, in practice I find that my intelligence, my experience and my common sense argue for something different; and I should be free to take responsibility for my decisions.

There was another perspective:

> I cannot recall anything that challenged me. However, there have been a few occasions when patients of mine have left therapy in an illegitimate way, which has prompted me to fulfil my professional obligation (to them) by having to go through the unpleasant procedure of making contact with them and making clear that they have behaved unethically.

The actual dilemmas reported were analysed with reference to the orientation of the psychotherapist, as shown in Table 1.1.

Given the size of the sample, some caution needs to be exercised before making judgements about any of the claimed theoretical approaches and their collective appreciation of ethical dilemmas in psychotherapy, therefore readers are left to ponder the implications of these figures for themselves.

Table 1.1: Orientation by type of response

Orientation	N	Dilemmas			Type of response No dilemmas			Unable to say		
		Freq	% total	% in orientation	Freq	% total	% in orientation	Freq	% total	% in orientation
Psychoanalytic	107	77	36.2	72	25	11.7	23.4	5	2.3	4.6
Cognitive behavioural	13	11	5.2	84.6	1	0.5	7.7	1	0.5	7.7
Humanistic/integrative	61	46	2.6	75.4	14	6.6	23.0	1	0.5	1.6
Systemic/relationship/sexual	19	14	6.6	73.7	4	1.9	21.1	1	0.5	5.2
Experiential/constructivist	4	4	1.9	100	0	0	0	0	0	0
Hypnotherapy	4	1	0.5	25	3	1.4	75	0	0	0
Not stated	5	3	1.4	60	1	0.5	20	1	0.5	20

The analysis of types of ethical dilemma, reported and compared with findings of earlier studies of BPS psychologists follows.

Confidentiality

The largest category of ethically troubling incidents reported was that of confidentiality. Indeed, the categorisation of these dilemmas was problematic as a number clearly overlapped with other categories, and are discussed here as examples of the other type of dilemma. For example, many issues with respect to training and supervision (e.g. of junior colleagues) were reported as concerns regarding confidentiality.

The dilemmas reported could be grouped as follows:

- risk to third parties — sexual abuse, other child abuse and neglect, threatened violence, HIV
- risk to the client — threatened suicide
- disclosure of information to others — particularly to medical agencies, other colleagues, close friends, relatives
- careless/inappropriate disclosure — by the psychotherapist or others.

The most numerous were those concerned with child abuse, in particular sexual abuse. There were 17 such dilemmas that tended to concern the appropriateness of reporting disclosure in psychotherapy. In some cases the clients revealed their knowledge of an alleged perpetrator. For example, one client, sexually abused herself while living in a children's home, had had two previous children fostered owing to sexual abuse by her partner. She disclosed information which indicated a third child was now at risk, but felt,

> it was safer to tell me than tell social workers, since I didn't have the power to take the child away. The dilemma concerned the need to protect the child versus the woman's need for help. If I were to break confidentiality it would destroy her trust in me.

In other cases the clients disclosed their own abuse of children:

> How much confidentiality to give a young man who has probably sexually abused a young child. I feel that I'm essentially saying, 'don't tell me how unsafe you are without being prepared for me to tell others'. Many of my dilemmas involve confidentiality and its uneasy coexistence with child protection issues and the law.

Respondents were concerned both about the relationship between psychotherapy and the need to meet child protection requirements, and the issue of evidence – should one 'bring allegations of sexual abuse to the attention of Social Services when the basis for these allegations appeared to be slender', asked one respondent.

This dilemma may also relate to the time since the alleged abusive behaviour took place. For example, one client had offended at the age of 15, twenty years previous.

The dilemmas regarding risk included the client,

> male, homosexual patient who said he was diagnosed as HIV positive and who described his active attempts to infect others through unprotected sex

and the male patient who chose not to tell his female partner that he had

> a sexually transmitted disease, which is uncomfortable for the man, but could have rendered his female partner infertile before she was aware of symptoms.

The psychotherapist worked with this young man for 3 months before he disclosed his condition and the woman had treatment.

Minority dilemmas included working with non-professional interpreters and 'the relentless pursuit by the media of high profile patients'. Concerns about disclosure included accidental revelations by the therapist and being inappropriately in receipt of information.

> I was a member of an observing team behind a two way screen and became aware in interviewing a new client that I had a personal connection with the client outside the role of therapy. I was able to leave the team immediately and had no further contact . . . but I had been made aware of the client's problem . . .

Psychologists also reported dilemmas regarding the appropriate passing on of information to other colleagues, especially GPs. One put this simply:

> when the interest of the patient requires contact with GP despite breach of confidentiality.

Another was concerned to be asked by a psychiatrist for information about a former client. Although some reported their means of resolving this dilemma was by seeking the client's consent, others reported instances where consent may not be given or the client may not be in a position to give *informed* consent,

> . . . where a borderline person's condition means disregarding their opinion and actually making a referral without their permission.

These concerns are similar to those experienced by the psychologists in both the BPS and the APA samples. They represent dilemmas in a fundamental domain of practice for psychotherapists and psychologists working with clients, namely the need to reconcile the benefits of maintaining confidentiality to ensure trust and hence effective psychotherapy and intervention, compared with the need to protect the client and others from harm. There was one report of a psychotherapist's concern that managers are, inappropriately, seeking information:

Working in a community child and adolescent mental health team funded by the NHS, there is ongoing pressure from third party interests – especially those who hold purse-strings – to 'know' what is happening in the therapy room . . . I fear that many patients, aware of this, may find it impossible to risk relating their most disturbing states of mind for fear of 'leakage' out of the therapy room.

Dual relationships

The second most prevalent category was that of dual relationships (excluding those involving sexual behaviour) with 11.8%. The main types of ethically troubling incidents were:

• social relationships with clients
• working with two separate clients who have a relationship.

The former mainly comprised situations where an existing or past client may be encountered in a social setting.

I lead a development group at . . . a community facility . . . which is open to any interested person. About six months ago a former training patient started to attend. My dilemma was the change in relationship, and could a person who had been a patient become a member of a group run by her former therapist?

This may be a particular problem in small communities.

Small provincial town raises issues of boundaries – 'who knows who' difficulties: social circles – a bit incestuous at times!

In other cases the respondent was concerned about the behaviour of others who appeared to transgress appropriate boundaries. In some cases the psychotherapist had to respond to social invitations by clients:

A person met during a first assessment for psychotherapy invited me for a social relationship. The invitation was declined, although I felt there were areas of mutual interest.

Male patient who dresses in my company as a woman wanted me to accompany him to buy a wedding dress.

In other instances, the psychotherapist reported an ethically troubling incident involving a client encountered inadvertently. One met the wife of a patient he knew to be unfaithful at a social function. Or inadvertently, a person known in a non-therapeutic setting might be encountered in a professional situation. One respondent reported:

> Professional discomfort when a daughter became friendly with a female client. Boundaries were difficult to hold.

The second set of dilemmas concern therapists involved with two clients who have a close relationship.

> Working with two clients repeatedly who also have a personal and professional relationship. Troubling in a sense of needing to be as free as possible to work with each without distorting information and carrying inaccurate assumptions because of my prior knowledge.

> Three weeks into starting a new female patient I realised that she was the sister of an existing male patient. I asked the brother if he was willing for me to tell the sister that I was seeing both of them (which would at least have placed them on an even footing). The brother was adamant, however, that his sister must not know he was having therapy. I would have liked to tell the sister that I could not continue to see her, but this seemed unfair and I could think of no good reason if I was not allowed to mention the brother . . .

Minority reports of ethical dilemmas with respect to dual relationships include a psychotherapist reported by a patient as wanting to enter a business relationship with the patient; whether to provide support for a colleague subject to disciplinary procedures; and how to deal with the wife of a client who:

> is convinced I am undermining their marriage by, as she has it, condoning his affair with another woman, has been seeking out and reporting to him my own infidelity in my marriage, and the difficult relationship I had with one of my children, and my (relatively) newly discovered lesbian sexual identity. . . . This faced one with the dilemma of sticking up for myself as a person about whom the truth was being vastly distorted, versus standing in my role as a therapist, and dealing with it as all part of his story. I chose the latter.

Conduct of colleagues

A total of 8.9% of dilemmas fell into this category. The most prevalent type of troubling incident with colleagues concerned inappropriate sexual behaviour and other dual relationships, both dealt with in separate sections. If these are aggregated, it is the second largest category. Otherwise, the psychotherapists reported a variety of ethically troubling incidents including:

- competence
- unprofessional comments
- professional conflict regarding referrals
- charging contracts
- inappropriate disclosure.

It is not always clear what to do when a psychotherapist is not competent, so leading to an ethical dilemma,

> . . . being aware that some other practitioners working with what I see as incompetence that is culpable and damaging.

The respondent went on to provide an instance of a trainee therapist they considered 'was being very ineptly handled by her therapist'.

Several respondents noted what they considered to be inappropriate comments by other colleagues or psychotherapists:

> On two occasions, clients told me of a colleague of mine making under-mining remarks about my clinical abilities due to my sexual orientation. The matter was serious enough to follow up, which I did. However, I felt I had to keep it quite separate from my clients and clinical work . . .

In this instance the psychotherapist considered the outcome was beneficial to their clinical work. Others reported denigration from colleagues with respect to the school of psychotherapy:

> Lack of respect – and denigration from colleagues from different training schools with different or same orientation towards trainees, etc. Due to lack of mutual contact and rivalry and ignorance.

Another type of dilemma concerned difficulties with referrals, where one professional referred a client/patient to more than one colleague, e.g. a psychotherapist, and a medical practitioner for ECT. There were also dilemmas regarding reports of colleagues amending contracts with clients – probably for financial reasons – and making inappropriate disclosures.

Sexual issues

Concerns about sexual issues accounted for 8.3% of the dilemmas reported. In this category, the sexual relationship between a psychotherapist and a client comprised the overwhelming proportion of the dilemmas reported. Six main issues arose with respect to these dilemmas:

- the fact that a therapist had a sexual relationship with a client
- the type of relationship, in particular whether it was long-term
- the timing of the relationship – did it start during or after psychotherapy
- who was considered to be taking a lead in developing the relationship
- the vulnerability of the client
- other sexual relationships such as between students and staff/supervisors.

Respondents reported a number of instances where they became aware of a colleague, or another psychotherapist, having an unethical sexual relationship.

I have had very painful experiences of finding out that my co-therapist had had sexual relations with our clients. This he did behind my back instead of asking me for help. Eventually I learned about it from others or from the clients themselves. Some people thought, of course, that it had been going on with my consent.

Disclosure of sexual abuse of clients and supervisees by a previous therapist who is still practising and has a high profile within the field.

In the majority of cases, no reference was made to the type of relationship, but in two instances the respondent specifically mentioned this was long term, for example:

Another colleague appeared to be living with a former patient, it seemed, but was not appropriate for me to establish, or was it? They began cohabiting when they were in a professional relationship.

The third issue, namely the timing of the relationship, is also raised in this dilemma. Where this was mentioned, the psychotherapist was understood to have started the intimate relationship during the period of psychotherapy, then the clinical relationship had stopped but the personal had continued. Within these respondents' reports there was no example of a psychotherapist starting an intimate relationship after therapy had stopped.

The fourth characteristic was the identity of the person taking the lead in developing a sexual relationship. In fact, in no case was it suggested that the client had been proactive. Rather, either explicitly or implicitly the respondents stated that the psychotherapist had been the active party.

A colleague has had in therapy someone who has been sexually molested by another (male) colleague, it is alleged.

Client telling me that a previous therapist had sex with her, and does not want to make a complaint.

Fifthly, some respondents made specific reference to the vulnerability of the client at the time of the relationship (e.g. 'a history of sexual abuse' or 'a very damaged and vulnerable woman').

In all of the above, the focus of the issue was the inappropriate relationship between a colleague psychotherapist and client. Other dilemmas regarding sexual behaviour included whether to disclose inappropriate sexual behaviour in clients most of which have been considered, with respect to sexual abuse (see Confidentiality p. 5). For example:

A supervisee had a client, a teacher, in a homosexual relationship with a 13-year-old pupil. The difficulty was deciding if this should be disclosed to the school authorities. After a lot of thinking one decided not to do this and continue work with the client towards ending the relationship.

The final category comprised overtly sexual behaviour by clients, e.g.

I worked with a male client who said he was in love with me and whilst working with him, in a dream he had started masturbating. He seemed unable to see anything past me (I am female)

or inappropriate intimacy, by a psychotherapist, allegedly governed by the psycho-therapeutic approach.

. . . inappropriate touching of that client was described and justified on the grounds that he was working in a client-centred way and the client needed to get in touch with feelings in her body.

Academic and training issues

The fifth largest category concerns training and supervision, with 6.3% of the dilemmas reported. The largest type of dilemma for psychotherapists within this category related to supervision:

Supervision of the psychotherapy of a patient who was herself in training with an organisation on the UKCP register. She was funding her life by prostitution. I felt torn between loyalty to the organisation and confidentiality – and too easy simply to advise the treating therapist to refuse to collude since, in the event, the patient simply changed therapist.

Other respondents who reported dilemmas arising from their supervision of therapists who they considered to be not ready to practice, or unsuitable.

. . . because of undealt-with issues in her own process, I did not think it appropriate for her to begin counselling.

Although in some cases the outcome was that the client changed from the respondent, in others the concern was that the training organisation sought no feedback on this area of training. Describing one trainee who first came in the second year of a two-year course, who had already left one psychotherapist, 'because he enraged her', one respondent reported,

. . . Her fourth session with me was spent entirely in a rage; she ranted for a full 50 minutes calling me, for instance, a stupid bitch who was as inconsistent and cruel as her mother had been. She cancelled the next appointment, taking the opportunity of ranting on the phone. Later she phoned to terminate the therapy. During the same period, she changed her doctor for being insufficiently courteous. Clearly she can't at present deal with her enormous transference problems. (She knew what transference is, but insisted that this wasn't anything to do with it.) My dilemma is that her course tutors want no feedback from her therapist(s). . .

In another example, however, the dilemma was:

> Being a therapist to a client who is also my student in training

and another respondent was concerned about having knowledge about individuals applying for training which could affect their acceptance on a course. Quite a number reported on knowing that trainees should not have been taken on training courses or should not be allowed to qualify because they were judged to constitute risks to clients seeing them for psychotherapy.

Competence

The final category to be considered in detail relates to respondents' concerns about competence (5.5% of dilemmas). Those reported concerned a variety of specific instances, without clear groupings of type of dilemma. For example, one psychotherapist was concerned about junior staff being referred cases by psychiatrists beyond their competence, while another reported a colleague who was drinking at work and not maintaining competence, whose contract was removed but:

> I have always wondered if I should have informed his professional association
> (not the same as mine)

Another psychotherapist did take action, but as the evidence was limited, felt vulnerable.

Other respondents referred to dilemmas regarding perceived lack of competence to undertake the work being addressed by counsellors at the beginning of their work,

> In the beginning of practice some, in ignorance, work entirely out of their
> depth, others with friends or even family members. Largely if not wholly this
> has been dealt with in supervision.

Issues to do with cultural difference

There were only four dilemmas reported with specific relevance to cultural differences. where clients because of cultural concerns were unable to get the right kind of competent help or supervision which they required.

Pedersen and Marsella (1982) wrote:

> A serious moral vacuum exists in the delivery of cross-cultural counseling and
> therapy services because the values of a dominant culture have been imposed
> on the culturally different consumer. Cultural differences complicate the
> definition of guidelines even for the conscientious and well-intentioned
> counselor and therapist. (p. 498)

and Korman (1974) is of the opinion that:

> The provision of professional services to persons of culturally diverse backgrounds by persons not competent in understanding and providing professional services to such groups shall be considered unethical. (p. 105)

> If we truly believe that multiculturalism is central to our definition of a competent counsellor, then monoculturalism can be seen as a form of maladjustment in a pluralistic society. (Szapocznik et al., 1983)

Comparison of psychotherapists with psychologists

The ethical dilemmas reported by our psychotherapist sample were compared with those given by members of the BPS and the APA (Table 1.2). Each of these samples contains a number of subgroups. For example, both the psychologist samples comprise randomly selected members of national associations of psychologists, and include academics and researchers as well as practitioners of various types (e.g. educational, clinical and occupational psychologists). However, both samples included psychologists who practised as psychotherapists.

The present sample were all psychotherapists in practice, many of whom were also supervisors and/or teachers on training courses. They each claimed adherence to one or more of a variety of schools and, while some were also psychologists, others had other backgrounds.

The most prevalent type of dilemma reported by each group comprised matters of confidentiality, with similar major sub-types: disclosure of child abuse and potential risk to others were the most frequent concerns. In each case the respondents reporting such dilemmas were faced by the need to respect confidentiality, as a keystone of professional practice, in conflict with responsibility to other members of society.

After this item, however, the ratings for each sample diverged. For psychotherapists the major dilemma concerned dual relationships, the conduct of colleagues and sexual issues. These three categories primarily encompassed inappropriate relationships, which conflicted with the practice of psychotherapy; for example, where psychotherapists, often in

Table 1.2: Ethically troubling incidents: A comparison of UKCP, BPS and APA samples.

Category	UKCP (%)	BPS (%)	APA (%)
Confidentiality	31	17	18
Dual relationships	12	3	17
Colleagues' conduct	9	7	4
Sexual issues	8	6	4
Academic/training	6	3	8
Competence	6	3	3

error, find they had a professional relationship with clients who had a close personal relationships. This is particular to the psychotherapeutic process and so would not apply to psychologists not involved in such work, whereas issues of competence, for example, are potentially common across all in each sample. Sexual relationships between the psychotherapist and client, whether seen as abusive or long-term and therefore, arguably, by mutual consent, were reported as ethical transgressions. Concerns about non-sexual dual relationships were also second highest ranked (17%) for the APA sample, but not for the BPS (3%, ranked ninth). On the other hand, conduct of colleagues ranked higher for BPS respondents (7%, ranked fourth) than APA (4% ranked seventh); sexual issues was similar: 6% ranked sixth for BPS, 4% ranked seventh for APA.

Ethical dilemmas arising from training were relatively infrequent in the BPS sample, (at 3%) whereas for psychotherapists these were more common. Psychologists in the APA reported proportionately more ethical dilemmas concerning academic/training issues (8%). It is also important to note that, on the whole, training dilemmas for the psychotherapists were also concerned with aspects of supervision, and the distinction in our analysis between these two categories was consequently problematic. In common with the psychologist samples, there were dilemmas arising from the resources and arrangements for training courses, particularly with respect to the cavalier approach to professionalism considered to be shown by some colleges and training institutions.

Unlike the ethical dilemmas reported by members of the BPS, the clear preponderance for psychotherapists were of the type termed 'traditional' by Lindsay and Colley (1995), that is concerns which are the focus of ethical codes in psychology, medicine and other similar professions. There were very few dilemmas of the second type identified in that study namely those arising from the pressure of employers (e.g. the National Health Service Trusts, or local education authorities) for psychologists to conform to particular guidelines concerning finance, for example, rather the professional judgement or evidence. Even in cases where dilemmas concerned a client in training, the majority related to traditional questions of competence, inappropriate relationships and the like, with rare exceptions. It is possible that this may be due to the fact that psychotherapy in the UK is a much younger profession than psychology and thus less aware of organisational issues at this stage of this development.

Consequently, the dilemmas of the psychotherapists tended to be addressed by the ethical codes of professional bodies. However, as with the psychologists this does not diminish the difficulties faced by the respondents when ethical principles were in conflict. This was particularly the case with the majority of dilemmas in the confidentiality category. On the other hand, psychotherapists reported more concerns regarding various types of inappropriate relationships of colleagues, with the dilemma of determining whether to take action, and if so what to do.

In some cases the respondent considered harm was clearly being caused, but in others they were not sure or, often, lacked direct evidence, receiving the information from a client in therapy or supervision. Some clearly felt vulnerable themselves (e.g. to losing referrals from colleagues) if they reported such allegations, and there were reports of relief when the psychotherapist concerned left practice for other reasons. Psychotherapists, therefore, reported a range of situations including taking action, welcoming unplanned events which resolved their dilemma, and feeling helpless that they did nothing – 'I feel strongly that my colleague should have done something about it then. He is my boss' – or they felt unable to act themselves, bound by confidentiality.

Finally, it is of interest that in all three studies, a significant minority of those who responded reported that they had had no ethical dilemmas. In the present study of UKCP psychotherapists this was reported by 22% of the respondents. Although in some cases this was explained by the respondent being very new to practice, or having retired, the majority made statements similar to this respondent:

> I do not consider I have had to face any ethical dilemmas.

Is it really the case that such a large minority of psychotherapists have not faced ethically troubling incidents? This is more easy to accept from the psychologist samples which contained many respondents whose work would have been less frequently likely to pose ethical challenges. Or is it unawareness? Or a reframing of the issue as with this respondent:

> I have not had any troubling ethical dilemmas in the past 10 years. But I suppose having spent 40 years as a GP, I am used to dealing with them before they became a problem – also I have learned to keep my mouth shut! Something I know is a problem for some therapists.

Our study has revealed ethical dilemmas that arise out of conflicts between accepted, competing ethical principles, where the essence of the dilemma is the resolution of the weight to be placed on each principle as a guide for action. In addition, a second set of ethical dilemmas, which interact with the first category, concern behaviour believed to be inappropriate (e.g. sexual relationships between psychotherapist and client) but where the dilemma is whether, and how, to take action. These are frequently not easy to resolve, but whereas the first group may be seen as intrinsic to the nature of psychotherapeutic and psychological practice, the second group represent behaviour violating the code of ethical conduct. Hence the former, being always with professionals in these fields, indicate the need for training and supervision at both initial and the post-qualification levels, whereas the latter imply the need for clearer guidelines on procedures to be followed when transgressions are suspected or known.

The BPS and the member organisations of the UKCP have codes of conduct, but the investigatory and disciplinary procedures vary in effectiveness. The need for effective regulation of psychotherapists is clearly shown by this study. The progress of the BPS towards the accreditation of chartered psychologists specialising in psychotherapy will aid its own regulatory system, but this process will not offer the degree of protection to the public available from appropriate statutory regulation, hence the Society's activity in attempting to persuade the government to implement a Psychologist Act which would give statutory power to disciplinary procedures. It is clear from the present study that the need for the effective regulation of psychotherapists is also evident.

References

Antikainen, J. (1997) Ethical dilemmas for psychologists in Finland. Chapter presented to the Vth European Congress of Psychology, Dublin, July.

Colnerud, G. (1997) The patient died but we did not break the principle of confidentiality. Paper presented to the 5th European Congress of Psychology, Dublin, July.

EFPPA (European Federation of Professional Psychologists Associations) (1997) Meta-Code of Ethics. Leicester: The British Psychological Society for EFPPA.

Hekman, S. J. (1995) Moral Voices, Moral Selves: Carol Gilligan and Feminist Moral Theory, Cambridge: Polity Press.

Korman, M. (1974) National conference on levels and patterns of professional training in psychology: major themes. American Psychologist, 29, 301–13.

Lindsay, G. (1995) Values, ethics and psychology. The Psychologist, 4, 493–8.

Lindsay, G. and Colley, A. (1995) Ethical dilemmas of members of society. The Psychologist, 8, 448–51.

McGee, H. (1995) The importance of being ethical. The Irish Psychologist, 18(6), 45–6.

Odland, T. (1997) Colleagues' conduct: The double dilemma. Chapter presented to the Vth European Congress of Psychology, Dublin, July.

Pedersen, P. B. and Marsella, A. J. (1982) The ethical crisis for cross-cultural counseling and therapy. Professional Psychology, 23, 492–500.

Pettifor, J. (1996) Ethics: virtue and politics in the science and practice of psychology. Canadian Psychology, 37, 1–12.

Pope, K.S. and Vetter, V.A. (1992) Ethical dilemmas encountered by members of the American Psychological Association. American Psychologist, 47, 397–411.

Sinclair, C. (1997) Ethical dilemma of psychologists: Canada and Columbia. Chapter presented to the Vth European Congress of Psychology, Dublin, July.

Szapocznik, J., Kurtines, W.M., Foote, F.H., Perez-Vidal, A. and Herris, O. (1983) Conjoint versus one-person family therapy: some evidence for the effectiveness of conducting family therapy through one person, Journal of Consulting and Clinical Psychology. 51: 881–99.

Vetere, A., Newell, A., Watts, M. and Kosviner, A. (1997) The registration of psychologists specialising in psychotherapy. The Psychologist, 10, 269–71.

Wassenaar, D.R. and Slack, C. (1997) Ethical dilemmas of South African Clinical Psychologists. Chapter presented to the Vth European Congress of Psychology, Dublin, July.

ITEM 1
The Psychotherapy and Counselling Oath

MARK AVELINE AND PETRŪSKA CLARKSON

Oaths and codes of ethics and practice

Each professional organisation for psychotherapy and counselling is elaborating codes of ethics and practice. These are important, but essentially they serve the needs of the organisation. They usually do not address the most deeply personal commitments of the individual practitioners. There is a significant difference between a code and an oath.

The form of an oath is very different from any codification of ethical principles. An oath goes directly to the heart of the personal undertaking and possesses a felt dimension which reserves issues of interpretation. The enunciation of an oath is a different order of process from legalistic issues of interpretation, being binding in conscience in the first instance. A codification of ethical rules may acquire the same ultimate value and moral imperative as an oath, but is neither a contract nor is it binding in conscience; it merely regulates a relationship by means of specified sanction. The behaviour of the therapist may become directed towards the avoidance of sanction in order to preserve the benefits that arise from subscribing to the code and, hence, retaining membership of the profession. The tendency, therefore, could be to obey the letter of the code at the expense of upholding spirit of the rules.

An oath is not a contract, but a profession in the sense of a public declaration of allegiance; the attitudes that the oath embodies are professed in the act of making it. A specific moment is reserved for its inception as a defining act in the formation of a therapist. It is a threshold in a rite of passage. A resonance is set up within the personality of the person giving oath. It becomes part of the way they define and present themselves in the world. A broken oath is a breach in the personal integrity of an individual, whereas a breach in an ethical code may be experienced as something less serious, possibly a mere failure to

17

comply with certain regulations which at some point have come to comprise freedoms relinquished, in order to obtain the benefit of inclusion in a particular professional group. The words 'agree to be bound' which often describe the relationship of a person to an ethical code are apparently silent on matters of individual integrity outside the perimeters of the contractual instrument.

An oath, also, represents a commitment to the principles of natural justice which imbed the action of the oath in the narrative and supra-individual dimensions of professional rules of conduct. It demands more than mere adherence to a code of ethics or practice. It demands commitment to the integrity of the oath as a whole, as well as to the honouring and enhancement of its professional purposes.

In the hallowed tradition of the Hippocratic oath, we offer an oath for the professions of psychotherapy and counselling.

The psychotherapy and counselling oath

I swear to uphold the good practice of my art during my lifetime as a therapist.

I will enter every therapy primarily for the good of my client*, keeping myself from all intentional ill-doing.

I will accept responsibility for my actions and seek to advance the field through critical reflection and research. Throughout my lifetime in this work, I will maintain my skills and seek to improve them. My attitude will one of learning from those with whom I work professionally and from wise colleagues. I will pay due honour to my teachers and the wisdom of the profession. I will pass on my learning through the teaching of others.

I will not claim or imply that I have greater experience or knowledge than is mine. I will recognise the limitations of my knowledge and skills and will call upon the expertise of others whenever necessary.

To my work, I will bring attitudes of humility and tolerance, respecting the decisions of others, the struggles that they have had in their lives and the compromises that they have made. I will be modest about both the power to influence of my therapeutic model(s) and the limits of its capacity to depict and explain the complexity of human nature and life. I will recognise that I am the product of my time and my culture with its biases and ideals. In this, I am not a first born, but part of a tradition which has shaped me and which I continue to influence. I will seek to be aware of my personal traditions and respect the traditions of those with whom I work professionally.

I will behave ethically in accordance with my conscience, even when I am in a minority or risk opprobrium and sanction.

I will endeavour to act in good faith, prizing truthfulness and tempering candour with respect for the client's situation and wish.

I will appreciate my client's circumstance, being aware of the interrelationship between responsibility and freedom, and will adapt my work and expectations in accordance with the client's capacity to exercise choice as it changes over time and condition.

My primary duty of care is to those with whom I work professionally. At times, I may also owe a duty of care to others, either because of legal or contractual requirement or ethical or moral duty. I will keep the secrets entrusted to me and explain where and when it may be necessary to share them with others.

I recognise that I came into this work with complex motivation and that I have a dual responsibility to the client and myself to maintain my well-being in order to offer the best service to my clients. I will not abuse my privileged position as therapist to exploit clients for my own pleasures and fears, recognising the need to lead a fulfilling life of my own.

If I keep this oath faithfully, may my craft and joy in this work increase to the benefit of all those whose lives are touched by it.

*Users of this oath can use either client or patient as suits their own practice.

Our grateful acknowledgement to Vincent Keter for his contribution to this work.

CHAPTER 2
Ethical Relationships

PETRŪSKA CLARKSON

> Reason cannot help the moral self without depriving the self of what makes the self moral: that unfounded, non-rational, unarguable, no-excuses-given and non-calculable urge to stretch towards the other, to caress, to be for, to live for, happen what may. . . [morality] can be 'rationalized' only at the cost of self-denial and self-attrition. From that reason-assisted self-denial, the self emerges morally disarmed, unable and unwilling to face up to the multitude of moral challenges and cacophony of ethical prescriptions. At the far end of the long march of reason, moral nihilism waits: that moral nihilism which in its deepest essence means not the denial of binding ethical code, and not the blunders of relativistic theory – but the loss of the ability to be moral.
> (Bauman, 1993, pp. 247 and 248)

As Hillman and Ventura (1992) pointed out in the title of their best-selling book: We've had a hundred years of psychotherapy and the world's getting worse. Of course, we have also had a hundred years of other things, and a conviction that the world is getting worse has been the opinion of parents at least since the time of Socrates. Psychotherapeutic work of some kind has probably existed since the dawn of time – patients were paying attention to their dreams on the kline (sleeping couch – from which the word 'clinic' is derived) of Aesclepius. But we stand in the light of that dawn and draw from those roots today whether we are aware of it or not. A hundred years is certainly a good span of time for reflection. And the next millennium is with us.

We know little of the ancient training schools for healers. Initiation ceremonies, segregation from the ordinary social group to live in priestly or Shamanic enclosures, temples, caves and personal journeys into hallucination (as in Siberian 'magician' circles) and culturally sanctioned possession as (as in Brazilian candombles) seem common across many cultures. As far as we know the first human explanations of the

emotional lives of men and women came from the notion of animism –
the belief that the world is controlled by god or gods, spirits, demons
and supernatural beings of different kinds. The beliefs of the class in
power – whether it be the Shamanic priests, Stalin's psychiatrists or
eurocentric child developmental theory – usually determines not only
the definitions of mental health and mental illness, but also the spiritual,
emotional and often physical fate of the mentally ill and the psychologically disturbed. It is salutary to remind ourselves that psychology's
original roots are from philosophy and religion and deeply coloured by
this vein of mysticism from many traditions.

At this point in history we also have to cope with the thought that,
despite fundamentalist convictions of some of the different theoretical
schools of psychoanalysis and psychotherapy that they possess the one
and only truth, in a growing body of research (e.g. Seligman, 1995),
none of them has been found to be particularly better than any of the
others. On the other hand, the very proliferation of approaches – some
450 at last count – suggests more a desperate search than the discovery
of certainty. I often wonder what trust we would place in a surgeon who
offered us 450 very different procedures to choose from for our heart by-
pass and the opportunity to take 'responsibility' for how the operation
turned out! But then perhaps psychotherapy is not really much like
medicine – in which case perhaps there should be less talk of 'standards
of practice', and as many psychotherapies as there are individuals who
seek such help? One enduring thread, however the standards may have
changed over the centuries, is the ethical heart of the Hippocratic oath –
to enter into the healing relationships to help and – in the first place –
not to injure (*primum non nocere*).

This makes it perhaps dangerous and irresponsible to regard 'ethics'
as something supplementary to the practice of psychotherapy when it is
a concession to consumer culture, an attempt to be seen to be politically
correct or an enactment of compliance to an external authority. In the
absence of any reliable evidence (outside of our own beliefs) that the
knowledge of a body of theory makes much difference to the outcome of
our work, the only rational justification for valuing psychotherapy
(financially or otherwise) as a profession, appears to be the presence of
ethics as the *sine qua non* of the relationship whose only purpose is
'therapeutic'. It is our commitment and express undertaking to further,
wherever possible and to the best of our knowledge, the growth and
well-being of our patients, and to refrain from doing anything adverse to
this goal, that sets us apart and gives a special value to our work.
Arguably, the boundary which divides ethical practice from quackery or
abuse is the degree to which any of us can maintain an unceasing critical
reflection on this undertaking in our own therapeutically intended
relationships. I am paraphrasing Plato when I remind us of what was
said to Thrasymachus: 'no one . . . in his capacity as therapist, considers

or enjoins his own advantage, but the advantage of this patient, the person for whom his practises his expertise. Everything he says and everything he does is said and done with this aim in mind and with regard to what is advantageous to and appropriate for this person. (Plato, 1974, Bk. I, 342e, written c. 390 BCE).

So, several trends are characteristic of the *fin-de-siècle* psychotherapy scene:

- psychotherapeutic approaches have proliferated *ad libitum*
- there are no consensually agreed discernible outcome differences attributable to theoretical orientation
- there is integration within schools – a kind of virtuous contagion
- there is integration between schools – not least as they begin to acknowledge that certain commonalities such as the centrality of the therapeutic relationship outweigh doctrinal disputes
- there is an attempt to reach consensus on certain issues such as standards, training procedures and professional ethics and practice – even to the extent where the differences in core syllabi is disappearing and trainees from very different schools share essentially the same core of reading and practice expectations.

As I've cautioned, one of the profound disadvantages may be exactly that the distinctiveness, uniqueness and individuality of different voices may be lost in this scramble for respectability, accountability and commonly agreed recognisable standards, bureaucratically defined standards of accreditation of component competencies, and auditing rules and regulations. Not that the latter are not honourable objectives and well worth pursuing – only that they too have a shadow which can obscure more fundamental principles. The solution to any one problem so often contains the seeds of the next problem like invisible succulent shoots of virulent weeds under the pristine surface of the newly ploughed field.

We also find that individual psychotherapists or psychoanalysts rarely fit into neat categories, particularly the more experienced they become. Already in the 1950s Fiedler, for example, studied the differences between exponents of three different schools of psychotherapy – Freudian, Adlerian and humanistic. He found that the differences in actual practice between more experienced people were considerably smaller than between beginners of different schools and their more senior colleagues from the same approach. That is, it appears that which theory is followed is much less important than the experience of therapeutic relationships. In 1953 Heine found that it was not possible, from a description of therapist activity, to determine to which theoretical school a psychotherapist belongs.

Of course it is also always possible to contest or question research results – and the good reasons/justifications are infinite. They range from methodological criticisms on the one hand to a treasuring of the essentially ineffable mystery of the therapeutic encounter which intrinsically cannot (and should not?) be measured. However,

> the meta-analyses mostly fail to show any difference between different forms of treatment, no matter how different in philosophy, e.g. psychodynamic or behavioural, or how different the procedures, e.g. group or individual, and no matter what the disorder being treated. This lack of appreciable condition treatment interactions is confirmed by a much smaller number of well-controlled comparative studies (e.g. Sloane et al., 1976). The only exception to the apparently non-specific effects of psychotherapy is the slightly greater success of behavioural methods in treating obsessions and phobias. But even they can be treated with almost equal success by psychodynamic methods. The lack of specificity is also shown by the comparative effectiveness of many treatments which are neither psychodynamic nor behavioural nor indeed psychological in any sense. (Prioleau et al., 1983 in Howarth, 1989, p. 150)

There appears to be no significant evidence that a theoretical approach is relevant to the successful outcome of psychotherapy – no matter how hard people have tried in the last hundred years and – no matter how measured (Norcross and Goldfried, 1992; Barkham, 1995; Elkin, 1995; Seligman, 1995; Parry and Richardson, 1996; Roth and Fonagy, 1996; Shapiro, 1996; Arundale 1997; Norcross 1997; Clarkson 1998).

There is, however, substantial evidence that it is the psychotherapeutic relationship rather than diagnosis or technique which potentiates the beneficial effects of psychotherapy. (See Fiedler, 1950, Clarkson, 1990, 1995b, 1998 and Norcross, 1997 as well as Chapter 12 for more detail.) It has further been found that different kinds of relationship are required for different kinds of patients and this factor is more important than diagnosis in predicting effectiveness of psychotherapy (Norcross, 1997).

On the other hand, evidence does exist that there are experiences of psychotherapy by which people feel harmed. One of the most salient facts here is that the harmfulness seems to have to do with the extent to which a psychotherapist entrenches into a theoretical position when challenged or questioned by their client (Masson,1989; Winter, 1997).

So, the evidence for the relationship as the common factor across different psychotherapeutic approaches therefore exists in:

- the bulk of the psychotherapy outcome research literature
- an extensive qualitative study of the literature of psychotherapy (Clarkson, 1995a, 1996b) – surveying some 1000 publications in psychoanalysis, psychology and psychotherapy published over these last 100 years
- anecdotal form – in subjective, phenomenological reports in informal research in which clients or colleagues were asked what had been the most important factor in their psychotherapy: clients tend not to report, for example, on the effectiveness of insightful interpretations

or elegantly facilitated catharsis. They report the significance of the relationship – that someone was there – that someone cared – that it mattered (Howe, 1993)

• finally, of course, it has been well documented throughout history that an important relationship – whether with God, an idea or another person – is what has facilitated major and permanent life changes in crisis, education, religious/political conversion or falling in love (see Clarkson, 1989).

We are born of relationship, nurtured in relationship, and educated in relationship. We represent every biological and social relationship of our forebears, as we interact and exist in a consensual domain called 'society' (Cottone, 1988, p. 363). Workers such as Goodwin (1994) at the frontiers of the new sciences bear out the centrality of relationship to human life:

> And we are biologically grounded in our relationships which operate at all the different levels of our being as the basis of our nature as agents of creative evolutionary emergence, a property we share with all other species. These are not romantic yearnings and utopian ideals; they arise from a re-thinking of our biological natures that is emerging from the sciences of complexity and is leading towards a science of qualities which may help in our efforts to reach a more balanced relationship with the other members of our planetary society. (p. xiv)

Relationship is at the heart of life. Human beings live and breathe in relationship. Relationship brings us some of our greatest joys and our greatest agony. Solitary confinement is one of the worst punishments available to man and the restoration of relationship one of its greatest rewards (as John McCarthy testified again at a 1998 conference of the International Association of Group Psychotherapy in London). The relationship is common – and crucial – to most approaches to psychotherapy. As psychotherapists we are at core professionally concerned with being in a relationship that is therapeutic. Of course our manner of being there will be the end product at that moment of our entire past, as well as present contact and future fears or aspirations.

The five therapeutic relationships: a framework for psychotherapy, training and supervision

If indeed the psychotherapeutic relationship is one of the most, if not the most, important factor in successful psychotherapy, one would expect much of the training in psychotherapy to be training in the intentional use of relationship. Some psychotherapies claim that psychotherapy requires use of only one kind of relationship, or at most two, for example, the ' therapeutic alliance' and the transference. Some specifically exclude the use of certain kinds of relationship. For example,

Goulding and Goulding (1979), transactional analysts, minimise the use of transference, whereas Moiso (1985), also in transactional analysis, sees it as a central focal point of classical Berneian psychotherapy. Gestaltists such as Polster and Polster (1973) and the existentialists such as May (1969) focus on the existential nature of the therapeutic relationship. Some psychotherapeutic approaches pay hardly any theoretical attention to the nature of the relationship and they may attempt to be entirely free of content (for example, in some approaches to hypnotherapy or NLP, therapeutic changes are claimed to be made by the patient without the practitioner necessarily knowing what these changes may be). In most approaches, of course, stated policy and actual practice often diverge. Even the actions of Freud (speaking perhaps louder than his words) often belied the assumed orthodoxy of psychoanalytic practice (see for example, Malcolm, 1981).

Of course, it is quite possible for an observer of a video of a session to see the skilful use of the therapeutic relationship – whether or not the practitioner is overtly or theoretically acknowledging the importance of the relationship. Milton Erickson (1967), for example, reveals a consummate master at work. Gee (1995) in a different context, displayed a willingness to consciously integrate different theoretical and ideological positions in his research on supervision delivered at a British Association for Psychoanalytic and Psychodynamic Supervision conference in London in 1995. He also emphasised that what unifies and makes integration possible is the centrality of the relationship in all approaches to psychotherapy and psychotherapy supervision.

Considering psychotherapy from the vantage point of the different kinds of relationships focused on by exponents of different orientations, it was thought that all approaches to psychotherapy would find their respective voices within the universe of discourse encompassed by the notion of 'the therapeutic relationship'. Therefore, depending on the scope and range of the practitioner, a comprehensive relationship framework could be more comprehensive, theoretically hospitable and practically compatible with almost all known approaches to psychotherapy. From my qualitative research, also reviewing that of others (Clarkson, 1990 and researching the therapeutic relationship) I identified five kinds of therapeutic relationship – *five universes of discourse* across all the major approaches to psychotherapy about the therapeutic relationship. These five modalities emerged as:

- the *working alliance* – the aspect of client-psychotherapist relationship that enables the client and therapist to work together even when the patient or client experiences strong desires to the contrary
- the *transferential/countertransferential* relationship – as the experience of unconscious wishes and fears transferred on to or into the therapeutic partnership

- the *reparative/developmentally needed* relationship – as intentional provision by the psychotherapist of a corrective, reparative, or replenishing relationship or action where the original parenting (or previous experience) was deficient, abusive or overprotective
- the *person-to-person* relationship – as the real or core relationship, the subject relationship as opposed to object relationship
- the *transpersonal* relationship – as the timeless facet of the psychotherapeutic relationship, which is impossible to describe, but refers to the inexplicable or spiritual dimensions of the healing relationship.

It is important to remember these are not stages but states in psychotherapy or psychoanalysis, often subtly 'overlapping', in and between which a client construes his or her unique experiences. This framework, whether called 'the five modes of relationship', or the five aspects of the therapeutic relationship or the five facets or the 'five-relationship framework' has been quite extensively used to form the inspiration or the basis for integration between approaches or to deepen one's understanding of any one approach. (It is not correct to call it the five 'levels' of relationship, since levels connotes another universe of discourse – the seven-level model of epistemological discourse [Clarkson, 1975] and skews my meanings into a misleading philosophical context.)

The then editor of the *British Journal of Psychotherapy* wrote about my original paper on the multiplicity of co-existing potential therapeutic relationships in any therapeutic encounter (Clarkson, 1990) that the framework of five therapeutic relationships exists in all psychotherapies – even though different psychotherapies prioritise different levels. 'This offers a way of circumventing the inherent contradictions and incompatibilities that exist between different psychotherapies; instead of incompatibilities we have different priorities and emphasis' (Hinshelwood, 1990, p. 119).

Practitioners may privilege one or more of these in their work, and clients, whether patients or organisations, may actually need different kinds of relationship at different times during their therapeutic journey. Hauke (1996) described my intentions for my *Therapeutic Relationship* book very well when he wrote that:

> It is a postmodern text that is clearly comfortable with the pluralistic 'universes of discourse' that exist in psychology and psychotherapy today, and which require of us a tolerance and a revaluation of fragmentation, a fresh look at old essentialisms. What is 'right' in psychology is what is right in each particular context, person or treatment. (p. 407)

Emphasis on each kind of relationship draws in specific universes of discourse, encompassing different worlds of values, perspectives on human nature, assumptions about free will and determinism, individuality and commonality, prejudices, blind spots and particular gifts of caution and vision. There are of course errors of confusion, conflation, abuse and neglect which can affect the responsible and effective use of all therapeutic relationships. Any or all of these can be used constructively and creatively or act as vortices for the violation of relationship.

Ethics and morality permeate every therapeutic relationship. Indeed, there may be no 'response-able' place for the psychotherapist to posit social responsibility or cultural and ecological awareness different or separate from therapeutic work (Samuels, 1989). In my way I have tried to say – whether explicit or implicit – they are the same. Because, being human, we are in relationship – with each other, the rhinoceroses in Africa, the billboards, the planet itself (Clarkson, 1989). Context is everywhere. In its original Merleau-Ponty sense:

> Intersubjectivity . . . describes the fact that our being is predicated on being in a world with others. [It] is a condition of human existence and not a specific quality of relating. Although there are types of relating within the intersubjective field which are important to identify and distinguish. This differentiation between modes of interaction are essential for the greater development of clinical understanding.' (Diamond, 1996, p. 322)

In some particular ways including entanglement theory from the new physics (C. Isham, personal communication, 1995), we can never be truly separate from each other, never not communicate with each other (even when we're not speaking), never disengage from relationship as long as time lasts.

Issues of ethics, morals and values should ideally not be seen as being an 'add-on' to any of the therapeutic relationships, but an intrinsic and inextricable part of every relationship, including the five modes that I have identified (Clarkson, 1990). As soon as 'culture', for example, is subject to such a state of 'apartheid', the distance may increase – and we know from personal experience and psychological studies that proximity can sometimes even help to reduce prejudice. A separation of content and context on these matters may be seen as equivalent to tacking on 'a module' on race or ethics in counsellor education or organisational development – instead of inviting such awareness to scent the very air we always breathe together.

Being ethical is not an additional relationship, it permeates all our relationships – and all kinds of therapeutic relationships. My plea is exactly for inclusion, not an artificial separation. I know, of course, that I do not succeed in this. I hope for recognising that the theoretical and professional separation often reflects both the origin and the continuation of the problem of denial of human relationship. The recognition of our interrelationship could begin to restore and enliven the dualistic Newtonian/Cartesian fractures in our sensibilities as well as in our professional lives.

It may be tempting to view the sociocultural-planetary context as a relationship mode in its own right. However, this view is philosophically flawed. This is because the purpose of isolating the five different kinds of discourse about therapeutic relationships is primarily to assist the practitioners in the relationship in identifying the task or the work to be done. It is often not possible or useful to isolate the sociocultural context in this way separate from the people in the relationship. I think this can result in an artificial stripping of the ethical from the theoretical and the practical – and at least since 1945 we should know better than that.

Here follow selected highlights on some of the polarities which can guide thinking, critique and theory-building, as well as strategies and interventions in using the five relationships as a framework for thinking and developing ethics in practice, supervision and training psychotherapy. These categories can also be applied in any psychotherapy or approach to applied psychology which seeks to take account of perspectives more inclusive than single secular, ideologically provincial concerns. This section is not designed to be a comprehensive overview of ethical considerations in clinical practice, but to indicate ways in which the five relationship framework can be used. It is merely a reflection specifically on the relationships and their ethical implications as an example of the kind of thinking and questioning which I trust readers will themselves take much further and deeper.

There are, of course, errors of confusion, conflation, abuse and neglect which can affect the responsible and effective use of all therapeutic relationships – particularly when they are not differentiated and distinguished. Emphasis on each one in turn draws in specific universes of discourse, encompassing different worlds of values, perspectives on human nature, assumptions about free will and determinism, individuality and commonality, prejudices, blind spots and particular gifts of caution and vision. I hope I have pointed out at least a significant number of these throughout this book to inspire and alert readers to their own most favourite and their own most avoided concerns.

The selected core themes for ethical focus are divided into pairs of polarities. Neither extreme is advocated, but since we are never permanently 'in balance', the question is asked: with which patient at this time am I tending to move in either direction – and why? Of course there are many other possibilities for readers to explore and rediscover, but those below are frequently foregrounded in training and supervision of students in psychotherapy training, supervision courses and collegial peer discussions of these issues.

Ethical issues around the working alliance: coercion or defensiveness

The continuum which ranges from defensiveness to coercion is quite a prevalent consideration in considering the ethical implications of the working alliance. When can it be said that a person has given informed consent?

> I challenge any psychotherapist to say directly to a client: 'I can probably make you feel better, but I am unlikely to be any more effective than a friend, a priest or a good variety of less qualified persons. Moreover, there is a real possibility which we must choose to ignore, that I will reduce your chances of promotion and make you more likely to become physically or mentally ill.' At the present time that is the honest thing to say and the only statement which can elicit appropriately 'informed consent'. (Howarth, 1989, p. 151)

Is it informed consent when a client is in despair, *in extremis*, and the psychoanalyst says that he or she is to lie down on the couch if they want to be helped? When a client is admitted to hospital and the 'doctors-in-white-coats-who-know-in-authority' decide that electric shock or a leucotomy is the best remedy? Or that short-term cognitive-behaviour therapy is indicated? Or that a client necessarily wants or needs a 'talking cure' which 'helps them to help themselves', rather than the provision of good guidance and advice based on better knowledge and experience – which is what many people may wish, and perhaps should have access to if that is what they do want?

The therapeutic working alliance can of course be used to focus on issues of social justice, client/therapist matching, choice of treatment, equal access to services, availability of information, cultural biases in testing and diagnosis, rights and responsibilities, differential confidentialities and so on – as in the example of the black man who was given ECT in South Africa for 'psychotic aural hallucinations' until a young psychiatrist discovered that the 'voices' were those on the intercom in the mental hospital (B. Dobson, personal communication, 1969).

I am thinking particularly of traditional models of healing, where a shaman, witch-doctor, guru or elder can be expected to prescribe a course of action which, if undertaken, is most likely (for whatever reasons) to lead to an amelioration of the problem and a reinstatement of the person's confidence and connection with the healing forces of their life and those of the world they inhabit. Paracelsus for example vowed:

> To give to each nation its own type of medicine best suited to it, as it behoves. For I can well realize that my prescriptions may turn out to be ineffectual among the foreign nations, and that foreign recipes may turn out to be ineffectual in our nation. (1958, p. 5)

As pointed out in my paper 'Despair Before Change' (Clarkson, 1991), the particular situation of counsellors in South Africa at that time was characterised by a hunger for appropriate knowledge and models.

They need money . . . and they also need people, but we need to be humble
and let them teach us. Importing European psychological models of
counselling based on the nuclear family for example can be destructive . . . it
is a visceral kind of counselling that is needed. Counselling needs to be
undertaken in the way that is most relevant' (p. 11).

In the UK, for example, there is overwhelming evidence that working-
class patients are, or certainly were, less likely to be offered
psychotherapy than other social classes (Bromley, 1995). At the moment,
it is not possible in the UK to find a list of black counsellors or
psychotherapists – and many Afro-Caribbeans, one of whom is now
doing her doctoral research on this theme, have complained to me
about this (Burrell, personal communication 1998).

In *Uncommon Therapy* Haley (1973) describes onerous and
sometimes painful and difficult preconditions prescribed for clients in
order to establish the working alliance. This is also the case in some
approaches to family therapy, for example the Milan School (in Cooklin,
1990; Gorell Barnes and Cooklin, 1994). Such procedures can and often
do enhance and stabilise the working relationship, but they are sometimes
based on what can be experienced as paradoxical trickery, mercurial so-
called therapeutic deceptions and the deliberate exercise of procedures to
which a client has perhaps given some verbal consent in terms of the
working alliance having asked for help, but not to the specifics of dignity,
truth and respect in particular aspects of the treatment.

One of the polarities of coercion is letting be, but in a negative sense
– ignoring or refusing to get involved. This can be a turning away or
withholding of information, help or succour in cases where the practitioners suspect it may be of help. The defensive practitioner may decline
the inclination to act because of concerns or fears about reputation,
ideological purism or a habitual and ill-considered disinclination to take
reasonable risks and opportunities. It is perhaps also both an insult to
the client and a demonstration of unthinking introjection of someone
else's discoveries on the part of the clinician if, after years, a desperate
person turns to a psychotherapist in hope of finally being helped – and
this person rejects the hopeful if naive expression of faith by some
psychologically knee-jerk reflex reaction which proclaims routinely that
'I do not have a magic wand'.

Then again there are the many instances where psychotherapists,
counsellors, psychologists or psychoanalysts turn patients away. They
reject them or refuse to work with them in case they are 'diagnosed' as
'difficult', borderline', 'psychopathic', 'overly dependent' with a bad
prognosis, the catch-all fashionable 'narcissistic', acting out, and so on.
Reluctance to get involved, prescribe, give information, provide
guidance, say what you believe is morally wrong and ethically unsound
can all be justified on the basis that the practitioner is simply 'taking
good care of themselves' by not rescuing, not getting involved,

maintaining the boundaries, etc. They may be, as I have even heard advocated in such circumstances 'protecting themselves'. However, what may be missing is the simple humanity of helping. Naively I have heard practitioners say, not once, but habitually about everybody: 'I never do more than 50% of the work'. On the contrary, sometimes I believe it is important for the regressed schizoid person or for the inhibited and traumatised child to have someone else such as a helper provide not only 50%, but even 100% of the work. This may be the only necessary and appropriate way to establish the working alliance where so often the sheer instillation of some hope or reasonable expectation is the *sine qua non* of seeding fruitful beginnings.

Ethical issues around the transferential/countertransferential relationship: reductionism or betrayal

For the purposes of our discussion here ethical issues around transference and countertransference are highlighted in terms of the polarity of reductionism or betrayal. The reductionism polarity may represent all those ethical transgressions or assaults where individual patients are reduced to the simplistic dynamics of transference interpretations no matter what the reality of their experience may be. These are the many instances where the client may protest at certain kinds of treatment – for example that 'There was at least one psychoanalyst who was regularly crocheting (!) in the sessions'. When the patient questioned this, the analyst referred it back to the client in terms of an interpretation of the client's pathology and forced her to choose between a lesbian lover and continuing in analysis. (This is in fact based on a real example of a psychoanalyst who claimed to be Kleinian.)

Many other instances concern cases where any criticism of the practitioner is (usually) seen as a sure sign of what is wrong with the patient in terms of the transference, thus de-legitimising and invalidating the serious and valid concerns of the client about the therapy or analysis itself. I have most frequently heard of this when colleagues have after some time (sometimes many years) attempted to terminate psychoanalysis or psychotherapy. Any indication that the treatment is not fully satisfactory is referred to, for example, the patient's resistance, their lack of ego-strength, the prevalence of their destructive envy. Given the uncomfortable dependency and trance-inductive elements of psychoanalysis and psychotherapy and some other forms of working, it is extremely hard for distressed or disturbed individuals to continue to trust their own judgement in the face of authority figures who know better than they interpreting all their objections, doubts and uncertainties as evidence of unresolved or unworked-through transferences emanating from an 'unconscious' in themselves to which they could never even have access. This kind of reductionism is an ethical concern in whatever theoretical language it is couched.

Furthermore, Little (1986) (amongst others) identified patients:

> . . . whose reality sense is seriously impaired, who cannot distinguish delusion or hallucination from reality, cannot use transference interpretations because the transference itself is of a delusional nature. Transference interpretation calls for the use of deductive thinking, symbolization, and the acceptance of substitutes. It is not possible to transfer something that is not there to be transferred, and in these patients their early experiences have not enabled them to build up either what needs to be transferred or a picture of a person on to whom transference is possible. They are still living in the primitive world of early infancy, and their needs have to be met on that level, the level of auto-eroticism and delusion. . . . In the early days of analysis no analyst had much personal analysis or much experience (either his own or other people's) to draw on, and in those days 'wild analysis' did in fact lead to danger situations which could not be dealt with. But conditions are different today, and the assertions that certain things are dangerous, or impede the analysis, can be tested out. Many such assertions seem to me to have the mythical or superstitious quality of superego judgements. (1986, pp. 75–6)

Equally at stake are the many explicit and implicit issues to do with neglect or ignorance of the person's wish to project or enact the transference drama and *the loss of the opportunity* to work through the transference with a psychodynamically skilful interpreter. Some therapists simply reject such a possibility. Thus their clients' capacity for and yearning for just such a transferential relationship possibility may be betrayed by destructive countertransferential contaminations which are neglected or ignored in the psychotherapy, the psychoanalysis or the course of psychological counselling – however they are dressed up as disciplinary, theoretical or differences of 'flag statements'. To use our clients for our own dramas, to stand in the way of their yearnings, to cure us of our madness (see Searles, 1975), to become dependent on being 'attractive' to our clients or supervisees in the absence of being 'attractive' to friends or lovers, is to betray the trust traditionally placed in healers of all descriptions. Even Hippocrates vowed by Apollo the physician, by Aesculapius, Hygeia, and Panacea, all the gods and all the goddesses:

> In every house where I come I will enter only for the good of my patients, keeping myself far from all intentional evil-doing and all seduction, and especially from the pleasures of love with women or with men. (Dorland, 1965, p. 680)

It is vitally important to acknowledge the presence in the consulting room – in or out of awareness – of far-reaching, powerfully violent and seductive forces of love and erotic attraction (Mann, 1997 is an admirable recent exploration of this theme). On the other hand it may be essential to consider the implications of the fact that some form of betrayal of the primal trust (Hillman, 1975) is a vital part of existential and personal maturation and that it is as important for the therapist not to provide a false, utopian, secure haven from the vicissitudes of real life (Samuels, 1993). Winnicott (1958, 1986) and Kohut (1977) also draw attention to the importance of 'failure' on the part of the therapist. This does *not* mean intentional evil-doing – merely the recognition that in the humanity of the physician there are many flaws – not all to the detriment of the patient. The most effective work may lie in the interstices of working through these failures rather than in the promise or provision of everlasting 'holding' in some womb-like Utopia – which means nowhere.

Of course, transference or countertransference issues may not always be as the therapist or supervisor perceives them. In psychotherapy of any kind (as in life) it is essential to question all our assumptions as culturally biased. This therapeutic dimension can highlight or bury particularly issues of prejudice including the psycho-physiological or emotional/olfactory bases of intuition, judgement, attraction, repulsion and culture-based assumptions; for example, the process of projective identification in an analyst's subtle rejection, shaming or minimisation of the sexuality of a person who is paraplegic, in a destructive arranged marriage or homosexual. For many women from certain African cultures the fear of being rejected by marriageable men outweighs the dangers of contracting AIDS. Airhihenbuwa et al. (1992) show that, for the women, to be rejected as a result of their insisting on condom use is a more immediate and palpable danger than potential death from the disease. To the inexperienced and economically dependent psychotherapist, transference or countertransference issues to do with money, real or perceived financial danger regarding the mortgage and children's education may additionally result in an ill-considered rejection of brief therapies, a refusal to confront ethical and professional misconduct in professionals who might make referrals to them, and also keeping on clients who actually need far more experienced or specialised care than they can actually provide.

Ethical issues around the developmentally needed or reparative psychotherapeutic relationship: dependency or deprivation

The major dimension of ethical concern which I encounter most frequently around this kind of relationship is that between dependency and deprivation. All the time-honoured admonishments against giving advice or information to clients or supervisees is grounded in the frequent and sometimes disastrous errors when deficit-filling interventions (for example, a transitional object over a holiday) are delivered without having a sound enough working alliance and within a distorted and unresolved transference or countertransference dynamic.

Sometimes the 'corrective or reparative experience' may result in some superficial beneficial change, but not the desired deep improvement, because the intervention did not address the problems as phenomenologically experienced by the supervisees. Another common mistake is to 'do it' for the therapist/client system rather than enabling clients and supervisees to find, use or discover their own resources.

However, on the other hand, to deprive clients or supervisees of information, guidance or advice when it is clear that they need it and likely that they will be able to use it well if carefully delivered, can be simply an unethical prolonging of ignorance and distress (Boadella, 1987). A married man needed only one session to relieve him of incapacitating guilt he felt for masturbating, by the practitioner providing him with the statistical information available on how normal and ordinary it is for many married men to do this – even happily married men. For a supervisee worried about whether the client complaining of persecution was psychotically paranoid, a call to the GP and the local race relations office was all that was needed to confirm that there had been many corroborated reports of vicious harassment on the client's housing estate.

Several court cases in the USA and a number of enquiries have led to a heightened awareness, both public and professional, of the destructive effects of dependency relationships forged in the name of psychoanalysis or psychotherapy. These can have disastrous, if not catastrophic or chronically limiting, effects on an individual's autonomy, freedom and capacity to heal and grow independently. Therapies are intrinsically no more or less dependency-evoking that encourage or welcome the kind of dependency associated with the reparative or developmentally-needed relationship than with certain types of transference relationships – they may evoke the same kind of dependency, with the exception that the client or patient is not 'gratified' in any way, but consistently frustrated.

Practitioners who favour the reparative or developmentally-needed relationship may indiscriminately engage in the same kind of dependency-provoking situation, but with slightly different repercussions. In the transference/countertransference relationship with an emphasis on deprivation, withholding and abstinence on the part of the therapist, there is the possible unethical outcome of a patient abandoned in their greatest need, deprived because of the dictates of the training institution, and/or neglected in obvious and necessary ways because of adherence to doctrinal mandates rather than the spontaneity and flexibility which is more commensurate with the approximations of real life.

Developmental theories, however useful otherwise, can also be abused within this mode of the therapeutic relationship for institutionalised infantilisation in therapy and in the training of therapists to support the *status quo* and compliance and delegitimise dissent or difference. Junior trainers on humanistic psychotherapy programmes, for example, have complained that their 'readiness' to teach or supervise was to be decided by their 'elders' on dubious, unknown and undisclosed grounds.

Ethical issues around the person-to-person or real relationship in terms of over-intimacy versus isolation: invasion or anomie

The person-to-person relationship is also referred to as the existential relationship, the core relationship, or the dialogic relationship. According to Merleau-Ponty (1962):

> In the experience of dialogue, there is constituted between the other person and myself a common ground; my thought and his are interwoven into a single fabric, my words and those of my interlocutor are called forth by the state of the discussion, and they are inserted into a shared operation of which neither of us is the creator. We have here a dual being, where the other is for me no longer a mere bit of behaviour in my transcendental field, nor I in his; we are collaborators for each other in consummate reciprocity. (p. 354)

This is the sense in which the practitioner is also changed by every important therapeutic relationship. Ethical dangers contingent on the over-disclosure or over-intimacy in the psychoanalytic or psychotherapeutic relationship have been very well documented (for example, Rutter, 1989). It has been shown that whenever there have been breaches in the boundaries of the relationships, for example, when practitioners have engaged in sexual or semi-sexual relationships with their clients, there has usually been some undue laxity of the boundaries which separate out the person as a professional (in a specified place for specified times) from the person as a private individual with a separate life, desires and naturally selfish needs and yearnings. I never returned to the hypnotherapist I once consulted to help me with my then 10 year 'writing block'. This man saw fit to tell me in this session – for reasons which I cannot recall – that his cat had died of throat cancer! Many clients have complained about hearing more about their therapist's private lives than they've ever wanted to know. I estimate that there is rightfully considerably more caution and clinical forethought before personal information is used in psychotherapy – or how it is used when it is staring you in the face – e.g. someone of a different colour. Yet, some of my most important personal therapeutic experiences in analysis have been when my analysts have shared their own personal feelings and experiences with me.

The opposite of invasion is the pretence or the denial of a real presence and natural undulations of life, love and existence and their impact on the course and the conduct of a psychotherapy or psychoanalysis. The reality of the person-to-person relationship and at least some minimal acknowledgement of it has been recognised in most practitioners from Sigmund to Anna Freud, from Langs to Casement, from Pavlov to modern-day cognitive-behavioural practitioners. It has also often been shown to be possible that the therapeutic person-to-person relationship can be used to explore the inescapability of valuing as part and parcel of every therapeutic moment, every perception, every intervention (or non-intervention), every disclosure as well as every non-disclosure, as well as the fundamental meanings of 'working with difference' – the unavoidable 'otherness' of another, any other.

Elsewhere (in *The Bystander*, Clarkson, 1996a), I explore in far greater detail the physical, emotional, phenomenological, cultural, rational, mythological and spiritual necessity for health and growth for human beings to experience, acknowledge and enact their relational connectedness with all other forms of life on this planet. When the reality of person is denied, another psychotic world is construed that I do not believe can be the basis for an ethical practice based on the core principles of the Hippocratic oath or the foundations of the practice that is the healing of souls. The origin of the word psychotherapy is, after all, the healing (therapy) of the soul (*psyche*). Sometimes the psychoanalyst or psychotherapist really is tired, bored or burgled (Herman, 19??).

Winter (1997) has shown from careful research that psychotherapeutic casualties are more likely to result from psychotherapists' retreat into rigidities and dogmatics of theory when they are challenged by their clients. This represents the polarity where practitioners isolate themselves from the human condition, often behind their ideologies which may be presented as 'theories'. This is where belief in the value of 'attachment', for example, can (and has) involved physically lying on (usually) attractive younger female clients. One of the worst situations I have ever come across of adherence to theory – in this case transference – was of an trainee in psychoanalysis who refused to respond humanely when the patient arrived at the door – she just been raped on her way there. The supervisee felt that if she went with the patient to the police station, she would be breaking the boundaries! Another more humorous example concerned a trainee at a conference who assured me that someone famous had published something about the particular issue we were discussing. When I enquired about the reference, she dismissively informed me that since she was more orthodox 'psychoanalytic' than me, she would not break the confidentiality boundaries of her source! (The much-published author was not her patient.)

Ethical issues around the transpersonal relationship: in terms of 'meaning from the mount' versus 'the despair of neglect' (bibles or illiteracy)

The transpersonal relationship refers to the spiritual, numinous or inexplicable dimensions of the relationship in psychotherapy and psychoanalysis. At the simplest level any experienced psychotherapist has discovered with Hamlet that ' There are more things on heaven and earth, Horatio, than are dreamed of in your philosophy.'

If one approaches this relationship dimension from a strictly scientific point of view we must also take account of the numerous inexplicable mysteries of science from Schrödinger's cat and entanglement theory to the indeterminism of chaos and complexity – as well as the inextricable relationship of observer and observed.

> Galileo was the first of a race of modern experimental scientists convinced of the infallibility of their 'exact empirical methods'; in fact he created the type. It comes as a surprise to hear him talk about things 'not only unknown but unimaginable'. But this ultimate modesty, derived from a sense of wonder close to mysticism, is found in all great scientists – even if hidden by an arrogant facade, and allowed to express itself only on rare occasions. (Koestler, 1989, p. 683)

If we approach it in the tradition of the great physicians (the word comes from *physis*, the life force) we hear time and time again that the doctor may prescribe the medicine, but it is Nature (or God) who heals. For many religious, spiritual or Jungian practitioners – by whatever name it is called – it permeates our work as Grace, as the Numinosum, as the Atman, Allah or Amen.

The transpersonal relationship is, I think, ethically most vulnerable to two extremes – too much and too little. If a psychotherapist is persuaded of a Zen perspective on life or a Christian patriarchal code of living, it is probably impossible for them to keep their own consulting work free of being influenced by their convictions. The practitioners who claim they can easily do this may well be in unethical practice far sooner and with more urgency than the psychological counsellor who searches during their supervision hours for the ways in which the religion of their childhood, the passing despairs of their own dark nights of the soul, the fleeting fancies of interest in things astrological or archetypal influence and permeate their practice. It is as always the naive assumption of scientific neutrality and objectivity that is of concern, rather than the self-questing and self-questioning individual helper who knows that it is impossible for us to interact without influence; who seeks to know the nature of those forces which influence us from each other, from the world, nature, the seasons, the undulations of history, the eager and potent psyche and the ancestral spirits of the person who sits (or dances) in front of us in the therapy session.

On the other hand, neglect, ignorance, denial or rejection of the transpersonal sources of meaning, the human yearning for awe, wonder, amazement, for transporting of the soul, is a travesty of our potential, whether it is still 'ethical' or not. To tie the human being to the mundane, to normalise only those adjustments which keep us manacled to blandness, to ordinariness, to mediocrity and conformity is to do violence to the madness, the excess, the spiritual expansiveness of the soul in the world and the world itself. However understood, it is a tragedy when the healers of soul cannot speak the language of the soul any more. The worst injustice is when they, without proper self-searching, prevent others from speaking this language or call it the language of the blind, the sick or the bigoted.

The therapeutic transpersonal relationship implicates the nature of the universe and our place in it – the creative order found at the edge of chaos, the way in which every thing is relationship, the interpenetration of observer and observed; of I and Thou; Physis rising and hiding, as living and dying, the paradoxical identity of wave and particle, self and other; the culmination of antimonian thought; the mystery of a quantum universe; the *conjunctio* of responsibility and freedom, justice and mercy, passion and compassion.

References

Airhihenbuwa, C.O., DiClemente, R.J., Wingood, G.M. and Lowe, A. (1992) HIV/AIDS education and prevention among African-Americans: a focus on culture. AIDS Education and Prevention, 4, 267–76.

Arundale, J. (1997) Editorial. British Journal of Psychotherapy 13(3), 305–6.

Barkham, M. (1995) Editorial: Why psychotherapy outcomes are important now. Changes 13(3), 161–3.

Bauman, Z. (1993) Postmodern Ethics. Oxford: Blackwell.

Boadella, D. (1987) Lifestreams: An Introduction to Biosynthesis. London: Routledge & Kegan Paul.

Bromley, E. (1995) Social class and psychotherapy revisited. British Psychological Society Psychotherapy Section Newsletter.

Clarkson, P. (1975) Seven-level Model. Paper delivered at University of Pretoria, November.

Clarkson, P. (1989) Gestalt Therapy in Action. London: Sage.

Clarkson, P. (1990) A multiplicity of psychotherapeutic relationships. British Journal of Psychotherapy, 7(2), 148–63.

Clarkson, P. (1991) Despair before change. Counselling News, March, 11.

Clarkson, P. (1995a) The Therapeutic Relationship. London: Whurr.

Clarkson, P. (1995b) Vengeance of the victim. In The Therapeutic Relationship, pp. 53–61. London: Whurr.

Clarkson, P. (1996a) The Bystander: An End to Innocence in Human Relationships? London: Whurr.

Clarkson, P. (1996b) Researching the 'therapeutic relationship' in psychoanalysis, counselling psychology and psychotherapy – a qualitative inquiry. Counselling Psychology Quarterly, 9(2), 143–62.

Clarkson, P. (1998) Beyond schoolism. Changes 16(1), 1–11.

Cooklin, A. (1990) Therapy, the Family and Others, in H. Maxwell (ed.), Psychotherapy: An Outline for Trainee Psychiatrists, Medical Students and Practitioners, pp. 73–90. London: Whurr.

Cottone, R.R. (1988) Epistemological and ontological issues in counselling: Implications of social systems theory. Counselling Psychology Quarterly, 1(4), 357–65.

Diamond, N. (1996) Nicola Diamond replies to Dennis Brown. Group Analysis 29(3), 320–3.

Dorland's (1965) Illustrated Medical Dictionary, London: Saunders.

Elkin, I. (1995) The NIMH treatment of depression collaborative research program: major results and clinical implications. Changes 13(3), 178–85.

Erickson, M.H. (1967) Advanced Techniques of Hypnosis and Therapy. New York: Grune and Stratton.

Fiedler, F. E. (1950) A comparison of therapeutic relationships in psychoanalytic nondirective and Adlerian therapy. Journal of Consulting Psychology, 14, 436–45.

Gee, H. (1995) Supervision: relating and defining (the essence of supervision). Talk delivered at Spring Conference and Special General Meeting of Group for the Advancement of Therapy Supervision (now the British Association for Psychoanalytic and Psychodynamic Supervision), London, 20 May.

Goodwin, B. (1994) How the Leopard Changed its Spots. London: Weidenfeld and Nicolson.

Gorell Barnes, G. and Cooklin, A. (1994) Family therapy. In P. Clarkson and M. Pokorny (eds.), The Handbook of Psychotherapy, pp. 231–48. London: Whurr.

Goulding, M.M. and Goulding, R.L. (1979) Changing Lives Through Redecision Therapy. New York: Grove Press.

Haley, J. (1973) Uncommon Therapy. New York: Norton.

Hauke, C. (1996) Review of The Therapeutic Relationship by P. Clarkson. British Journal of Psychotherapy 12(3), 405–7.

Heine, R.W. (1953) A comparison of patients' reports on psychotherapeutic experience with psychoanalytic, nondirective and Adlerian therapists. American Journal of Psychotherapy, 7, 16–23.

Herman, N. (1999) Sister Mary. London: Whurr.

Hillman, J. (1975) Loose Ends: Primary Papers in Archetypal Psychology. Dallas, TX: Spring Publications.

Hillman, J. and Ventura, M. (1992) We've Had a Hundred Years of Psychotherapy and the World's Getting Worse. San Francisco, CA: Harper & Row.

Hinshelwood, R. (1990) Editorial. British Journal of Psychotherapy, 7(2), 119–20.

Howe, D. (1993) On Being a Client. London: Sage.

International Association of Group Psychotherapy (1998) 'Annihilation Survival Recreation', 13th International Congress of the IAGP, London, 24–8 August.

Koestler, A. (1989) The Act of Creation. London: Arkana (first published 1964).

Kohut, H. (1977) The Restoration of the Self. New York: International Universities Press.

Little, M. (1986) Toward Basic Unity: Transference Neurosis and Transference Psychosis. London: Free Association.

Malcolm, J. (1981) Psychoanalysis: The Impossible Profession. New York: Knopf.

Mann, D. (1997) Psychotherapy: An Erotic Relationship: Transference and Countertransference Passions. London: Routledge.

Masson, J.M. (1989) Against Therapy. London: Collins.

May, R. (1969) Love and Will. New York: W.W. Norton.

Merleau-Ponty, M. (1962) Phenomenology of Perception (trans. C. Smith). London: Routledge & Kegan Paul.

Moiso, C. (1985) Ego states and transference. Transactional Analysis Journal, 15(3), 194–201.

Norcross, J.C. (1997) Light and shadow of the integrative process in psychotherapy. In Psychotherapy in Perspective, post-conference seminar at the 7th Annual Congress of the European Association for Psychotherapy, Rome, 29 June.

Norcross, J.C. and Goldfried, M.R. (1992) Handbook of Psychotherapy Integration. New York: Basic Books.

Paracelsus (1958) Paracelsus: Selected Writings, ed. J. Jacobi (trans. N. Guterman), 2nd edn. New York: Pantheon.

Parry, G. and Richardson, A. (1996) NHS psychotherapeutic services in England. London: Department of Health.

Plato (1974) The Republic (D. Lee, trans.) London: Penguin.

Polster, E. and Polster, M. (1973) Gestalt Therapy Integrated: Contours of Theory and Practice. New York: Random House.

Prioleau, L. Murdock, M. and Brody, N. (1983) An analysis of psychotherapy versus placebo studies. Behavioral and Brain Sciences, 6, 275–310.

Roth, A. and Fonagy, P. (1996) What Works for Whom? A Critical Review of Psychotherapy Research. New York: Guilford Press.

Rutter, P. (1989) Sex in the Forbidden Zone. London: Mandala.

Samuels, A. (1989) The Plural Psyche. London: Routledge.

Samuels, A. (1993) The Political Psyche. London: Routledge.

Searles, H. F. (1975) The patient as therapist to his analysist, in P. L. Giovacchini (ed.) Tactics and Techniques in Psychoanalytic Therapy, Vol. II, pp. 94–151. New York: Aronson.

Seligman, M.E.P. (1995) The effectiveness of psychotherapy. American Psychologist, 50(12), 965–74.

Shapiro, D.A. (1996) Foreword to What Works for Whom? A Critical Review of Psychotherapy Research (A. Roth and P. Fonagy), pp. viii–x. New York: Guilford Press.

Szasz, T. (1999) Discretion as power: Language and money and status in the situation called psychotherapy. Universities Psychotherapy Association Review No 7: 1–14.

Winnicott, D.W. (1958) Collected Papers: Through Paediatrics to Psycho-analysis. London: Tavistock.

Winnicott, D.W. (1986) Home is Where We Start From. Harmondsworth: Penguin.

Winter, D.A. (1997) Everybody has still won but what about the booby prizes? Inaugural address as Chair of the Psychotherapy Section, British Psychological Society, University of Westminster, London.

ITEM 2
A Decision-making Hierarchy Regarding Ethical Issues

Novice and experienced psychotherapists of any approach have often expressed the need for a reasonably simple structure that can help them to sort through the vast amount of information, both conscious and unconscious, which we are processing as psychotherapists. When there is no time pressure in the situation, we can, of course, wait for supervision or a consultative discussion with colleagues, illuminating dreams, looking something up in reference texts or an appointment with a specialist such as a neurologist or a an orthodox rabbi – as the case may require. Unfortunately the most serious ethical situations often don't have the benefit of leisure and decisions of ethical priority need to be taken, sometimes at speed and always with the client's benefit in mind – even when the welfare of others (or self) are seriously judged to be under threat and thus should take priority.

For many years I have noticed a particular and invariable sequence of problem-solving in emergency situations which appear to be an intrinsic and generalised pattern used by people used to dealing successfully with complicated and even life-threatening situations. Since I identified it, it has been generalised and applied to supervision, organisational consultancy, child protection, decisions about house repairs, preparing for examinations, facilitating couples' counselling (or a divorce) and many other situations. It is based on phenomenological observation of effective behaviour under stress, so you may already be consciously or unconsciously aware of it.

An example is simply this: when the ambulance people stop at a road traffic accident they first of all pay attention to whether a life is in *danger* and act to safeguard this by pulling people free from the wreckage if there is a danger of the vehicle catching fire, or someone choking to death, for example. The next step seems to be to sort out *confusion* – what the matter is. If someone is bleeding – is this from a surface skin wound, a deep injury or dangerous internal bleeding – where?; if they are still, are they in a coma, coming round or dead; how many people were travelling in the car, etc.

41

If one can isolate steps (for the sake of analysis and learning) in what often seems a seamless sequence, the next focus of attention appears to be in resolving *conflict* of some kind. There may be a choice, for instance between moving the person free of the car and risking their spine being further broken, or which child needs to be attended to first. Then only does the bandage go on, or the injured person placed on a stretcher and moved, or oxygen delivered or whatever. So the provision of the deficit is made only after danger has been assessed and attended to, confusion clarified and conflict (of decisions or priorities, for example) resolved.

The equivalent sequence in law is 'The *injunction* – to take immediate action against danger, the pleadings to sort through the *confusion* and to purge the issues for the *trial* where the conflict is heard and argued before judge or jury; finally, the judgement is made which supplies what was needed in the particular case, whether punishment or an order for reconciliation or community service. In an ideal situation there would be post-trial counselling where people have an opportunity to learn from their experiences and perhaps live better lives in future. This sequence can, of course, unfold over a great length of time or be lightning fast. In an emergency skilled operators may look natural and spontaneous, and they have probably become so unconsciously competent that they won't even be aware of it at all. However, we can learn from it so that the structure can be available and practised at leisure in supervision and training until it is available as a reflex resource in our general psychotherapeutic work – and for the time we might need to make the best and most ethical decisions urgently.

The other reason the sequence is so important is because when people do not naturally or because of learning follow the steps in sequence, many avoidable and often serious clinical and ethical mistakes are made.

- Organisational consultants are called in for 'conflict resolution' and are puzzled that nothing can be done – until they discover that the staff are paralysed from fear of being 'made redundant'.
- Trainers are employed to teach race awareness techniques (deficit interventions) without clarification of danger, confusion or conflicts around such issues.
- The marriage counsellor tries to facilitate the couple's communication through the use of various interpretations or techniques and misses the fact that the man is battered and bruised.
- The group analyst or psychotherapist focuses on transference dramas of inter- and intra-personal conflict in the group and misses the fact that the patient is dementing.
- The psychospiritual guide provides meditation techniques and exercises in forgiveness when the person is angry with mother for

abusing them, and does not pay attention to the rage not yet felt (and perhaps buried) against a father who did not protect them and which is feeding a cancer which the client is ignoring.

- Sex education is provided to children who are being bullied beyond endurance or worried that their parents are divorcing and may leave them forever or, like Jude's son in Hardy's *Jude the Obscure*, may even commit suicide by misunderstanding some overheard remark – and we are aware of the increase of suicides among the young – particularly young men.

Examples obviously proliferate. This idea may only make useful sense when applied to specific problems – which are *not* being resolved by other means. You may wish to skip it now and only return to it when you are experiencing some problem in your work or your supervision. It may also be useful for considering and exploring all the dimensions of the ethical dilemmas – optional exercises in moral imagination – which follow.

Ethical dilemmas for practice and discussion using the decision hierarchy – or any other useful framework

- A client who was sexually abused while living in a children's home had previously lost her first two children, who were taken into care and fostered, after she found out that they were being sexually abused by her partner, and she found she was unable to cope with or care for them. She later had another child, but during a breakdown, during which she was hospitalised, the third child was also fostered. On her recovery, the woman is referred to you and the child came back to live with her, in the hope that she would now be able to manage her. The client is desperate to make a go of it, and says she would kill herself if the child was taken away again. After some weeks, she disclosed information to you which indicates that the child could well be at risk. She felt it was safer to tell you than to tell social workers, since she knows that you do not have the power to take the child away. Experiment with unpacking the factors to be taken into account as if for student psychotherapists.
- Several clients tell you about a colleague of yours implying or saying that you are not a trustworthy psychotherapist or supervisor because you have made a complaint about the organisation. The colleague who was attacking your reputation is well-liked and exerting professional pressure in the society to which you both belong which is interfering with your work with your clients and supervisees. What do you do?
- Patient (who is a psychoanalyst) disclosed her having had an affair with her patient – they set up home together and your client now

wanted to disclose this but was being blackmailed not to. What are your options?

- Adult disclosure of childhood sexual/physical abuse with perpetuator still potentially having access to children. Client refusing to act or make further statements. Conflict with local child protection guidelines and social services need to have 'case' that they could take forward of evidence.
- Discharging someone (borderline personality disorder) knowing this would be perceived as rejection, with no one to refer on to whom the patient would find acceptable.
- You discover that you know much more about the patient from personal friends than they knew you knew, after group psychotherapy had begun.
- The decision about whether or not to inform a GP about a patient's suicidal feelings and past history of sexual abuse and torture at her mother's hands, given that she was due to have a very serious operation, was terrified of the physical intrusiveness of the operation and in the grip of psychotic fears and phantasies about how she would deal with convalescence on her own at home. If you call the GP she might think that you are inadequate to the task of bearing her pain.
- A young woman presented in assessment tells you that she had been sexually abused three times as a child adolescent. She tells you that these incidents had been completely unknown to her before they were remembered under hypnosis with a previous therapist and that it had taken her a long time to accept that it could be true. You feel very unsure about whether the incident had taken place or had been suggested by the hypnotist.
- An Asian woman had an abortion. She was suffering from continuous bleeding but in seeking medical help was unable to inform them of her previous history. What would you do?
- A patient asks you to report to their solicitor in order to gain financial advantage in a divorce settlement. What do you need to consider?
- A patient brings you an expensive gift in gratitude for the good work you have done with her. Under what conditions would you accept it, and how would you reject it if you did?
- Finding a patient sexually attractive to such an extent that it is interfering with concentration. What are your options?
- Finding a patient sexually attractive to such an extent that you can no longer work with her effectively – and then she starts telling you that she wants you to make love to her because she knows that you want to do it.
- A male, homosexual patient tell you he was diagnosed as HIV positive and describes his active attempts to infect others through unprotected sex. Another patient, also with HIV, tells you that he cannot tell his wife of his condition and that they are desperately trying to

conceive a baby because that is his wife's heart's desire. How would you deal with these in therapy?

- My own continuing concern with the matter of how to provide genuine confidential treatment for those in training to become psychotherapists when one does not think they are going to be able to achieve a sufficient standard in their own clinical practice.
- Male patient tells you he feels distressed and then gets out his penis and masturbates right there in front of you.
- You have a client who was sexually abused by her stepfather when she was 7 or 8 years old; 20 years later her stepfather is being prosecuted for this abuse and the abuse of her four siblings. Your client has blocked off from the memory of the abuse and finds her level of distress at recalling the memories aversive. She tells you she has to give your name to her father's barrister.
- You know that your clients have the right to ask to see your records about them and write them in such a way as to take this into account. However, there is certain information which, in the hands of a lawyer, can be turned against your client, e.g. she had had a history of promiscuity and periods of drinking heavily, and has attacked and smashed up hotel rooms.
- After some months in therapy your client discloses that she is having a very passionate sexual affair with a member of a terrorist group. He has asked her whether he could leave some weapons at her flat for safekeeping. She is very much in love with him and wants to do this. She is also afraid that his friends will take violent vengeance on her if she does not agree or hurt her boyfriend. What do you do?
- You have a longstanding practice with patients who have had serious 'psychiatric illness' in their lives and are quite dependent on you when you discover that you have a life-threatening illness which will gradually reduce your competency – although you may not neces- sarily be aware of it. What do you do?

Table 2.1: The decision-making hierarchy

Priority of focus in descending order of importance and urgency	Examples of important questions	Examples of interventions from a variety of perspectives
Priority 1: DANGER	Who may be at risk? Where?	Call ambulance
Some threat, e.g. making psychodynamic interpretations while patient is dying of brain tumour	What *may* be at risk? Of what? When – immediately or perhaps later? What are the grounds for the assessment? Could it be prevented? Could it be justified later upon investigation, e.g. in court?	Make no-suicide contract Phone GP after consultation with client or – when not?

(contd)

Table 2.1: (contd)

Priority of focus in descending order of importance and urgency	Examples of important questions	Examples of interventions from a variety of perspectives
	Consequences of action - or non-action? Consider legal, organisational, professional, contractual and personal dimensions – any others?	

Priority 2: CONFUSION

Some loss or lack of clarity of focus, e.g. confusion between loyalty to training institution and client confidentiality in a case where clients are being abused by a colleague.	Having dealt with any danger, from the perspective of each party or organisation: What are the issues involved? (Define or specify) What may the neglected or avoided issues be? What would others with a different opinion consider most crucial? Why? Could you make a diagram or drawing of the situation?	Diagram the system showing all involved parties' interests? Brainstorm or mind-map issues 'Complexify' before simplifying – use divergent thinking first, before convergent thinking. Interpretation.

Priority 3: CONFLICT

Some split, polarisation or conflict, e.g. client returns to therapy and only after some months does the psychotherapist discover that client's abusing ex-husband is another of her patients. They may meet and discuss this.	Having clarified the issues, what are the conflicts involved in the dilemma? Between who and whom? Between what and what? Which of these should take priority? By which set of criteria? Can you be specific about these for yourself?	Identify two or more conflicting ethical values or conflicts between legal, ethical and moral values and test these against value hierarchies and defensibilities and consequences for self, others, organisations, larger culture/s. Role play, enactment, active imagination dialogue.

Priority 4: DEFICIT

Some experience of need or lack of information or action, e.g. patient suffering from spinal injury and failing to find adequate medical attention.	Having identified the conflicts and resolved or managed them some other way: What remains to be done?	Give information or find or provide access to information or resources, e.g. list of gay organisations in library, books/references

Table 2.1: (contd)

Priority of focus in descending order of importance and urgency	Examples of important questions	Examples of interventions from a variety of perspectives
Psychotherapist has personal experience of specialist who has excellent reputation and experience of just such problems.	What remains to be understood, taught, found out, documented, recorded, supervised? How will you go about fulfilling this deficit – or facilitating the other parties to fulfil it? How will you know this stage has been completed?	Give health information on the issue, referrals to legal helpline, AA?

Priority 5: DEVELOPMENT

Some increase depth, breadth or complexity required, e.g. client discovers that some years ago they had defrauded customers through being misled by their then employer.	Having fulfilled the deficit or provided the necessaries or enabled where and how to find these: How can this issue be turned into a developmental opportunity for most of the parties involved – including yourself and the profession – or the wider world?	Expand the issue to consider wider values, organisational or cultural contexts, historical perspectives, adjacent psychodynamics or ultimate concerns; creating space for intuition, synchronicity, quantum creativity – the cultural evolution of morality.

© P. Clarkson, 1998

Further reading

Clarkson, P. (1998) Supervision in counselling, psychotherapy and health: An intervention priority sequencing model. European Journal of Psychotherapy, Counselling and Health 1(2): 195–212.

Clarkson, P. and Kellner, K. (1995) Prioritising organisational interventions – a diagnostic framework: What goes wrong in management consultancy and some pointers to how to minimise it. In Changing Organisations. London: Whurr.

CHAPTER 3

Values in Counselling and Psychotherapy

PETRŪSKA CLARKSON

> How is it rational to respond to the claims of different moral traditions? It will depend upon who you are and how you understand yourself [and others]. This is not the kind of answer which we have been educated to expect in philosophy, but that is because our education in and about philosophy has by and large supposed what is in fact not true, that there are standards of rationality, adequate for the evaluation of rival answers to such questions, equally available, at least in principle, to all persons, whatever tradition they may happen to find themselves in and whether or not they inhabit any tradition. When this as a belief is rejected, it becomes clear that the problems of justice and practical rationality of how to confront the rival systematic claims of traditions contending with each other in the agōn of ideological encounter are not one and the same set of problems for all persons. What those problems are, how they are to be formulated and addressed, and how, if at all, they may be resolved will vary not only with the historical, social and cultural situation of the persons whose problems these are but also with the history of belief and attitudes of each particular person up to the point at which he or she finds these problems inescapable. (MacIntyre, 1988, p. 393)

Counselling and psychotherapy are disciplines which emerged on the one hand from religion and philosophy and on the other from the scientific laboratories. In the academic towers they attempted to think through the issues of good and evil: in the laboratories they tried to circumvent it by so-called objectivity. There are three men credited with parenting the rivers from which counsellors and psychotherapists drink, and forge our ephemeral sieves for the sorting of psyche's seeds today (Clarkson, 1994a). These are the people who shaped our attitudes and blindnesses, our hubris and our humilities, our engagement with or recoil from the regions ruled in previous times by the pastors, and the mythical and magical healers for whom the issues of right and wrong were divinely ordained, and not the painful, wet, overheated clumsiness that we so often bring to bear upon them. Each one brought with him his own world-view, his beliefs about the limits and reach of humankind, his ideals and disappointments.

Three heritages and their position on values

The ideological grandfather of the cognitive-behavioural therapy and rational-emotional therapeutic approaches that we know today is of course Pavlov – a white-coated scientist who apparently did not show too much concern for the dogs driven mad by scientific experiments in his care. He studied their psychotic terrors dispassionately, seeking to find principles which might be of value elsewhere.

Being what they are, it seems that the more human beings tried to keep the laboratory clean and ordered, the more it also spewed forth the shadows – the unpredictable and the gruesome. The mould on the saucer which the assistant forgot to clean was noticed by chance, and gave us life-saving penicillin. The imaginative outbreak of the shadow fears of the mad scientist, Frankenstein, Dr Jekyll and Mr. Hyde, the monstrous playing-out of our most macabre vision – the world destroyed in the brilliant light of a skin-searing, eyeball-melting, mushroom sun. This thing was made by boy scientists who had no thought, when they played in the desert sun, of the havoc their objective scientific invention would wreak.

The second ideological grandfather, Freud, is directly in line with most approaches to counselling and psychotherapy that call themselves psychoanalytic, psychodynamic or a similar variant name. This prototype approach to human distress also emerged from scientific neurological studies. But soon Freud found himself enmeshed in the vicissitudes of *fin-de-siècle* middle-class Vienna's hysteria, in which sexual desire and repressed fantasy mingled with the horrors of child abuse and professional respectability in almost indistinguishable ways. He tried throughout his career to find and keep an idiom of scientific acceptability for psychoanalysis. Arguably he failed in this quest. Even today it is most likely that practitioners and students from this school may resist the implementation of the outcome of research measures and tape-recording of their sessions. Often they are vociferous in questioning the validity of other attempts to quantify what is essentially unquantifiable and unmeasurable, for example, by claiming that shorter, cheaper more effective 'cures' are 'just' symptom substitutions. This *may* be true.

Is it perhaps also true that issues of respectability, status and economic concerns infect the regions devoted to the study of the forces of sex and death? Can we tolerate the thought that Freud made interpretations about how a woman was transferring her hostile feelings onto him? Yes, but – while she was actually rotting away from a suppurating wound in her nose, bandages gone septic from an operation conducted by his friend because she masturbated too much? What is to be said of Jung, who saw in Hitler a new Messiah? Of the analyst who treats a woman while she is engaged in a political movement against

pornography but only confesses after many years that he really likes
Playboy? The ones who keep taking the money while they use the couch
for purposes other than Freud intended? The financial impossibility of
serving any substantial proportion of the population except the most
élite in the profession or the independently wealthy? The school
psychologist who supports the scapegoating and shaming of a
homosexual teacher on 'theoretical' grounds?

We can consider that the third ideological grandfather is Moreno –
the doctor of souls who wanted as an epitaph, that he had brought
laughter back into psychiatry. Most of the existential humanistic
approaches owe a debt of allegiance, origin or familial affinity to his
conviction, his methods and his vision. This includes existential,
phenomenological, gestalt, transactional analysis, integrative arts and
many group therapy and other integrative approaches. He at least made
no pretence of being 'objective' or free of values. He stated and
celebrated the telling and enactment of stories, the freedom of
spontaneity, the energy of playfulness as major values. Moreno (1975)
also entitled a major work around a crucial ethical question: 'Who shall
survive?'

Of course I do not speak of all people in all approaches. However, I
think we all stand in the shadows of the goodness of those from whom
we inherit and pass on this complicated legacy in a similarly double-
edged way. When we talk about values, no one theoretical approach has
particularly emerged as *better* than any other in alleviating human pain,
providing for all who need help, keeping itself free from the corrosive
discarded acid of the very chemicals with which it sought to cure. Is this
failure an embarrassment or a liberation? An omen to throw it all away or
an invocation to think and feel and question again for ourselves again
and again?

> And there is undoubtedly something to learn, food for thought, in writings
> that do not accord with our views, as psychologists, of what is scientifically
> respectable. It would be presumptious and naive scientism to dismiss such
> work out of hand. Psychotherapy, although by no means totally beyond the
> reach of the scientist's grasp, nevertheless reminds us of the primitive state of
> psychological methods and knowledge. In particular, how much can we
> claim to know about the origins of personality, or about the formation, devel-
> opment and impacts of intimate human relationships? These are the central
> concerns of psychotherapists and their clients. Scientific psychology must
> continue to innovate, grow and change if it is to further our understandings
> of these pervasive aspects of the human condition. (Shapiro, 1988, p. 154)

Psychology as value-free science?

Interestingly enough, as psychology continues to seek a scientific logical
positivistic objective kind of validation for itself as science, science has
itself moved well away from objectivist delusions, the hope for a

constant reality, the simplistic modernist notions of the Enlightenment Project. Physics – once the stamping-ground of Newton and the wellspring for Cartesian dualism – stands open-mouthed before its own progeny, asserting that one particle is in two places at the same time, that 'light is both a particle and a wave, two mutually exclusive entities depending on how you look at it, and when' (Bragg in Zohar, 1990); that the cat in a cage filled with cyanide gas is dead or not depending the moment of opening; that the objective, impartial observer always interferes with the field; that there are currently eight different authoritative scientific versions of the nature of physical reality, all of them 'weird' to common science and positivism (Herbert, 1985): and that the places at the edges of imbalance, disorder and chaos are often the optimum conditions for healing, creativity and evolution on earth (see Gleick, 1988; Briggs and Peat, 1989; Zohar, 1990).

At about this point at the start of a new century we also have to cope with the thought that, despite the fundamentalist convictions of the different theoretical schools of counselling and psychotherapy, none of them has particularly been found to be better than any of the others on most measures. The very proliferation of approaches – some 450 at last count – seems to spell out more a desperate search than a certain, solid rock. There is research indicating that theoretical orientation makes no difference to the effectiveness of outcome in counselling and psychotherapy, that training makes no difference – a beginner may well be as effective, if not more so, than an experienced practitioner; even that personal psychotherapy makes no discernible difference to successful outcome! The fact that we can hold as firmly to our convictions of what 'works' in the face of all this scientific objective evidence, and continue to market our version of this discipline, is a credit to our faith in the ineffable, the unsaid and the unproved – hardly a thorough scientific positivistic or rationalist basis from which to operate. The jury is out, but it seems as if neither the marketplace vendors nor their customers have heard the verdict yet.

A brochure for a particular respectable psychotherapy training organisation states that 'It is expected that the trainee will come to share the theoretical orientation of their training analyst'. Well, this is quite clear. The Humanistic and Integrative Section of the United Kingdom Council of Psychotherapy also are quite clear about the place of values in their combined approaches. An approach which specifically adheres to Buddhist values sits comfortably along with those of a more specifically psychosynthesis persuasion in the transpersonal grouping of schools in this section. However, it is required that one subscribes to the 'flag statement'.

In contrast, most of the commonly available and read books on psychology, counselling and psychotherapy deal with the issues of values, social justice and ethical questions either by simply ignoring them (check the indexes of your favourite textbooks) or by referring it to consensually agreed codes of ethics and professional practice – all of which are shot through with unanswered ethical dilemmas and profoundly serious questions to the profession itself.

However, even when we acknowledge the shaping and influencing role of values in the work of counselling and psychotherapy, probably the most frequently heard admonition to which most training schools would agree is the warning dictum: 'Do not impose your values on your clients or patients!' This is a grievous and probably unforgivable professional sin, leading to charges of exploitation, zealotry, missionary urges and the like. It is very unprofessional. Yet what else are we doing? And can we truly deny this? To me it seems not so much as a matter of 'Do not impose your values' – because you obviously will, but rather 'Be aware of what values you are indeed imposing and become conscious of this importation of the world of ethics and aesthetics, which you inevitably do when you engage in a healing encounter with any other human being.'

The ubiquity of values in human life

Scientific findings indicate that we hardly ever perceive any stimulus without experiencing it as better or worse, more or less beautiful, more or less important, more or less valuable than another. Just look at a sharp corner or a rounded one – which do you prefer? Perhaps you cannot say which; or why. To be human is to make value. This finding corresponds with our own common sense and everyday subjective experiences. Some kind of constantly changing selection according to criteria of value is clearly the only way in which the central nervous system switchboard can keep some kind of prioritising in process; especially given the bombardment of a multitude of competing demands for our perceptual and emotional attention. Whenever any one stimulus becomes figure, another inevitably becomes ground and is thus less important than the first one.

Whenever my first analyst, safely ensconced behind me (out of my field of vision) made a note, I heard the scratching of his pencil on the paper and knew in that moment that my particular utterance had special value. I may well have been wrong, but I felt that I had just said something very important. Of course I sought to replicate the stimulus which made him move. Many people have since told me similar stories from their own experiences. Clinical lore tells that Jungian patients have Jungian dreams, Freudian patients have Freudian dreams and gestalt patients, gestalt dreams.

The principles of operant conditioning explain how when the Rogerian counsellor says 'Uhm' after a particular expression of emotion but sits still during an intellectual exposition, it is more likely that the person will repeat the expression of emotion. So the 'Uhm' of the Rogerian counsellor, the interpretation or the shuffle of the psychoanalyst all give constant selective reinforcement to the patients in the position of supplicant. 'This is what makes him yawn; if I do this she goes to sleep; if I do this I can hear his breathing increase and his body animate with feeling – I can smell his fear', and so on. I can have these effects on my psychoanalyst or psychotherapist and in this process condition and be conditioned not too dissimilarly from rats who learn to stabilise certain learning best when intermittent reinforcement schedules are implemented. The occasional sympathetic hum is more indicative and more powerfully so for long-term learning about how to be the client the psychotherapist wants, than regular and predictable pellets of attention of movement or interest.

This is really not very strange. Who has not dreamt of the movie seen the previous night, the office dispute the previous day, the family problem upon which we were racking our imagination just before we went to sleep? Of course we are influenced by and influence others in this selective attention paid to some aspects of an interaction and not others. Each one carries a statement of value even if only implicitly. Indeed each statement carries a value charge more powerfully, the more implicit its value messages are, hidden or embedded out of conscious awareness.

It seems that experimenter expectation apparently influences the speed at which rats learn mazes (Feather, 1982); we know that children perform better academically if their teachers (falsely) believe them to be more intelligent (Rosenthal and Jacobson, 1968); we know the measurements of atoms are influenced by the person of the physicist – do we really think that in the close and intimate space of the therapeutic consulting room we can keep a value-hygienic environment which no one has been able to successfully and repeatedly accomplish anywhere else in the universe?

At the very least each communication message in human interaction carries along with its overt content, also a covert content – a meta-communication which is a statement about the relationship between sender and receiver or a message about the context in which the communicative message is being delivered (Satir, 1967). Apparently 85% of the meaning of a communication is visual – the words alone count for a measly 15%. It is the context of the question: 'Where have you been?' which makes it either friendly interest, a genuine enquiry or the restart of a long-smouldering marital fight teetering on the brink of a messy divorce. It is not the words of mother saying 'I love you' which declare the emotional truth – it is the look in her eyes, the gentleness or roughness of her hands, the willingness to be attentive or neglectful when others and other things are calling that fundamentally conveys the value of the persons in the message.

Avowed and enacted values

Of course, there is a difference between avowed and enacted values. A true value is enacted as well as avowed (Severin, 1965). This is one of the biggest problems that has to be faced by schools of thought, psychotherapy or pastoral counselling that are willing and able to enunciate their values explicitly and do not rely on the covert transmission of these. Fletcher (1966) explores this as situational ethics. Freud prescribed the importance of the analyst being a blank screen, yet shouted at his patients, lent them money, and gossiped to them about other patients. Melanie Klein treated her own children (how blank can you get?) and some Kleinians currently alive have been known to touch their patients, allow between-session phone calls, and participate in conferences where patients and analysts, supervisors and trainees engage in politically sensitive and ethically delicate and controversial decision-making meetings. How do you reconcile what you say with what you do? Do the discrepancies between your walk and your talk outweigh the congruencies? The explicit statement of values immediately (and necessarily) moves the ethical debate to another level of questioning. Not only are there values in here, but which are those values? And if these are they, how do they work in the everyday living, teaching and practice of this work?

In humanistic and existential psychotherapies there has always been an open and espoused position about the importance of values and their exploration in counselling and psychotherapy. This had not been free from abuse. A tradition which began with Moreno, working in the parks of Vienna with latchkey children and prostitutes, has continued through the radical psychiatry movement of the 1960s (ably assisted by many transactional analysts), to recent involvement with Eastern European problems today by several members of the psychotherapeutic communities in Britain. Gradually also in other areas there is an awakening to the issues of social responsibility, moral relevance and responsible engagement. Mostly this is a tentative walking on eggshells so as not to challenge the avowed legalistic (but perhaps spurious) supremacy of the 'Don't impose your values on your clients' caveat.

A theoretical door from psychoanalysis opens when we consider the issues in terms of countertransference. Surely we bring to the analytic encounter our prejudices about men and women and what they each can achieve in our society? Our discrimination against the disabled, the black, the different? Of course, these countertransferences have an impact on the treatment, but if we do not own them as values open for being stripped naked, how can they change or grow as all ethical systems do and continue to do over time and across place?

The imposition of values in counselling and psychotherapy

Of course you should not berate, preach and exploit clients to adopt your religious, political or psychotherapeutic beliefs. Of course, you do impose your values even when you try not to. And to the extent that you are unaware of this, it is probably most dangerous. Saying it out loud may be fairer, because then a client may be in a better position to give informed consent to working with a counsellor who believes that a gay lifestyle will always show genital immaturity. Any helper models a certain way of dressing, of speaking – it is not too difficult to change an accent and intonation. This is the way of speaking you have valued above all others. You could pretend to be class-deaf or colourblind. You could deny or unduly emphasise the difference in experience, you don't comment on it. When the client asks your position on homosexuality or mothers who give artificially assisted birth past their menopause, you can speak or you can explore what these issues mean for the patient. You are complicit whatever you do in supporting or suppressing values or value-clarification in yourself and your client. You may think that you're truly neutral but to the extent that they are healthy, your client knows you're not.

You have or do not have certain pictures in your room. Your furniture proclaims a whole cultural world of values reverberating as strongly around the psyche of your client as the living rooms of their childhood (Rowan, 1988). Are there flowers there or is it a bland beige and brown space, so as not to interrupt the transference? What makes transference the higher value? Or is it like the consulting room of the person who first suggested this 'neutrality' – a riot of a fantasy space imbued with ruby-red and terracotta Persian carpets, lusciously shaped sensuality of Egyptian figures and ancient evocations of the past in sculptures, prehistoric rocks, much-loved books, the traces of ongoing intellectual labour and figurines which hark back and forward, above and below?

After several months of fruitless endeavours to establish a mutually satisfactory supervisory relationship, the supervisor asked the trainee (who was from Asia): 'Please tell me what the matter is – I know I may be doing something wrong for you to block your learning and growth – please tell me what it is?' She replied shyly, saying that in their culture they would never criticise a teacher and now she was being asked to do so. This was already too difficult. After much more prevarication she said that it was the books. What about the books? 'The books in your office. They make me feel inferior. They make me feel stupid. I can't think with those books in your bookcase sitting there judging me.' Another value confronted, another lesson learned, another adjustment to be made, another awareness to metabolise.

Of course we impose our values. But how? And which ones, when? Where do we learn to investigate this imposition, this teaching by example, this conversion through the adoption of the particular way of talking of the person in 'authority' – the person being paid? Farrell (1979) pointed out some years ago in a comparative study of different approaches to organisational groups and systems, that a person is often declared as having 'insight' when they have adopted the 'WOT' – the *way of talking* of the consultant. Is this very different from the way oppressed nations learn the language of the conqueror, but the ruling class rarely learns the language of the slaves, the victims or the blatantly needy of the vanquished country? Is this metaphor too strong or can we honestly say that a meta-narrative, the white, male, capitalist, eurocentric, able-bodied, heterosexual storyteller (author) of the history of our professions leaves a full, free voice for alternative narratives? For other stories equally possible, equally privileged, equally worth listening to and being silent for? And when we do not explicitly say this, what are we saying with our silence? A woman told me that when she told her first counsellor that she had attacked her husband, the therapist simply ignored it – not once, but several times. In this way we write our stories, give our lives meaning and the applause, catharsis or denial of the other define and rework these values. In the end, since being human is such a value-constituting enterprise the conduct of counselling or psychotherapy without meaning-giving values is impossible.

That's inside the consulting room – but what about the profession as a whole in the outward turned profile of its Janus head? Clinical psychology has been accused of 'ethical irrelevance'. Masson (1989) says that the non-abusive practice of counselling and psychotherapy is impossible. Hillman and Ventura (1992) charge the profession with interiority, narcissism, self-absorption; Olivier (1991) with falling between the stools of privatisation and professionalisation. Samuels (1993) calls us to face the need for political development of the psyche and mature involvement in the affairs of *polis* and state. He reckons this is the work of analysts and counsellors. Fox (1983) exhorts us to look to our organismic oneness with the whole of the living planet – its plants, her stories and its rhythms of coming into being and dying, again and again. I have written and spoken (Clarkson, 1994b) about the incursion of 'defensive psychotherapy' (how can I prevent being sued by my client or their family, challenged by my supervisor, criticised by my colleagues?).

Legitimisation in this profession has moved from the hand-on-the-shoulder 'knighting' by founders or second-generation followers to legitimisations by groups of people – none of whom really own the responsibility for deciding who's in, who's out and who's in charge, but all of them guardians of standards and ethics – as long as these are theirs. Elsewhere (Clarkson, 1995) I also take our profession to task in its commitment to, examples of and complicity with bystanding in clients, colleagues, the profession and our culture as a whole. Bystanding is an active choice of non-involvement in a situation where someone else is in danger or being treated unjustly. The major bystanding rationalisation of counsellors and psychotherapists is their much avowed putative scientific neutrality. Yet neutrality always favours the aggressor – and can we not see it in the distribution of resources within our society? In the practice of our laws? In the genocide around us?

These conversations all rely on a universe of discourse where values can be articulated, explored, clarified (Smith, 1977). I submit that it is psychotherapy's task to do so whether these values are explicit – counselling in a pastoral setting (Catholic, Adventist or Buddhist) or implicit – psychotherapy in a Brixton refuge for battered women or psychoanalysis in a middle-class home in a leafy North London suburb. Whether these are the values we bring to the enterprise, the values the clients bring or those the circumstances impose and with which we comply. Where the explication and exploration of these values are hedged, dodged or excused, they exist nonetheless – probably more virulent in neglect than in the careful monitoring of their pervasive potency for good or ill.

References

Briggs, J. and Peat, F.D. (1989) Turbulent Mirror. New York: Harper & Row.

Clarkson, P. (1994a) The nature and range of psychotherapy. In P. Clarkson and M. Pokorny, M. (eds.), Handbook of Psychotherapy, pp. 3–27. London: Routledge.

Clarkson, P. (1994b) In recognition of dual relationships. Transactional Analysis Journal, 24(1), 32–8.

Clarkson, P. (1995) The Bystander. London: Whurr.

Farrell, B.A. (1979) Work in small groups: some philosophical considerations. In B. Babington Smith and B.A. Farrell (eds.),Training In Small Groups: A Study of Five Groups, pp. 103–15. Oxford: Pergamon.

Feather, N.T. (ed.) (1982) Expectations and Actions: Expectancy-value Models in Psychology. Hillsdale, NJ: Lawrence Erlbaum.

Fletcher, J. (1966) Situation Ethics: The New Morality. London: SCM.

Fox, M. (1983) Original Blessing. Santa Fe, NM: Bear & Co.

Gleick, J. (1988) Chaos: Making a New Science. London: Heinemann.

Herbert, N. (1985) The New Reality: Beyond the New Physics. London: Rider.

Hillman, J. and Ventura, M. (1992) We've Had a Hundred Years of Psychotherapy and the World's Getting Worse. San Francisco, CA: Harper.

MacIntyre, A. (1988) Whose Justice? Which Rationality? London: Duckworth.

Masson, J.M. (1989) Against Psychotherapy. London: Collins.

Moreno, J.L. (1975) Who shall survive? In I.A. Greenberg (ed.), Psychodrama: Theory and Therapy. London: Souvenir Press.

Olivier, G. (1991) Counselling, Anarchy and the Kingdom of God. The 1990 Frank Lake Memorial Lecture. Oxford: Clinical Theology Association.

Rosenthal, R. and Jacobson, L. (1968) Pygmalion in the Classroom: Teacher Expectation and Pupils' Intellectual Development. New York: Holt, Rinehart & Winston.

Rowan, J. (1988) Counselling and the psychology of furniture. Counselling, 64, 21–4.

Samuels, A. (1993) The Political Psyche. London: Routledge.

Satir, V. (1967) Conjoint Family Therapy. Palo Alto, CA: Science & Behavior Books.

Severin, F.T. (1965) Humanistic Viewpoints in Psychotherapy. New York: McGraw-Hill.

Shapiro, M. K. (1988) Second Childhood: Hypno-play Therapy with Age-regressed Adults. New York: W. W. Norton.

Smith, M. (1977) A Practical Guide to Value Clarification. La Jolla, CA: University Associates.

Zohar, D. (1990) The Quantum Self. London: Bloomsbury.

ITEM 3
Discovering your own Values

Questions for psychotherapists and others

- What values are you communicating to your clients or patients with the clothes you wear – the colours, the quality, the state of cleanliness or repair, the appearance of tidiness or casualness, the make, types and condition of your footwear, the make of your watch, your other jewellery such as a cross or a Star of David or a wedding ring?
- What values are you communicating to your clients or patients with your physical appearance – your posture, your skin colour, your gait, your pace of moving or speaking, your accent, your mode of speech, the metaphors you use, your haircut, the state of your fingernails, your perfume or aftershave or smell of soap, your face – make-up or shape or whether or not you wear a beard?
- What values are you communicating to your clients or patients with the physical surroundings to your consulting room – the car in the drive, the state of the office, the address and location, the pictures (or not) on the walls, the presence or not of tissues, the presence or not of flowers or plants, what books, papers, journals or periodicals are on your shelves to be seen?
- What values are you communicating to your clients or patients through membership of your professional organisation – how many black people are in positions of authority or leadership in this organisation, does the council and executive board reflect the gender distribution of all members of the organisation, has this organisation ever actively or passively supported discrimination or has it taken positions on issues such as publicly objecting to the pathologising of homosexuals?
- Spend one week keeping track of the phrase you use most often in sessions with clients or patients – what are you communicating to your clients or patients when you use this phrase, what else could you say, what would someone say who held an opposing theoretical

position from yourself, what would be the objections to this?
- What values are you communicating to your clients or patients when you don't answer their questions – or when you do? How often do your clients criticise you and have you ever apologised to a client or patient? Have you ever cancelled an appointment and do you charge patients for missed sessions even when they (or their children) are ill? What values are you modelling by your behaviour?
- What values are you communicating to your patients or clients by identifying with the particular theoretical position your hold – or not? Are you aware of the public perception of this approach and what clients or patients may strive for as result?
- What values are you communicating to your patients or clients by your fee structure?

If you don't know the answers to all these questions, ask a colleague to give you honest and useful feedback – you might just learn things about yourself you may wish to change. In any event, becoming conscious of how we as psychotherapists live our values in every action or non-action we commit in our work, enhances our clinical awareness and therapeutic acumen.

CHAPTER 4
Bystanding in Counselling and Psychotherapy

PETRŪSKA CLARKSON

> The problem of the professional shadow touches other fundamentals of psychotherapeutic activity. As analysts we constantly deal with severe suffering, with uncommon and tragic destinies. Often what is required of us is to help a troubled person to understand himself as far as possible, not only to take up contact with the unconscious but also simply to bear the tragic aspects of life in all their incomprehensibility. In order to help an ailing person in a tragic life situation – in a situation which remains tragic even if contact with the unconscious improves – we must also be able to face our own tragic situation, the tragedy that, the more we try to be good psychotherapists and to help our patients to broader consciousness, the more we repeatedly slip into the opposite of our bright professional ideal.
> (Guggenbühl-Craig, 1971, pp. 30–1)

- A man is viciously attacking a woman with a knife by an English roadside. Several people see this and drive past. The woman says later in therapy that many of the drivers 'looked right into my eyes'. No one helped.
- Children who had been horribly abused for many years say: 'What has always hurt me more than anything else was the fact that nobody helped me.'
- Victims of torture in the home or in prison tell the same when they meet therapists.
- A young woman is dragged screaming from a Birmingham shopping centre in broad daylight to a brutal rape. Dozens of people see and hear her distress, and do nothing – they did not even call the police after the event. Some of these are in therapy.

In a recent survey on ethical dilemmas faced by psychotherapists some 34% (a third!) expressed concern about unethical behaviour of their colleagues toward clients, but say, 'Well, you know that kind of thing goes on, but no one wants to risk making trouble about it.'

Definition

In everyone's life there are experiences of not helping or not being helped. Every day we hear the devastating effects of bystanding described in the consulting room. The act of turning away from someone who needs help can be called 'bystanding'. A *bystander* is someone who does not become involved when someone else needs help.

Studies indicate that three out of four people will not step in even when a child is being publicly abused. Nine out of ten people will not act if they witness someone being given wrong instructions for a bus or train. Many people will rather act against their principles than risk speaking up against authorities – even to the point of inflicting damage on others – as we all know from the Milgram (1974) experiments and the compliance experiments. Therapists are subject to the very same psychological pressures as the subjects in these experiments.

Motivations for bystanding

There are many reasons why people do not act on behalf of someone else whom they see is in trouble: fear of being injured or killed; fear of being laughed at for 'interfering', or being called a 'have-a-go hero'; or fear of not 'conforming', of doing something different from the crowd. (It has been shown that the greater the number of people there are witnessing an atrocity, the less likely any one individual is to step in and take action.) Sometimes these fears are very real and sometimes they are skewed for the sake of convenience. It is very hard, if not impossible, to know which is which.

For the therapist – particularly the therapist seeking ideological acceptance or scientific respectability of the Newtonian kind – the biggest reason for bystanding is often fear of ridicule, fear of being sued, fear of not being objective or 'neutral'.

Some of the reasons for bystanding apparently becoming more prevalent in our time are that we are so overloaded with media information about injustice, cruelty and violence in the world, that we become numb to empathy with others; or we suffer from charity fatigue owing to the multitude of requests for help; or we feel so alienated from ourselves, our bodies, our relationships with others and our natural world, that atrocities no longer quite register with us in the same way as they might have in the past. We have become morally and empathically desensitised. Yet there is so much we could do – or teach.

Rationalisations for bystanding

People say things like: 'It's none of my business', 'She brought it on herself really', 'I don't want to rock the boat', 'I don't know enough about the situation', and so on. Everyone has a reason for passing by 'on the other side of the street' – often without even trying to find out more about the situation. Whether such reasons are called 'good explanations' or 'immoral excuses' depends on who is making them and why.

The power of bystanders

Whether in Nazi Germany or a local playground, there are usually many more bystanders than there are bullies or victims. These bystanders usually have the greatest power to stop (or call someone else to stop) the wrongs being committed. There were only *three* rapists in the Birmingham example; here were *dozens* of people watching. Often one person alone – causing a distraction by shouting 'fire!' or keeping close records of events – can make a great and important difference to situations in which an individual client is being maltreated (in your hospital) or hundreds of needy people are denied services (in your community). *Schindler's List* (Keneally, 1994) showed the power of one accountant, Itzhak Stern, who memorised the names of the employees under threat. It was only one person who first took the chains off the mentally ill patients – Pinel (Davison and Neale, 1986, pp. 15–17).

The myth of neutrality as a value

When bystanders do not act or involve themselves, they are in fact supporting the perpetrators. 'Neutrality' in the face of evil is not really possible, because neutrality always favours the aggressor. Bullies – Hitler, or a sexually abusive psychotherapist, to give a couple of examples – are almost always psychologically supported in their behaviour by people who 'do not want to get involved'. Sometimes the wrongdoer actually wants to be stopped; sometimes the *apparent* wrongdoer has simply been misunderstood; sometimes the wrongdoer is falsely blamed – for example, some bosses are called 'bullies' by dishonest staff, and many of the claims made against teachers for sexual harassment actually turn out to be false. No man (or woman) is an island and we can never claim *not* to be involved while we remain human on this planet – particularly not if we claim to be trying to help other humans.

Counselling and psychotherapy are currently coming under increasing attack both from within the profession and from without. There are many articles being written in the popular press against psychotherapy, such as Weldon (1994), as well as from within the profession. For example, Hillman and Ventura's (1992) delightfully provocative book title – *We've had a Hundred Years of Psychotherapy and the World is getting Worse* – encapsulates a gnawing uneasiness amongst both professionals and consumers that the 'helping professions' failed in very important ways. As Hillman correctly points out, psychotherapy has had a hundred years with which to grapple with its role and function and at the end of the century we are in a position to assess its impact on the state of the world – and it does not look good.

When religion and the meta-narratives of modernity have eroded, there appear to be no truths outside of man. In this relativist culture with no fixed and fundamental rules, the moral guide for life is sought in a scientific psychology. The new psychology took over religion's task of providing guidelines for human life. The priests as confessors were replaced by therapists as paid companions. With an economy of production being replaced by an economy of consumption, the Protestant work ethic is gradually replaced by a psychology of need gratification and indulgence. With the erosion of a comprehensive frame of meaning, of traditional values and communal bonds, individual self-realisation became the goal of life. 'In the United States, at least, psychology has become a new religion establishing an inner quest for self where before there had been an outer quest for God' (Leahey, 1987, p. 479). It should be noted that the religious roots of psychology are not confined to the humanistic versions. Thus Watson's scientific behaviourism was almost a literal translation of the Baptist theology that he studied while training for the ministry (see Birnbaum, 1964; Kvale, 1992, p. 54).

Of course, we cannot hold psychotherapy or psychology responsible for all social ills, but we can hold its practitioners responsible for their abuse of power as well as for their lack of involvement in social issues. *An insistence on a spurious 'neutrality', a lack of appreciation for the role of values, the development of professional and regulatory societies and the preoccupation with competency* all seem to be driving practitioners further and further away from dealing with real people in the real world and more towards a self absorbed overly rigid somewhat hyper-vigilant kind of defensive practice.

As someone working on quite a number of professional investigation and ethical adjudication panels I am, of course, bound by very strict rules of confidentiality, but I can speak freely about certain general patterns that have emerged, not in single cases but repeatedly in different professional organisations. Rarely are these bad people doing intentionally bad things. Usually it is ignorance, fear, temptation, confusion and lack of support which lead to ethical problems. Anyway, the first resort should always be conversational, dialogic and enquiring rather than judgemental legalism on the one hand, or pubescent tittle-tattle on the other.

With the increase in consumer education and public awareness and the development of counselling and psychotherapy as a growth industry, there has been an concomitant explosion of concerns about not making mistakes, insuring against client claims of damage, an unprecedented rise in complaints and ethics charges against practitioners. The increasing need for a professional psychotherapist to anticipate every kind of possible measurable outcome, professional audit or performance review may well result in a proliferation of contracts to be countersigned or even legal advice being taken before a client even starts to tell their story.

What I see, unfortunately, among many practitioners is this rather regrettable attempt to be more and more careful, more and more conscious of third parties listening, interpreting and judging on degrees of reality which can only ever be mediated by the two (or ten) people in the confines of the consulting room. There seems to be an increasing preoccupation with being 'error-free', with avoiding spontaneity and intuitive authenticity.

Of course, it is vitally important that the profession has grown up to seriously question its criteria for inclusion, membership, ethics and so on. Certain kinds of bad practice (for example, sexual relations with clients) are justifiably ameliorated or exposed as a result of these efforts of professionalisation. Going from free-for-all encounter groups led by unqualified practitioners to adjudicating five different levels of National Vocational Qualification competencies in terms of showing empathy has solved some problems but has created and is creating many more. Whyte also expressed his disquiet about this in a recent issue of the *British Journal of Psychotherapy* (1994, p. 568). In some circles I have heard the phrase 'the bureaucratisation of sadism' as a way of describing the ever-increasing professional demands for certification, qualification and documentation.

Unfortunately a preoccupation with these kinds of details – which may or may not be relevant to ethical practice – seems to lead more and more to professionals seeking to protect themselves rather than their clients. Two recent cases have shown this: the Slade and Bromley case heard by the British Psychological Society, where a psychologist sexually abused a patient and was merely reprimanded and given an undertaking not to practice clinically in future. He had actually referred this patient to another psychologist who colluded with him against the interests of the patient to 'contain' the fact that his colleague had a sexual relationship with her. What is particularly worrying and caused widespread concern in some circles was that this was the second time he had been found guilty of such misconduct.

The other case concerns the unfortunate situation of the United Kingdom Council of Psychotherapy's Governing Board which had to be taken to the High Court for judicial review because of acting improperly and with the appearance of bias in avoidance of their duty to the public and professionals to oversee psychotherapy complaints procedures. The fact that an executive officer of the UKCP attempted to prejudice the due course of justice by putting pressure on a complainant fortunately resulted in a public apology of profound sorrow and hopefully a return to integrity in this sector of British psychotherapy. (See Appendix 1 for more details of this case.)

Much of the contemporary literature reveals an almost prurient preoccupation with an ideal, if not mandatory, hermetically sealed therapeutic relationship. Lloyd (1992), for example, refers to a 'dual relationship phobia' abroad in counselling education. Freud (1912a) advocated that the analyst should refrain from allowing his personality to intrude into the analysis and introduced the simile of the analyst being a 'mirror' for the analysand (p. 108). In 1912 he proposed that the psychoanalyst model himself on the surgeon, put aside his human sympathy and adopt an attitude of emotional coldness (1912b, p. 115). However, in my recent research of some eminent psychologists, psychoanalysts and psychotherapists (Clarkson, 1998b) it was also clear that emotional coldness, absolute neutrality and total abstinence is more a figment of the profession's imagination than a reality encountered by the average patient.

Four major charges are being made against psychotherapy:

* *Manipulation and abuse* are inevitably part of psychological treatment whether it is psychoanalysis or 'befriending' those diagnosed as having HIV.

  It might be argued that therapists, even if they are not more likely to show a sense of social justice, are not less likely to do so than any other professional. That there are individual therapists who feel outrage over social injustice I am certainly prepared to believe. But has any particular group of psychotherapists ever taken a stand against abuse? Did Freud? (Masson, 1989, p. 44–5)

  Certainly a few people from the anti-psychiatry movement and others such as Smail (1987), Mair (1988), Newnes (1990) and Rowe (1990) have spoken out on many important issues. The founding of the organisation Psychotherapists and Counsellors for Social Responsibility in London in 1995 also heralds a new willingness for engagement in social relationship by British psychotherapists. Much of the current impetus for this movement can be credited to the work of Andrew Samuels who, in his major book *The Political Psyche* (1993) opened politics as a legitimate issue for conversation and exploration in psychoanalysis and psychotherapy. Of course humanistic psychotherapists, from their grandfather Moreno (Greenberg, 1975), who first worked with groups of prostitutes and the latchkey kids of Vienna, to the anti-psychiatry work of Steiner (Steiner *et al.*, 1975) and the political anarchy of Goodman (Stoehr, 1991), have had quite a long and illustrious history of social engagement.

  The current emptiness and irrelevance of a psychological science to culture at large may be due to psychology's rootedness in modernity, in the study of the logic of an abstracted 'psyche', which is out of touch with a postmodern world. (Kvale, 1992, p. 52)

- The ideal of neutrality or non-involvement or 'not imposing your values on your client' is impossible, delusional and dangerous. Of course, I do not mean outright evangelising, I mean the subtle and inescapable ways in which psychotherapists, like all other human beings, convey their values, ideals and aspirations through the myriad cues in their being, doing and not doing. The defence or rationalisation of innocent (or neutral) bystanding as 'professional behaviour' is wearing thin.

  Although the counselor's moral and ethical standards may not be made clear to clients, or even to the counselor himself, they are influential in his reactions to the client's story, his emphases, his choice of objectives and counselling method, and in the techniques he uses to carry out the chosen method of interviewing. (Severin, 1965, p. 369)

- The interiority or unhealthy narcissism of psychotherapy has led to *a false and destructive rupture of the inevitable* and morally and ecologically necessary interconnectedness between the individual, society and the planet. If neither therapist nor client is explicitly acting on their values they are being complicit with evil and social injustice despite the fact that they may in other settings claim to be against it.

  This is a staunchly political message: as people become more absorbed in the psychological life, they become, on the average, less concerned about social dramas. After all, the same sensibility that drives one to seek ever deeper layers of truth in the psychological sphere might as easily drive one to seek an understanding of social tragedies and attempt to remedy them. The same quest for growth that drives one to change one's psychological makeup might as easily drive one to struggle to change the social arrangements. But because there seems to be no public forum to accomplish the latter kind of change, and little hope for real social progress, many people turn their attention inward where real gains seem possible. Even the 1960s generation of rebels and radicals has fallen prey. Many are just as committed therapy consumers today as they were activists then. As people get used to consulting therapists for help addressing more of their everyday problems – including unhappiness at work, problems raising children, domestic violence – they become less practised in social or collective solutions to these problems. And once we assume the unhappiness emanates entirely from a flaw deep within, we tend to seek more and better therapy whenever we experience more unhappiness. Clinicians are quick to devise new theories and new therapies. The endlessness of the quest explains the interminable nature of therapy (Kupers, 1988, pp. 139–40).

- Infantilisation in psychotherapy. A number of socially committed psychotherapists, psychoanalysts and psychologists are seriously questioning the tendency to infantilisation in psychotherapy and psychotherapy training and supervision.

There is little doubt that childhood experiences can in many cases lead to adult disturbance. However, an increasing chorus of workers in the field are beginning to question and criticise the infantilisation of clients, patients, trainees and even conference attendees. What is seen as an unhelpful and possibly even destructive and abusive overemphasis on childhood and the unremitting use of developmental models predicated on the idiom of mother and child perpetuates a hierarchical and power-based patriarchal division of knowledge and expertise.

When this model is furthermore applied to adults, particularly in training and supervision situations, the capacity of autonomous decision-making, capacity for risk and ability to question and challenge can be seriously undermined. Where the notions of 'holding', empathising and 'containing' hold sway and supervisors and therapists model themselves on ideal womb or mothering environments, the inner child runs a risk of being elevated to the overarching paradigm or archetype of our times. Titles such as *Rage for Utopia* (Conway, 1992) and *The Reluctant Adult* (Hall, 1993) and Hillman's poetic and iconoclastic tirades (1992) all in different ways explore how citizens become babies when 'the numinosity of sex has been replaced by the numinosity of feeding' (Samuels, 1993, p. 274). In the fable of the Grand Inquisitor encountering the returning Christ, Dostoevsky had already come to the conclusion that human beings would always choose dependency rather than freedom. This is rather a sad vision of humanity but it corresponds with the fear of freedom as Fromm (1991) and others have articulated it.

> Thou wouldst go into the world, and art going with empty hands, with some promise of freedom which men in their simplicity and their natural unruliness cannot even understand, which they fear and dread – for nothing has ever been more insupportable for a man and a human society than freedom. But seest Thou these stones in this parched and barren wilderness? Turn them into bread, and mankind will run after Thee like a flock of sheep, grateful and obedient, though for ever trembling, lest Thou withdraw Thy hand and deny them Thy bread. (Dostoyevsky, 1955, p. 299–300)

• The blank screen psychoanalyst is for the patient or client a model of an individuated person as someone who is neutral and not involved. Therefore he is above the turbulent counter-currents of moral decision-making, and free from the ebb and flow of human relationships. Because we are never free from conflict, from ambivalence, from pain and fear, even when we are involved with other people, our love for others is the human creature's greatest vulnerability. It is threat to a beloved spouse or kidnapping of a child which are the greatest levers for blackmail in our world. The pain of those close to us is often experienced as greater than our own pain. How often has a parent, watching a child die, not pleaded with God to let them take over the pain rather than to have to witness its ravages in the body of the other.

- The rhetoric of 'professionalisation'. Frank's (1973) argument that it has been impossible to show convincingly that one therapeutic method is more effective than any other for the majority of psychological illnesses (p. 2) has been impressively substantiated by the Smith et al. (1980) meta-analytic study which further added an emphasis on the success of placebo groups. There are literally hundreds of other studies coming to the same conclusion (Clarkson, 1996, 1998a). Yet – in the face of a virtual avalanche of such evidence – we still see the proliferation of counselling, psychotherapy and psychoanalytic training courses and training in institutes which valorise single model approaches and credentialling systems which rely on 'theoretical adherence' or practice justified by congruence with theoretical orientation. This professional situation of finer and finer theoretical differentiation and accreditation procedures that rely on the replicated theory in action can only exist when a group gets together and labels others as outsiders – *less* than them for whatever reason. Then those who do not meet the conformity criteria (such as heterosexuality) can be excluded or allowed to be persecuted on the grounds that 'they do not meet the standards'. A profession dedicated to neutrality can then maintain a rhetoric – or a way of talking which is saturated with value judgements – sometimes on the flimsiest of grounds.

Weigert (1970) has explored the common characteristics of professional rhetoric.

They include a rhetoric of affiliation by which the profession aligns itself with higher status groups and distances itself from lower status groups; a rhetoric of special expertise that includes claims to valid theories and distinctive methods; a rhetoric of public service that simultaneously plays down careerist motives; a rhetoric of social passage that identifies and justifies credentialing requirements; a rhetoric of self-policing that defends against 'interference' from others; and a delegimitising rhetoric of the outsiders, including 'Psuedo-professionals', 'charlatans', 'Popularizers', and 'cranks'. (Simons, 1989)

Any resurrection of community values is bound to depend upon a shared morality. In contemporary society, no such shared morality exists. I know that this is an unpalatable opinion and I am saddened to have to state it so bluntly. The conventional view of today's Britain is that the overwhelming majority of its citizens agree about morality but for some mysterious reason

they are prevented from getting what they want. We are told that nearly everybody has the same view of the crime of murder. Similarly there is a shared
opinion about the institution of marriage, the obligations owed to parents,
the need to show uncomplaining fortitude and the importance of putting
social duties ahead of personal gratification. Life would be simple if all of this
were true, but one only has to look around to see that it is not. (Walden,
1994)

In effect, the members of this psychological and psychoanalytic community share that internalised therapist, much as a clan shares a totem. As
the therapist is internalised, so is a whole worldview. However neutral
the particular therapist feels she or he is, she or he is spreading a very
specific message about the proper conduct of lives. First, the therapist
confirms there is a flaw deep within that explains one's feelings of alienation and also calls for a course of psychotherapy. Then the therapist, in
conducting the therapy, presents the client with this prescription:
Analyse actions and fantasies, search for meanings instead of acting out
impulsively, try to be in touch with feelings, or, if the problem is a
tendency to be overwhelmed by feelings, always remember to think
things through and be confident there will be no falling apart. Whatever
the particular words therapists tailor for specific clients, the therapist's
maxim is always to give the inner life a place of priority in one's
conscious ruminations. Wisdom does flow from this way of thinking,
and for many the message is quite compelling.

It is this duality of good and evil, the good and the bad, the Christian
and the un-Christian, kosher or not, the ethical versus the unethical
practice that designate these discussions as predicated on a duality where
the world is one and the soul another, a left hand and a right, shadow and
light. And in most of human affairs these are the battles fought in the name
of love, the country, the flag, the cause: 'For England, Harry and St.
George'. It is in the name of such value divisions or disputes that entire
tribes are wiped out (Jew, Bosnians, Hutus or Tutsis). The names change,
the story of brutality, starvation, torture, rape by one group of another in
the name of a 'higher good' does not. In Miller's words:

And as long as human beings can sit and watch with hands folded while their
fellow-men are tortured and butchered so long will civilization be a hollow
mockery, a wordy phantom suspended like a mirage above a swelling sea of
murdered carcasses. (1941, p. 177)

And this applies to the 'helping' professionals as well.

Psychology, psychoanalysis, even psychotherapy and counselling
have attempted to become a science and modelling the discipline on
that of physics since Freud's Newtonian dualistic division into the
conscious and the unconscious realms of the mind, the blind positivistic
dedication of clinical psychology and the desperate devotion to

neutrality, impartiality and objectivity which are still held as ideals in much of psychology teaching at university and much of psychoanalytic and psychotherapy training outside in the practice of the professions.

> With the death of God, proclaimed by Nietzsche at the turn of the century, man came to be the measure of all things, and psychology became the secularized religion of modernity. In modernity the loss of belief in an absolute God had been succeeded by the modernist declaration of faith: 'I believe in one objective reality.' Religion as a truth guarantee was replaced by the new sciences, the priests as truth mediators were substituted by the scientists. (Kvale, 1992, pp. 53–4)

> We will have to come to terms, as we stagger into the postmodern era, with the hard-to-avoid evidence that there are many different realities, and different ways of experiencing them, and that people seem to want to keep exploring them, and that there is only a limited amount any society can do to ensure that its official reality is installed in the minds of most of its citizens most of the time. (Anderson, 1990, p. 152)

References

Anderson, W.T. (1990) Reality Is Not What It Used To Be. San Francisco, CA: Harper & Row.

Birnbaum, L. (1964) Behaviorism: John Broadus Watson and American Social Thought, 1913–1933. PhD dissertation, University of California, Berkeley, CA.

Clarkson, P. (1996) Researching the 'therapeutic relationship' in psychoanalysis, counselling psychology and psychotherapy – a qualitative inquiry. Counselling Psychology Quarterly, 9(2), 143–62.

Clarkson, P. (1998a) Beyond schoolism. Changes, 16(1), 1–11.

Clarkson, P. (1998b) The psychology of 'fame': implications for practice, in P. Clarkson (ed.) Counselling Psychology: Integrating Theory, Research and Supervised Practice. London: Routledge.

Conway, R. (1992) The Rage for Utopia. St. Leonards, NSW: Allen and Unwin.

Davison, G. C. and Neale, J. M. (1986) Abnormal Psychology (4th edn.). New York: John Wiley.

Dostoyevsky, F. (1955) The Brothers Karamazov (trans. C. Garnett). New York: Vintage.

Frank, J. (1973) Persuasion and Healing. New York: Schocken.

Freud, S. (1912a) The dynamics of transference. In J. Strachey (ed.), The Standard Edition of the Complete Psychological Works of Sigmund Freud, Vol. 12, pp. 97–108. London: Hogarth Press.

Freud, S. (1912b) Recommendations to Physicians Practising Psycho-analysis. In J. Strachey (ed.). The Standard Edition of the Complete Psychological Works Of Sigmund Freud, Vol. 12, pp. 109–20. London: Hogarth Press.

Fromm, E. (1991) The Fear of Freedom. London: Routledge.

Greenberg, I.A. (ed.) (1975) Psychodrama: Theory and Therapy. London: Souvenir Press.

Greenson, R.R. (1967) The Technique and Practice of Psychoanalysis, Vol. 1. New York: International Universities Press.

Guggenbühl-Craig, A. (1971) Power in the Helping Professions. Dallas, TX: Spring Publications.

Hall, J. (1993) The Reluctant Adult. Bridport: Prism Press.

Hillman, J. (1992) The practice of beauty. Sphinx, 4, 13–28. London: Convivium for
    Archetypal Studies.

Hillman, J. and Ventura, M. (1992) We've Had a Hundred Years of Psychotherapy and
    the World's Getting Worse. San Francisco, CA: Harper.

Keneally, T. (1994) Schindler's List. London: Sceptre.

Kupers, T.A. (1988) Ending Therapy. New York: New York University Press.

Kvale, S. (ed.) (1992) Psychology and Postmodernism. London: Sage.

Leahey, T.H. (1987) A History of Psychology. Englewood Cliffs, NJ: Prentice-Hall.

Lloyd, A.P. (1992) Dual relationship problems in counselor education. In B. Herlihy
    and G. Corey (eds.), Dual Relationships in Counseling, pp. 59–64. Alexandria, VA:
    American Association for Counseling and Development.

Mair, M. (1988) A psychology for a changing world. Psychotherapy Section Newsletter,
    no. 4. Leicester: British Psychological Society.

Malcolm, J. (1981) Psychoanalysis: The Impossible Profession. New York: Knopf.

Masson, J.M. (1989) Against Psychotherapy. London: Collins (first published 1988).

Milgram, S. (1974) Obedience to Authority. New York: Harper & Row.

Miller, H. (1941) The Colossus of Maroussi. Harmondsworth: Penguin.

Newnes, C. (1990) Counselling and primary prevention. Counselling Psychology
    Quarterly, 3(2), 205–10.

Rowe, D. (1990) A gene for depression? Who are we kidding? Changes, 8(1), 15–29.

Samuels, A. (1993) The Political Psyche. London: Routledge.

Severin, F.T. (1965) Humanistic Viewpoints in Psychotherapy. New York: McGraw-Hill.

Simons, H.W. (1989) Distinguishing the rhetorical from the real: the case of psy-
    chotherapeutic placebos. In H.W. Simons (ed.) Rhetoric in the Human Sciences, pp.
    109–118. London: Sage.

Smail, D.J. (1987) Taking Care: An Alternative to Therapy. London: J.M. Dent.

Smith, M.L. Glass, G.V. and Miller, T.I. (1980) The Benefits of Psychotherapy. Baltimore,
    MD: Johns Hopkins University Press.

Steiner, C., Wyckoff, H., Marcus, J., Lariviere, P., Goldstine, D., Schwebel, R. and mem-
    bers of the Radical Psychiatry Center (1975) Readings in Radical Psychiatry. New
    York: Grove Press.

Stoehr, T. (ed.) (1991) Nature Heals: The Psychological Essays of Paul Goodman.
    Highland, NY: The Gestalt Journal.

Walden, B. (1994) The Mail on Sunday (London), 30 October, p. 10.

Weigert, A. (1970) The immortal rhetoric of scientific sociology. American Sociologist,
    5, 570–3.

Weldon, F. (1994) Affliction. London: Harper Collins.

Whyte, C.R. (1994) Competencies. British Journal of Psychotherapy, 10(4), 568–9.

ITEM 4
Bystanding and Responsible Involvement in Psychotherapy, Organisations and Society

PETRŪSKA CLARKSON

- *Definition*: A bystander is someone who does not become involved when someone else needs help (see Latané and Darley, 1970).
- *Description*: Bystanding is to be differentiated from compulsive 'rescuing' on the one hand and from a phobic avoidance of 'interfering' on the other. People have many conscious and unconscious reasons for not getting involved in a responsible way with injustice, cruelty or scapegoating; for example, 'It's none of my business', 'I just want to remain neutral', or even blaming the victim for bringing it upon themselves. There may be real dangers in responsible involvement. Yet we also know that 'all that is necessary for evil to triumph is for good people to do nothing'.

From Kitty Genovese (Latané and Darley, 1970) to James Bulger people have bystanded situations where their intervention could have made all the difference. Abused children often discover their greatest pain is about the people who knew of their plight and did not intervene. Abusive scapegoating on the playground or in group therapy cause casualties. Consultants know that victims of a 'lynching' in the organisation report a similar incomprehension as former friends and natural associates turn their eyes away. The tragedy of the holocaust was largely dependent on the passivity of 'innocent bystanders'.

Psychotherapists and their clients have to deal with the wounds of bystanding committed or endured in the past, as well as with the existential reality that such moral and ethical dilemmas continue to face us as individuals and professionals all the time both in the present and the future. This workshop, drawing on substantial research on this theme, is about ethical and moral issues in our work. We will explore theoretically and experientially these issues as they affect us as group psychotherapists, supervisors, organisational consultants and as citizens every day of our lives.

- How has bystanding affected you personally?
- How has bystanding affected you professionally? (as a group therapist, supervisor or organisational consultant)
- How has bystanding affected you organisationally?
- How has bystanding affected you as a citizen of the world?

Please rank yourself in order from 10 (most used) to 0 (never used) the following kinds of 'bystander slogans'. You may of course have your own versions of these. Note if there is a difference between things you might say aloud in public and things you think or feel, but keep to yourself.

- It's none of my business (Pontius Pilate)
- It's more complex than it seems (Who knows anyway?)
- I don't have all the information (Ignorance is bliss)
- I don't want to get burned again (Let them fry!)
- I want to remain neutral (I don't want to take sides)
- I'm only telling the truth as I see it (Gossip is juicier than responsibility)
- I'm only following orders (It's more than my job's worth)
- The truth lies somewhere in the middle (Six of the one and half-a-dozen of the other)
- My contribution won't make much difference (Who? Me?)
- I'm just keeping my own counsel (I'm all right, Jack!)
- Victim blaming (The 'just world assumption')
- I don't want to rock the boat (I don't want to raise a difficult issue)

Reference

Latané, B. and Darley, M. (1970) The Unresponsive Bystander: Why Doesn't He Help? New York: Appleton Century Crofts.

CHAPTER 5
In Recognition of Dual Relationships

PETRŪSKA CLARKSON

Aufidius: Our virtues lie in th' interpretation of the time. (Shakespeare, Coriolanus, IV.vii.49)

This chapter examines some of the underlying asssumptions of the 'dual relationships' preoccupation in the current psychotherapeutic literature, questioning whether intellectual, moral and clinical effort should not rather be expended in educating psychotherapists and clients in how to deal with the unavoidable breaks and disruptions of boundaries of the precious but probably mythical 'single relationship' rather than fuelling a phobic, but unrealistic attempt to avoid all dual relationships in psychotherapy. In particular, the neglected issue of political exploitation of the psychotherapist trainee as client and supervisee in professional organisations is raised.

In recent literature and in the contemporary professional climate of counselling and psychotherapy there seems to be an increasing preoccupation with so-called dual relationships, exploration of boundaries and real or possible boundary transgressions (Stone, 1976; Gutheil, 1989; Epstein and Simon, 1990; Gutheil and Gabbard, 1993). The importance of clear boundaries in counselling and psychotherapy, the inviolate right of individuals to be treated with respect, confidentiality and the avoidance of professional exploitation of a sexual, financial or emotional nature has apparently been worked out and worked over thoroughly. In the ethical codes of every major counselling and psychotherapeutic society these concerns appear to be represented (ITAA Training Standards, 1991; BAC, 1992; UKCP, 1993). There has been a spate of books, papers and conferences on professional abuse of clients, and the power relationships inherent in counselling and psychotherapy (AHPP Conference, 1993; BIIP Conference, 1993). Organisations such as the Prevention of Professional Abuse Network (POPAN) have been formed in

75

Britain and elsewhere, which are specifically concerned with identification, prevention and amelioration of professional abuse by psychotherapists of their clients (Pepinster, 1993). This phenomenon has emerged concomitantly with the growing recognition of the prevalence of sexual (and other kinds of) abuse of children by their parents (Miller, 1983a, 1983b, 1985) and the important and serious questioning of the collusion, minimisation and cover-up of professionals to protect themselves, white male rights, the powers that be (Masson, 1989).

This chapter needs to be read in the postmodern context of our time. It is not meant in any way to minimise or reduce the importance of these other voices and activities – indeed in many forums I have spoken and written adamantly and passionately in favour of increased sensitisation, awareness and caution in terms of the potential harm involved in psychotherapists conduct towards clients (Clarkson, 1988, 1990, chaired panel of BIIP). However, there are some aspects and considerations in our cultures and these fields of our work which may be in danger of being omitted, neglected or denied. This chapter is intended to highlight these – not to exclude or minimise the other perspectives, but to widen, sensitise and differentiate some important aspects of the overall context of discussion which I believe are in danger of being ignored as patients and professionals risk becoming overly and perhaps exclusively aware of one polarity of concern at the expense of others. That this apparently public and professional overbalancing in one direction – that of the client – is also happening in the context of legal, political, financial and social considerations with their differential reward systems is particularly significant.

The ubiquity of dual relationships

It is a historical fact that many of the founding fathers of psychoanalysis, analytic psychology and psychotherapy conducted serious dual relationships with their patients (Freud, Fromm, Reichmann), their friends (Fleiss), their mistresses (Jung, Perls) and even their children (Klein in Grosskurth, 1986) which in today's climate would be considered unwise if not downright unethical. However, it could also be said that many of these dual relationships formed the very fulcrum and the breeding ground from which many of these important approaches originated and developed. Could Klein have developed her theories about the psychoanalysis of children without experiencing the envious assault of her own children while she was 'analysing' them for her own professional advancement? As has been pointed out by Cornell (1994) few of these people would meet the ethical standards of the professional societies that today embody their theoretical legacies. Yet, could they have achieved what they did without engaging in such dual relationships? In much of the contemporary literature there has grown an almost prurient preoccupation with an ideal if not mandatory hermetically sealed therapeutic relationship.

I have written about the multiplicity of psychotherapeutic relationships (Clarkson, 1990) but that work does not deal with dual relationships in this sense but refers to relationships within the therapeutic frame, whereas dual relationships usually refer to relationships within and outside the therapeutic frame.

Freud (1912a) went so far at one point as to suggest that the analyst model himself on the surgeon, put aside his human sympathy and adopt an attitude of emotional coldness. 'This means that the analyst must have the ability to restrain his therapeutic intentions, must control his urge for closeness and must "blanket" his usual personality' (Stone in Greenson, 1967, p. 389). Freud advocated that the analyst should refrain from intruding his personality into the treatment and introduced the simile of the analyst being a 'mirror' for the analysand (Freud 1912a, p. 118). This may not in fact be an accurate picture of what Freud had in mind. Perhaps he emphasised certain 'unnatural' aspects of psychoanalytic technique because they were so foreign and artificial to the usual doctor–patient relationship and the customary psychotherapy of his day.

For example, in a chapter written in the same year as the one where he cites the recommendations for emotional coldness and the mirror-like attitude, Freud stated:

> Thus the solution of the puzzle is that transference to the doctor is suitable for resistance to the treatment only in so far as it is a negative transference or a positive transference of repressed erotic impulses. If we 'remove' the transference by making it conscious, we are detaching only these two components of the emotional act from the person of the doctor; the other component, which is admissible to consciousness and unobjectionable, persists and is the vehicle of success in psycho-analysis exactly as it is in other methods of treatment.(1912b, p. 105)

Freud prescribed a mirror-like impassivity on the part of the analyst who should himself be analysed, who should not reciprocate the patient's confidences and not try to educate, morally influence or 'improve' the patient, and who should be tolerant of the patient's weakness. In practice, however, Freud 'conducted therapy as no classical Freudian analyst would conduct it today' (Malcolm, 1981), shouting at the patient, praising him, arguing with him, accepting flowers from him on his birthday, lending him money, visiting him at home and even gossiping with him about other patients!

The psychoanalyst Sechehaye (1951) was able to break through the unreal wall that hemmed in her patient Renee and bring her into some contact with life. In order to do this, Sechehaye not only took her on holiday to the seashore, as Ferenczi had done with one of his patients, but also took Renee into her home for extended periods. She allowed her to regress to the point where she felt she was re-entering her mother's body, thus becoming one of the first of those psychotherapists who have literally undertaken to 're-parent' schizophrenic clients. She allowed her to lean on her bosom and pretended to give milk from her breasts to the doll with whom Renee identified.

This preoccupation may have now reached its enantiodromic apotheosis. This polarity has been explored so well that its opposite may have become obscured and in need of emerging out of the shadow. Lloyd (1992), for example, refers to a 'dual relationship phobia' abroad in counselling education. Historically this may have been a necessity. Currently, a solution to a past problem may (as is often the case) breed the seeds of the next problem. The important professional and public concern about psychotherapist exploitation of clients has been necessary and important to highlight and prevent some most disturbing abuses – particularly the sexual exploitation of therapist-induced client dependence (Rutter, 1989) or the unethical sexual relationships between trainers and people in training or supervisors and their supervisees. Of course, so-called dual relationship issues incorporate a field much wider than sexuality or finance alone. Kitzinger (1987) was not the first to point at the aphrodisiac qualities of political power – and psychotherapy is becoming more and more political. Psychotherapy at this current time encompasses many multiple relationships – past, present, potential, historical and actual – a much more complex field than the putative simplicity of ethical codes or published directives for professional conduct can ever hope to encompass.

I think it is time to suggest, however unpopularly and uncomfortably, that it is impossible for most psychotherapists to completely avoid all situations where conflicting interests or multiple roles may exist – even if they tried sincerely and dedicatedly to do so. Furthermore, I believe that a profession that is built on the naive and utopian ideal that such dual or multiple relationships can indeed always be avoided does not equip trainee or experienced professionals with the awarenesses, attitudes or skills which can make it possible for them to deal with these situations if and when they do arise – as I believe they almost inevitably will. Such impossible ideals may lead to some equally false and impossible professional aims – to somehow be successful in avoiding all multiple relationships – dual seems simple compared to what most senior psychotherapists in any significant professional organisation have to cope with! I think it is an unfair and unkind myth to suggest to trainees in psychotherapy (what most experienced psychotherapists have discovered over and over to their cost to be untrue) that it is possible that the psychotherapeutic relationship can be purified from intentional or unintentional boundary disturbances. Of course there may be individual exceptions. For the sake of this chapter it is important to distinguish between

- clients seen in institutions such as large hospitals
- clients seen in private practice in a practitioner's home or office
- clients who are or who become trainees and/or members of the profession.

Obviously readers will have to modify some of what I have to say to suit these different situations.

Where the client is in training

There are, of course, particular complications when clients or patients are part of a training or professional institute or involved with a supervisory relationship with trainers or psychotherapists or supervisors who have professional interests in a particular professional society ('in contrast to private practice with clients outside the profession who do not or may never attend a public education event, dream seminar with films or whatever). This particular section of this chapter concerns the many cases where the client is or may become a trainee and thus eventually a fellow professional. (We never know what may happen when we take individuals into psychotherapy – and it is not uncommon for many patients at least to consider taking up psychotherapy as their profession sometime during their own treatment, whether or not they eventually act positively on this.) Which client eventually becomes a trainee psychotherapist or counsellor (and thus potentially a future colleague) can at no time be foreseen.

Psychotherapy conducted within a training or professional institute provides a peculiar amendment of the therapeutic frame. Any psychotherapist seeing a psychotherapy trainee as a client or patient must be influenced by this fact because it is (at the very least) imbued with ethical implications. Many psychoanalytic institutions require that the analyst support their continuation to graduation from training. It certainly has been a debatable issue whether the psychotherapy or analysis of a trainee or a supervisee who is preparing to enter the profession can ever be said to be the same as that of someone who does not need to 'be in psychotherapy' for their professional purposes (Freud, 1912b). At a professional conference I attended several years ago, a psychiatric resident who was in psychoanalysis was featured on the programme as an analysand to make a speech about how valuable they felt their psychoanalysis was, with their current analyst present! They both appeared unaware of the incredible contradiction between lauding the therapeutic objectivity of their purist psychoanalytic setting while manifesting such a blatant contradiction in their public presentation (perhaps as result of their objective and non-transferential desire?) to promote their own particular brand of psychoanalysis.

Conferences, meetings, professional associations – these constantly invoke and provoke us to deal with these recurrent and perhaps unavoidable vicissitudes of the psychotherapists' life. Many such examples may at best eventuate as studies in professional exhibitionism and politically managed exposure for the public relations of the institute with which the person trained. Training literature and supervision to avoid these kinds of situations are no doubt well meant. However, they give us (and our charges) no criteria, little guidance and therefore no validity or possibility for growth and development in managing these impossibly complicated, sometimes – no matter how well-intentioned we are – unavoidable enmeshments of our personal and professional matrixes.

A few years ago I attended, as usual, an annual professional gathering of a hundred or so of the major psychotherapeutic organisations in Britain. They were represented by some of the most senior people within each organisation. Gathered in this conference hall with an apparently common purpose and with many, if not all of us holding the ideal of 'not engaging in dual relationships', I could identify my current analyst, my current supervisor, someone who was currently in supervision with me, the wife of a current client, the lover of a past client, the ex-wife of a colleague, my partner's psychotherapist at the time, a colleague against whom there had been an ethics charge (I had sat on the complaints board during the case), the analyst of someone who was in supervision with me at the time, the friend of an old friend of mine who was at this time on the opposite side of the political fence. I know that most of the senior people in that gathering will have had versions of the same experience.

I also had the experience of seeing the psychoanalyst with whom I was in treatment at this time scapegoated in a professional setting. I heard gossip about the family of a psychoanalyst with whom I subsequently went into psychotherapy and had to deal with my supervisor stretched and impaired in their organisational role. A colleague was there whose patients had seen him on a nationwide TV programme which was variously received. A supervisor with whom I had had an unhappy relationship was there. I knew this person had had an unethical relationship with a supervisee who was also at this conference as an organisational representative. I remember being trapped on one unfortunate occasion in a residential setting from which I could not escape overhearing a violent fight between my therapist at the time and his wife; this changed my opinion about him forever.

I have been at conferences and professional associations with these ex-therapists, ex-supervisors and current colleagues and will be perhaps for the rest of my professional life associated with them (or similar others) in the same kind of ways. Supervisees and ex-clients who come into the profession will face the same situations if they are involved with any training organisation in any way. One of the greatest difficulties is not to try to avoid these situations, because we cannot; but to find ways of understanding and supporting ourselves and each other in these multiple role situations which are unbelievably demanding and challenging and potentially stressful to all concerned. If only they could be dealt with by a simple manageable prohibition of dual relationships.

At least in the consultation room in the psychotherapeutic hour there is frequently a contract to deal with positive and negative transference. Within the conference hall or the committee room both future and past therapeutic relationships are constantly being reworked and revised non-contractually, and sometimes at least retroactively spoilt or idealised. I don't think as a profession we have begun to deal with these multiple relational implications – I certainly have not read much in the professional literature which helps me or my trainees to negotiate these situations. I differentiate these from unethical or unprofessional abuses. These situations may all be basically ethical in the sense that they are not based on intentional professional exploitation but they are also mostly unintentionally, fundamentally, profoundly and unavoidably dual or multiple in essence.

This brings me to the ethical issue that I find most disturbing in the sense that it is ubiquitous in so many psychotherapy settings linked with training and professional institutes – that is, the political exploitation of clients. It is ordinary and normal and mostly left unquestioned that clients and/or supervisees are in a position where they have to vote for their psychotherapist or supervisor in terms of being appointed officers of the society, committee members, representatives at conferences, or agreeing annual accounts drawn up by the therapist or supervisor in their role as treasurer. This kind of democratic ideal is often held as sacrosanct and inviolate in these societies. This position seems to me often to be a direct contravention of the ethical code dictum not to exploit a client. I would challenge any psychotherapist or supervisor to make a waterproof case for the fact that their clients or supervisees can be untransferentially engaged in such voting procedures that carry direct gains or losses in terms of popularity, status, financial reward or assistance without being influenced by the other psychotherapeutic/supervisory relationships, or vice versa. It is unfortunately not unheard of that in some formal cases ethics investigators are appointed who are known political opponents and have actively canvassed for votes against the complainant!

For most professional societies, if they were to exclude dual relationships, they would need to prohibit all people who are still in psychotherapy, whether or not it is related to their training, to refrain from participation in the organising of conferences, the publishing of newsletters and the election of officers. What would it mean for the ITAA, or the Institute of Psychoanalysis for that matter, to avoid perpetuating such dual relationships? What does it say about congruence in terms of ethics that these issues remain (as far as I know) unaddressed? The consciously so-called democratic procedure that is therefore so highly valued in some professional societies and the sanctity of the 'single role' of the psychotherapeutic relationship are apparently ethically in unavoidable contradiction in practice. Ignoring this particular kind of dual relationship, perhaps the most pernicious one in terms of collective discounting of exploitation, is perhaps most dangerous to client, patient, psychotherapist and psychotherapeutic society alike.

I hope that I have raised enough questions for people to consider if they are involved with training institutions or training psychotherapists whether they are indeed within the strictures of the ethical codes for not exploiting dual relationships. My hope is that if professional people have become less desensitised and less habitually blinded in certain directions they will consider means, ways and educational tools for helping us all to deal with what is a clearly ubiquitous and perhaps unavoidable demand on us as professionals to learn how to become easy, graceful and fluent in the multiple relationships that are the unavoidable consequences of our work.

Clients who are not in training

As has been said before, we may know some people as trainees or as purely private clients at the time we initiate the psychotherapeutic process with them. However, it is practically impossible to know whether someone may in future become a trainee. We think this is a much simpler case, of course. Kottler (1986), for example, says

> If we run into a client at a social gathering, etiquette requires us to fade into the background unless the client chooses to recognize us. If a client's name comes up in conversation, we must pretend indifference so as not to give away our involvement. It is as if we were conducting secret affairs with fifty people simultaneously! We even arrange our schedules and offices so clients do not accidentally meet one another. All of this results in a kind of sanctuary for the people we help and a kind of prison for ourselves. (p. 60)

Kottler goes on to say, 'All over the city there are restaurants and bars we cannot feel comfortable visiting because clients or ex-clients work there' (1986, p. 61). However, even this statement of Kottler's assumes that it is possible to avoid visiting places where clients or ex-clients may be if we know that they work there. But how can we know all the places our clients, their spouses, their children and their friends and lovers may go just for recreation or education, or by coincidence? There are many places where we may encounter current or past clients (their friends, colleagues or family members) without any idea, in fact with the ultimate hope that they would not be there at all. I shall relate three true incidents culled from my own experience and that of other colleagues to protect the identity of innocents (all).

- A supervisee of mine happily reported how 'secure' she felt to find her psychotherapist and the therapist's lover both naked in the Turkish baths on a day when she went there.
- A therapist/colleague from another country (say Hong Kong) met a colleague in (say New York) for a social visit on a holiday – a friend suggested that they visit a sex shop for fun since the colleague from Hong Kong had never done it. As the three psychotherapists were amusing themselves by looking round the sex shop at its various displays and equipment the visiting psychotherapist suddenly

recognised one of her clients – a man she had been seeing recently with his wife for sex therapy. The consulting room and the place of encounter were separated by some 3000 miles! The probabilities against this type of coincidence must be enormous. The impact of this kind of encounter on the unconscious process, however skilfully dealt with (shortly after the time of the accidental encounter), in terms of both transference and countertransference responses must be enormous, uncontrolled and potentially full of both damage and benefits. One can only hope training and supervision can equip psychotherapists for these kinds of inter-contaminated encounters. Do not think that you are somehow exempt from coincidences of this kind. I used to.

• At the end of one summer I was extremely tired, fed up with the world of psychotherapy and wishing to have some space within which I did not have to be so everlastingly 'care-full' about the trans-ferential implications of my life as I usually have to be while I am in practice on my premises as a professional psychotherapist and head of a prominent organisation. I got on the aeroplane to a city in (say Greece) and immediately pointedly ignored the passenger next to me – I feared that any involvement in a social conversation would lead to questions about myself and my profession from which at this point I wanted to escape. The passenger next to me made several overtures not withstanding my discreet but definite show of disinterest. At about attempt number six to engage with her saying, 'Where are you going?' I replied (to avoid appearing terminally impolite) that I was going to (say) Phatos. This opened the floodgates of interrogation. 'I am a teacher – What do you do?' she said. Conflicted between inauthentic dissimulation and surreptitious invitation, I replied that I was a writer. 'A writer about what?' she asked. This was difficult. I couldn't refuse to answer with any claim to courtesy. At the same time if I disguised the facts it wouldn't be that hard to find me out or feel that I had been unfairly withholding. 'On counselling and psychotherapy', I said. 'Oh' she said 'do you know a place called Metanoia? I am in psychotherapy with someone who said they trained at Metanoia and at the moment he is telling me about the games I play – do you know Metanoia and would you go along with this kind of way of treating people? I have been thinking about terminating my therapy with him. What do you think I should do?' I realised that the person to whom she was referring to as her therapist was in supervision with me. These facts would not be impossible for her to ascertain if she set her mind to it on her return.

I immediately flipped into therapeutic first gear. Bracketing my desire for peace, quiet and space, I related to her for the rest of the journey in a way conducive to facilitating the optimum therapeutic atmosphere in terms of encouraging her to discuss her difficulties with her psychotherapist. All in all I behaved as if I was being paid in my consulting room knowing that it was not only the reputation of the institution that I was protecting but also the integrity of the therapeutic frame between my supervisee and his client. It was not what I had expected to do on the flight to my holiday destination.

Kottler writes of psychotherapists: 'we live in glass houses on display' (1986, p. 61). We apparently also travel in a similarly exposed way. Another way of phrasing this is that there is no place to hide for the modern psychotherapist. It is probably impossible for the psychotherapist to be a guaranteed blank screen exempt from the vicissitudes and coincidences of all the revealing tendencies of life. Any dream to the contrary is just that. You may and will be seen in the supermarket and your patient will make facts and fantasies about the food in your trolley as much if not more than they would about the trolley of anyone else they met there. If not in the park relating to your children, clients will see you in the doctor's surgery waiting room and wonder why you are there. Can any one of us be sure to avoid our clients in all such situations even most of the time, without becoming monastic recluses? It seems to me far more important that psychotherapists learn how and where to get the education and modelling to deal with these occurrences which may be life events or incidental or purposeful invasions and intrusions.

There is always and honestly the unavoidable impingement of the psychotherapist's life on their practice (Orlans, 1993). It is hard to hide the physical effects of pregnancy – its psychological effects may be much more far-reaching than anticipated (Clementel-Jones, 1985; Gottlieb, 1989). It is not possible to hide the death of a spouse if the obituaries appear in the newspapers, marriage makes headlines or the rumour mill, moving house is publicly declared, illness can show through traces in the face, a bandaged leg or absences from the practice, births and deaths are publicly marked in chosen and unchosen ways, graduations and publications are celebrated with or without consent. Unavoidable and unplanned interruptions occur much more often than we would wish (the plumber, administrative emergencies, a car crash in the street outside, Mrs Klein ignoring her own daughter knocking repeatedly and despairingly at the door while she continues in an analytic session with a favoured patient, behaving as if the disturbance was not in fact occurring, Wright, 1988).

I submit that it is a myth that the psychotherapist can entirely protect their personal life from their clients. Like all myths, if we make them imperatives they become persecutory and oppressive – devoid of creativity, spontaneity and genuineness. When I complained about a client using her information about my marriage, my supervisor at the time said 'of course she is not supposed to know about this'. I chose that moment to confront her with the fact that I knew about a custody case being fought between one of her adult children and her ex-spouse since it had been all over the newspapers. I did not need to be told to avoid these types of cross-over. I needed to be helped by her to manage them. However much we wish we could live anonymous lives I don't believe we can any more. The desire for psychotherapists to be the new 'secular priests' is in my opinion profoundly based in grandiosity and naiveté with incalculable negative consequences for both the psychotherapists and their clients demanding new infallible but absolute self-sacrificing gods.

In addition there are occasions of accidental invasion. For example, my first Tavistock-trained Freudian psychoanalyst, scrupulous to the nth degree in avoiding any shape or form of conscious multiple relation-ships, happened to be sitting in the waiting room outside my doctoral thesis supervisor's office. I was shocked to find him there when I went for an appointment with my supervisor. Frankly, neither of us knew how to deal with it very well at all. I now think it was so painful, unexpected and unprepared-for that both of us pretended it had never happened. I still wonder what they could have been discussing although both are now dead. I have met colleagues who are acquaintances of my current psychotherapist when this person suffered the bereavement of her spouse. I hated the derogatory way in which they spoke of my analyst in her hour of need and have never yet found the right way to deal with it inside the therapeutic situation. However, I love her for this vulnerability as much as I retrospectively despise another (short-term) trainer who used to be publicly massaged by his female clients (deeply in idealised transference) while high on dope.

The impingement of the therapist's professional life (even when exemplary) on their practice is unavoidable and minimised only at the cost of maintaining a self-deluding rather solipsistic therapeutic avoid-ance of the accidents and serendipities of real life. It is as important to learn how to deal effectively and therapeutically with a disruptive fact of life as to discriminate this activity from not doing wrong or exploitative things. It is probably even more important to learn to question and differentiate moral categories than to tiptoe around legal niceties in service to an exaggerated psychotherapeutic fastidiousness.

Promotion at the hospital, change of office or address; publications, professional or popular, celebrate national and international fame; public position indicates popularity with implicit or explicit seduction, promises of connections, work recognition, glory by association with the famous – reactionary or revolutionary. The effects of being in therapy with a writing psychotherapist are at least as complex as being in therapy or supervision with a psychotherapist who is politically ambitious in the field. At the very least clients may say: 'you are not who I thought you were from your last book written some years ago' or 'you contradict what you said on page 94'! Naturally many are concerned about the basic questions 'will you put me in' or 'will you leave me out'? They feel

'This is me'! Often those aspects we believe are most unique to us are shared by many others, and composite case histories are too often just that – notwithstanding a client's persistent belief to the contrary.

I am sure that the clients of any psychotherapist of any eminence frequently struggle with the management of this kind of information (publicity, rumour, gossip, public appearances, ceremonial occasions) from sources outside the therapy room about their psychotherapist. We do not have well established ways of thinking about or dealing with these kinds of things in our profession yet. Pretending we can avoid it is likely to lead to more abuse through ignorance, embarrassment and preciousness than a sincere and humble personal and professional engagement with the probabilities of real life.

Many practitioners will privately admit that they have modified their practice in the last decade – taking fewer risks, fearing unjust collegial criticism for therapeutic 'errors' or concerned about avoiding unfair client persecution for unethical conduct by trying to play absolutely by the rule book without any space for misinterpretation – as if this were possible! However, the professional phenomenon of 'minding our backs' is well under way in psychotherapy training and peer support. I believe this is deeply disturbing and much as it may prevent some abuses, it may create others. An example of this is the phobia around touching. I am told that some US insurance companies will not insure a psychotherapist against malpractice suits if they touch their clients at all. Against this I would like to posit the question posed by Woodmansey (1988) 'Might we be depriving our clients by not touching them?' Does the emergence of defensive psychotherapy lead to a concomitant loss of spontaneity, novelty, experimentation and risk? Has it become more important to avoid error than to do whatever is thought necessary and important to help the patient rather than to protect the therapist from criticisms or lawsuits?

Recommendations

There is much to say in terms of recommendations and little space. Of course, we should uphold and improve the ethical consciousness currently developing to protect clients from the abuses of the exploitation of dual relationships. And then we should go further.

- Firstly – to face up to the fact that most of the profession is in a state of dual role denial, role confusion, and the unaware interpenetration of role boundaries (time and space).
- Secondly – the necessity and urgency of developing countertransferential awarenesses, methodological tools and conceptual and moral facility in developing 'role fluency' – that we train and supervise with the existential vicissitudes of the so-called single role therapeutic

relationship in mind and do not hold an ideal state as normal. We need to equip ourselves and our charges to deal with rather than avoid real life.

* Thirdly, that we stop over-idealising the therapeutic hour and the consulting room and take seriously the research on state-dependent learning (Baddeley, 1983; Eysenck and Eysenck, 1989) which mandates a thorough rethinking of what we believe makes most of the difference in psychotherapy to a patient's real life outside. Some years ago I researched my past patients to find what was the most significant intervention I made in terms of their psychotherapeutic journey. I was expecting appreciation for significant deep interpretations, for facilitating particular catharses, for my empathic presence. There were some of these. However, to my surprise many more replies attested to the so-called extra-analytic effect – shades of the following comment: 'it was the way you seemed pleased to see me at a conference where neither of us expected to see one another that really changed my life – nobody had ever been pleased to see me before.'

References

AHPP (1993) Association of Humanistic Psychotherapy Practitioners Conference, 1993. place??? [details to come]

BAC (1992) Code of ethics and practice for Counsellors/Counselling skills/Trainers/Supervision of counsellors (four leaflets). Leicester: British Association for Counselling.

BIIP (1993) Therapy and Power: The right to speak. Conference, British Institute of Integrative Psychotherapy.

Baddeley, A. (1983) Your Memory: A user's guide. Harmondsworth: Penquin.

Clarkson, P. (1988) Ego state dilemmas of abused children. Transactional Analysis Journal, 18(2), 85–93.

Clarkson, P. (1990) A multiplicity of psychotherapeutic relationships. British Journal of Psychotherapy, 7, 148–63.

Clarkson, P. (1992) Transactional Analyis Psychotherapy: An Integrated Approach. London: Routledge.

Clarkson, P. (19??) re state dependent learning???? – details to come

Clementel-Jones, C. (1985) The pregnant psychotherapist's experience, British Journal of Psychotherapy, 2(2), 79–94.

Cornell, W. (1994) Dual relationships in transactional analysis: training, supervision and therapy. Transactional Analysis Journal, 24(1), 21–30.

Epstein, R.S. and Simon, R.I. (1990) The exploitation index: an early warning indicator of boundary violations in psychotherapy. Bulletin of the Menninger Clinic, 54, 450–65.

Eysenck, H. and Eysenck, M. (1989) Mind Watching. London: Priori.

Freud, S. (1912a) The dynamics of transference. In J. Strachey. (ed.), The Standard Edition of the Complete Psychological Works of Sigmund Freud, Vol. 12, pp. 97–108. London: Hogarth Press.

Freud, S. (1912b) Recommendations to physicians practising psycho-analysis. In J. Strachey (ed.). The Standard Edition of the Complete Psychological Works of Sigmund Freud, Vol. 12, pp. 109–20. London: Hogarth Press.

Gottlieb, S. (1989) The pregnant psychotherapist: A potent transference stimulus. British Journal of Psychotherapy, 5(3), 287–99.

Greenson, R.R. (1967) The Technique and Practice of Psychoanalysis, Vol. 1. New York: International Universities Press.

Grosskurth, P. (1986) Melanie Klein: Her World and her Work. New York: Alfred A. Knopf.

Gutheil, T.G. (1989) Borderline personality disorder, boundary violations, and patient-therapist sex: medicolegal pitfalls. American Journal of Psychiatry, 146, 597–602.

Gutheil, T.G. and Gabbard, G.O. (1993) The concept of boundaries in clinical practice: Theoretical and risk-management dimensions. American Journal of Psychiatry, 150(2), 188–96.

ITAA Standards Committee (1991) Statement of Ethics. In Training and Certification Manual for the Training and Certification Council of Transactional Analysts, Appendix 28, pp. 115–16. San Francisco, CA: International Transactional Analysis Association.

Kitzinger, C. (1987) The Social Construction of Lesbianism. London: Sage.

Kottler, J.A. (1986) On Being a Therapist. San Francisco, CA: Jossey-Bass.

Lloyd, A.P. (1992) Dual relationship problems in counselor education. In B. Herlihy and G. Corey (eds.), Dual Relationships in Counseling, pp. 59–64. Alexandria, VA: American Association for Counseling and Development.

Malcolm, J. (1981) Psychoanalysis: The Impossible Profession. New York: Knopf.

Masson, J. (1989) Against Therapy. London: Collins.

Miller, A. (1983a) The Drama of the Gifted Child and the Search for the True Self (trans. H. and H. Hannum). London: Faber.

Miller, A. (1983b) For Your Own Good: The Roots of Violence in Child-rearing (trans. H. and H. Hannum). London: Virago.

Miller, A. (1985) Thou Shalt Not Be Aware: Society's Betrayal of the Child (trans. H. and H. Hannum). London: Pluto Press.

Orlans, V. (1993) The personal and the practical: the counsellor's life crisis. In W. Dryden (ed.), Questions and Answers on Counselling in Action, pp. 62–7. London: Sage.

Pepinster, C. (1993) Presence of mind. Time Out (London), 20 May.

Rutter, P. (1989) Sex in the Forbidden Zone. London: Mandala.

Sechehaye, M. (1951) Reality Lost and Regained: Autobiography of a Schizophrenic Girl (trans. G. Urbin-Rabson). New York: Grune and Stratton.

Stone, M.H. (1976) Boundary violations between therapist and patient. Psychiatric Annals, 6, 670–7.

UKCP (1993) Ethical guidelines. In the UKCP National Register. London: United Kingdom Council for Psychotherapy.

Woodmansey, A.C. (1988) Are psychotherapists out of touch? British Journal of Psychotherapy, 5(1), 57–65.

Wright, N. (1988) Mrs Klein. London: Nick Hern Books.

ITEM 5
Information for Prospective Clients

PETRŪSKA CLARKSON

Introduction to the psychotherapeutic relationship

Psychotherapy is a very personal, unusual and private kind of relationship. Your psychotherapist may get to know you better than many people will ever know you. This is, of course, so that you can know and understand yourself better, and change if you want to. For some people, their relationship with their psychotherapist is more intimate even than that which they experience in their marriage or their primary relationship, certainly more intimate and honest than most people experienced with their parents or early caregivers. Whatever theories or approaches practitioners believe in, research shows that the most significant factor in determining the success of psychotherapy is the *quality of the relationship* between client and psychotherapist. This is often hard to understand at the beginning, when you may feel it strange that you would want to pay to tell someone some of the deepest feelings, wishes and desires of your life. However, it is precisely because of the nature of this confidential relationship that people can and do share themselves in this way in order to achieve their goals. As children we are humanely entitled to love, affection, protection, education and the like. As adults, however, it is very often only within psychotherapy that we can re-experience the possibility of this kind of true entitlement (because of the fee or other consideration exchanged) to fully explore our feelings and attitudes about another person or people.

Protection of the boundaries

It is very important to safeguard the boundaries of the psychotherapeutic relationship. Spouses, lovers, employers, family members, may all have varying degrees of investment in the outcome of your psychotherapy. They may be frightened that you will change, or change

89

in such a way that you want to re-evaluate your primary relationships, your marriage, your choice of career or country. On the other hand they may wish that the psychotherapist would dramatically change you into someone else whom they would like or love better. There are thus often a great many open as well as hidden expectations from other people in your family, social and professional networks if they know that you are engaging in the journey that is called counselling or psychotherapy in our culture.

Many marital arguments have been started by 'My therapist says . . .', and much misunderstanding and pain has been caused when someone in all innocence tries to share the intimate moments of a group psychotherapy session, for example, with a spouse who feels painfully and jealously excluded or who cannot be 'made' to be interested. You must therefore think very carefully about whom you tell that you are going to enter into psychotherapy. You are also advised to think through clearly if you really do want to relate your intimate aspects of your process of self-discovery and/or change – and, if you do, it is then worth considering which of those aspects and how they should be handled. It is best to discuss this quite extensively with your psychotherapist, while understanding the deeply ambivalent (or double) feelings your nearest and dearest may have about your development and growth as a person.

Confidentiality

If you are going into group psychotherapy it is also important to safeguard the confidentiality of other members of the group and to insist that they protect your confidentiality. We actually live in rather a small world. Simply not mentioning someone's name when recounting a feeling or sharing a story is not sufficient protection to safeguard the privacy of others in the way that you would want them to safeguard yours. People so often put two and two together to make five. The presence of others – clients, parents, employers – in the consulting room is of course natural and important, whether that presence is psychological (hearing a father's voice within your head, for example) or symbolic (for example, how you relate to authority figures). However, to dilute your psychotherapy by taking the events or experiences that belong in the group or with your psychotherapist into your social or other arenas of your life can be extremely detrimental to the benefit which you can derive from psychotherapy. It may not be in your best interests for friends in the pub, the students in your evening class or your lover to be in a position to intrude upon this private space that you have created for yourself.

There are at least two important issues here. One is the ethical obliga-tion of your psychotherapist to insist that the group members protect one another's confidentiality, just as he or she undertakes to protect the confidentiality of all group members. The other issue is the extent to which it is advisable or even efficient to include other parties in this process in any but a *nominal* way. Perhaps couples or family therapy could be more appropriate. To the extent that other people's influences are carried into the consulting room without acknowledgement, the psychotherapy process itself may be limited in its effectiveness.

Confidentiality and outside relationships

Many group psychotherapists insist that group members have no relationship of any kind of with each other outside the group. In my experience this rule is honoured more in the breach than in the observance – no matter what people say. I personally know many people who have had both social and sexual relationships with other group members for many years under this rule system without the so-called group conductor ever finding out. Keeping such secrets from your practitioner is indeed a waste of financial and emotional investment. Often there is no adamant rule against social contact with other group members outside the group. However, external relationships are almost always a source for interested concern and caring investigation. This is because any relationship outside the group, even with other group members, has to be brought into the group if the person is to have the maximum benefit from their psychotherapy. There can be no beneficial confidentiality about such relationships which naturally and inevitably impinge on the group life. So, whereas obviously no one can be forced to keep the rules, it is important that you understand and that your psychotherapist explains the reasoning behind observing the cautions and roadsigns which he or she has learned over time.

Since the psychotherapy situation can partly resemble that of the confessional, it really works best if it can be a place in which people can say and explore whatever is in their hearts, minds or fantasies in safety, privacy and without fear of gossip, blame or punishment. You will notice that I am not including *physical behaviour*, for there are certain behaviours such as violence to yourself or others, and/or certain criminal acts, about which your psychotherapist may ultimately have to break confidentiality. But they should always request your permission or explain their reasons to you first, and this happens rarely if the ground rules are securely established at the outset.

Another exception to the limits of confidentiality is the regular discussion by the practitioner with other colleagues for supervision, consultation and accreditation purposes. All professionally responsible practitioners remain in supervision with senior colleagues where they regularly review their client practice. Such supervisory procedures are designed to improve the quality of their service to you and assist their professional development, and fundamentally are of greater benefit to you, their client. The primary reason for their asking permission to tape your sessions with them is to review such material personally or with their supervisor for improvement of their work with you. Colleagues consulted within these professional boundaries are, of course, always adhering to the same rules of confidentiality that your psychotherapist observes. As a client you have a right to know where and under what circumstances the confidentiality of the psychotherapeutic relationship is likely to be excepted. For instance, your psychotherapist must tell you that the work you do together will be reviewed in supervision, and also that they might consult a lawyer or participate in an ethics committee.

Creating space for growth and change

Often, within the safety of a group, people can become very intimate about feelings of rejection, anger, fear, love and sadness. This may include the verbal exploration of attraction towards one another or towards the psychotherapist. It is always better to explore such thoughts and feelings in the group in words first with the psychotherapist, before pursuing this kind of attraction outside the group in any way whatsoever. This advice is the outcome of the accumulated testimony of practitioners of the twentieth century. The damaging effects of sexual relationships occasionally formed within individual and/or group psychotherapy is well known. Sexual relationships formed within a group situation are almost always destructive of the psychotherapy process. It is usually potentially negative for the people involved; if not immediately, then in the long-term.

Psychotherapeutic groups indeed give us an opportunity to be close to other people and to explore our feelings about them to the extent that we can be sure that no one will take advantage and that we do not have to follow through the consequences of our fantasies into behaviour at all times. But we have to safeguard this space carefully in order to have this symbolic freedom. They can help us become more comfortable, both socially and with the specific psychological relationships within the psychotherapy group, so that we can pursue friendship or sexual relationships with other people.

Professional conduct guidelines

It is important to establish at the beginning whether your practitioner is in training or already qualified. If the latter, find out in what way, and on which professional register (BAC, UKCP, BPS) they are entered.

If you wish to change psychotherapist, it is not considered professional behaviour for a psychotherapist to start seeing a client who is already in psychotherapy elsewhere. It is common advice to finish with one before you start with another. If a psychotherapist encourages you to break off with a colleague, they are behaving unprofessionally. They must discuss this course of conduct, with your permission, with the other psychotherapist first. It is often difficult for someone not used to the world of psychotherapy to judge if you are simply going through a temporary (and important) difficult patch with your psychotherapist, or whether there is a definite lack of helpfulness towards you as client. Sometimes people just don't get on, sometimes they are ill-matched, sometimes the timing just isn't right.

If you have a particular concern, such as whether your new psychotherapist has values that could undermine your relationship with them or affect your work negatively do not hesitate to ask. Whether and how they answer your questions about their position on homosexuality, religion, race, pornography and so on is an important part of *you* interviewing *them*. You have the right to ask such questions and, on that basis, to make a decision about engaging with them or not. It is important to remember that you can choose your psychotherapist and that, as with doctors or hairdressers, you can see several practitioners until you feel comfortable enough with a particular person to embark on this important journey with them.

Usually discontent, irritation, fear and other uncomfortable feelings experienced in the psychotherapeutic relationship are very valuable and should be explored. Always try to talk about such issues before you take precipitate action, such as not returning to terminate the psychotherapeutic relationship with proper notice and due care to all parties – a minimum notice of three sessions is usual. You can always return to your original referring agency to help you relocate to a practitioner who may be more suitable for you at the particular stage of your development, or more suited to your preferences at the particular time. It is also a good plan (in most situations) to think very carefully about suddenly changing partners, jobs, medication or other significant parts of your life without discussion in therapy first. Most psychotherapists will explain their procedures for dealing with emergency calls out of hours. Though the service offered by the Samaritans is not intended as a substitute for individual psychotherapy, in a crisis, remember that when the therapist or a central number at the clinic is not available for some reason, you can always call the Samaritans, who keep a telephone line open around the clock and all the year. Their 24-hour phoneline (UK national Lo-Call number) is 0345 90 90 90.

In a similar way it is important to know that a psychotherapist is never to touch you physically without your permission, and that any sexual behaviour from them towards you while you are their client (and usually also afterwards) is always unethical. Seek the help of the psychotherapist's supervisor and the school principal or institutional ethics committee immediately if you are unsure about such behaviour. However, it is best always to talk to your psychotherapist first as openly as you can about anything that worries you or that you want to know about the process and conduct of psychotherapy. A couple of excellent books on the subject are listed at the end of Appendix 1. Professionals do disagree about many things, however – as in any established field of work. Get the best information you can, so as to form your own opinion; consult experts in the field, and then take responsibility for your decisions and commitment to the process.

Practical details

You will normally be expected to pay for all psychotherapeutic sessions booked but missed – for whatever reasons – if you are attending group psychotherapy. In some cases your psychotherapist will not charge you for a cancellation received with one week's notice for an individual psychotherapy session. But practitioners do differ, so make sure you ask about and understand the rules and conditions that govern the practice of which you become a client: how much they charge, how this is to be paid and how often fees are adjusted. Most psychotherapists carry a limited proportion of their practice at lower fees. Low-fee clinics are available for people in genuine financial need. Most psychotherapists will give you good advance warning of their own holidays and breaks whenever they can. When absences are unavoidable they will let you know as soon as possible or arrange for a stand-in service where appropriate.

Psychotherapy is not always the best option for people – sometimes a dating agency, healthcare programme, or specific education or training may be more helpful. There are no guarantees about the success or speed of psychotherapy, but many people have used it to become better and more creative individuals with enhanced compassion, potency and choice in the world for themselves and others.

Towards a Beginning

I have written these very brief preliminary guidelines to give you an idea of some of the issues involved in becoming a client. There may be many omissions, or different forms of expression. Please accept this as an attempt to be helpful, subject to your own personal exploration, and let me know of issues which you think are vital and/or ways in which these could be stated in a better or clearer way. Finally, whether you are entering, leaving or re-entering counselling, counselling psychology or psychotherapy, I wish you a fruitful, challenging and satisfying journey for the rest of your life.

Example of letter used for tape-recording training sessions

Professor Petrūska Clarkson, FBPsS, FBAC
12 North Common Road, London W5 2QB.

Dear Training Group Member,
Due to recent changes in various codes of ethics it has now become necessary to ask you for you for written confirmation of your verbal permission for me to tape-record our work.

As I have explained, you are always entitled to ask me to switch the tape off or even to erase anything subsequent to your having said this. Tape recordings are my major way of keeping records. Tapes are kept securely and there is provision in my will for their destruction should I become incompetent or die. They may also occasionally be used for supervision, qualification or re-accreditation purposes. In such a case the other professionals involved by necessity would be bound by the same rules of strict confidentiality as I am. Such activities are primarily to your own benefit seeing as they are concerned with monitoring and improving quality of my work for you.

I would also ask your permission to use our tape-recorded sessions for research should that become necessary or desirable in the future. Of course, I will protect identities and other identifiable material if I don't ask you for your specific permission to use your work first. You have all read the way I use client material or case studies in my work, so you have an idea of the respect and care I have shown for writing about anyone who embarks on this journey into the self.

Obviously the primary purpose of this permission is to advance the effectiveness and knowledge of psychotherapy, supervision and related activities in our world to benefit others. If, however, you wish to withhold your permission for any reason, you will not be disadvantaged in any way and I will specifically not use your work. It should be remembered that many people may feel something is unique to them, whereas many more people may share similar experiences, so identification of any specific individual is unlikely in any event. In any event, I do not consider research separate from my ongoing reflection on my own practice in order to do work of better quality.

Thank you.

Signed:...

Further Reading

Clarkson, P. with Carroll, M. (1993) Counselling, psychotherapy, psychology and applied psychology: the same and different. In P. Clarkson, On Psychotherapy, pp. 3–19. London: Whurr.

CHAPTER 6

Vengeance of the Victim*

PETRŪSKA CLARKSON

Whose truth is it anyway?

Here is a little anecdote that Rupert Riedl, the Austrian anthropologist
and biologist, recounted in a paper on causal thinking. He used it as an
illustration of how we make up causes to fit effects; I want to use it to
illustrate a couple of other points about the constructivist view of experience processing:

> People are getting on a streetcar in Vienna. Among the passengers is a
> working-class woman with her young son. The boy has an enormous bandage
> wrapped around his head. (How dreadful! What happened to him?) People
> give up their seats to the afflicted pair. The bandaging is not a professional
> job, it was obviously done at home and in a hurry; they must be on their way
> to the hospital (people secretly search the child's face for an explanation, and
> the bandage for traces of blood). The little boy whines and fusses (signs of
> sympathy from everyone). The mother seems unconcerned (how inappro-
> priate!); she even shows signs of impatience (that is amazing). The little one
> begins to fidget; his mother pushes him back in his seat. The passengers'
> mood turns to open confrontation. The mother is criticized, but for her part
> rejects all interference. Now she is criticized again and more openly.
> Thereupon she tells them to mind their own business and questions the
> competence of all those who criticized her. (That is too much! An outrage to
> human decency!) Emotions run high, and things get noisy and turbulent. The
> child is bawling; his mother, red-faced and furious, declares she is going to
> show us what is the matter and begins (to everyone's horror) tearing off the
> whole bandage. What appears is a metal chamber pot that the little Don
> Quixote has pushed so tightly on his head that it is stuck; they are on their
> way to get help from the nearest plumber. People get off the streetcar in great
> embarrassment. (Anderson, 1990, pp. 68–9)

*This material was first delivered as a keynote paper at the Annual Conference of the
Israeli Psychotherapy Association in February 1994.

96

This piece is written, not to review or rehash the familiar ground of client abuse by therapists, but to open some questions and considerations along the other polarity – client abuse of therapist. Is this at all possible? How is the profession dealing with its increasing manifestations and why is this happening now?

There is currently much self-critical questioning of psychoanalysis, counselling and psychotherapy practice. Concerted action, in terms of accreditation, professionalisation, and standardisation, has indubitably beneficially influenced the quality of clinical work. Most importantly, it has given consumers more information and greater choice. Lay members of the public have become more challenging about the views, accountability and assumptions of psychotherapy generally. In several instances I have been one of the exponents leading this movement towards increased consumer education, quality control and a more refined, nuanced and sophisticated ethical awareness. There is no doubt that patients are nowadays more conscious of their rights and more likely to challenge the therapist.

There is much justified concern about therapist sexual abuse of clients and an increased public awareness of the damaging consequences of such abuse. In the past few years, there has been a virtual explosion of conferences, papers, meetings, and books on this theme (Garrett, 1994). Some who may be victimised or feel traumatised by what happens in therapy are the partners and children of patients. Often the family or significant others are in a kind of non-contractual third-party transference relationship. They may experience the therapist as destructive to extant emotional relationships, and sue for alienation of affection, either on their own account or as a vicarious acting-out by the patient, who may coerce, manipulate or seduce the partner into taking such action. Or, as in the Tarasoff case (see Thompson, 1990, Chapter 12), people can be murdered, and the therapist seen as having failed to protect the victim or warn the family.

At the same time, there are certain developments in contemporary culture which indicate an increasing and escalating attack on the new secular priests of psychotherapy. The authority of many major twentieth-century figureheads is being challenged, including Freud's. There is also an apparent public backlash against psychology and psychotherapy as is evident in our newspapers, magazines, novels, and in increasing numbers of professional investigations, ethics complaints and litigation in the USA. In the UK too there is a growing number of lawsuits against counsellors, psychologists and psychotherapists.

Many of these revolve around differential constructions of reality. If these different constructions of reality were opened in the confines of the consulting room, it could provide fruitful exploratory and potentially healing space. However, when exposed to outside judgement they can become contentious issues of verifiable truth and consequently

exceedingly problematic. The verities of the consulting room are not
necessarily those of the court. The following randomly chosen three
disguised examples illustrate the diversities or interpretations of truth
around touch, alienation of affection and abandonment:

- For one person, a psychotherapist laying a hand upon their shoulder
  can be subjectively and phenomenologically experienced as rape, retraumatising a person who had been previously abused through a
  sexual assault by a teacher or a sadistic medical practitioner. For
  another the absence of such a touch may be a repeat experience of
  parental coldness, neglect and fear of physical contact – disgust for a
  child with a facial disfigurement. Are clients told that there are
  reputable and ethical therapists who would respond physically to
  them without being abusive?
- Psychotherapists have been accused of using 'mind control'
  techniques to alienate the affections of clients' partners citing the
  spouse's divorce settlement claims as evidence for intention to financially exploit the complainant's spouse. *Affliction* by Fay Weldon
  (1994), for example, tells the story of a woman whose husband left
  her, claiming that it was as a result of his psychotherapy. Many people
  may indeed start psychotherapy in order to find the strength or
  courage to leave unsatisfactory marriages. Some cults do prohibit all
  outside relationships and exploit their members financially. Who
  shall define mind control? Watkins (1954) argues that all transference
  in psychoanalysis is 'trance' – i.e. hypnotic induction; Mahrer (1985)
  showed how therapists' words are frequently more prescriptive than
  is usually acknowledged and a UKCP Guideline for psychotherapists
  on delayed memory shows how a simple question can be construed
  as having multiple implicit prescriptions.
- Several psychotherapists have been charged or sued for abandonment of one kind or another – in one case because the therapist
  terminated her clinical work as result of her pregnancy. It is not
  unusual for patients to feel abandoned when the therapist goes on
  vacation or is ill. Does this constitute cause for damages?

The emergence of 'defensive psychotherapy'

I speak from research findings, my own experience with clinicians who
are in supervision with colleagues and me, as well as talks and debates at
conferences on several continents. I also draw on my experience of
sitting on a number of professional investigation and ethical adjudication panels. Without breaching confidentiality I can say quite simply that
sometimes the complaints are justified on the evidence provided – as far
as we on the board can see – and sometimes they are not. However, I
also know that injustice can and does occur even where the best of

intentions are present. Courts of law founded on centuries of tradition and experience have sometimes made mistakes condemning innocents to death or life-long imprisonment. Psychotherapy complaints boards have virtually no training and few precedents, and are often composed of people who have chosen in their careers to privilege subjectivity leaving the objective assessment of evidence to those – like police and judges – trained to do it.

The climate of current public opinion is sometimes swinging against the professional psychotherapist and in favour of the genuine victims of these professions – those who have been exploited, abused or damaged. These victims need protection. And the judgements of the law are affected by public opinion. In some other cases, it is now sometimes the professionals who become the innocent victims of their clients. It is possible that the pendulum may now be swinging too far in the opposite direction. There are men who have been falsely accused of raping their daughters. There are innocent people who are framed by malicious gossip or planted drugs. There are professionals who are falsely pilloried – sometimes with an assist (through acts of commission or omission) from their professional peers.

These are the cases where the working alliance is destroyed and the psychotherapy ruined by legal action, ethical complaints and the assassination of professional reputations. The increasing need for a professional psychotherapist to be conscious of the possibility of litigation and to anticipate every possible outcome may well result in a proliferation of contracts to be countersigned by all parties involved. (And where does it end?) Legal advice is now sometimes being sought before a client even starts to tell their story – and this is only likely to increase.

Unfortunately, what I see among many practitioners is a rather regrettable attempt to be more and more careful, more and more conscious of third parties (for example, supervisors) listening, interpreting and judging what can only ever be mediated by those involved in specific interactions in the confines of the consulting room concerned. There is an increasingly anxious preoccupation to be error-free, with avoiding spontaneity and intuitive authenticity. There may even be a growing concern with safeguarding the letter of the working alliance which may already be eroding the spirit of a relationship – a dangerous mutual and unpredictable engagement.

A clinical practice is now developing which I would call 'defensive psychotherapy'. This is an appropriation of the term 'defensive medicine', which is used in North America to describe an ethos in which doctors and paramedics refuse to become involved, for example, with accident victims on the road, because they are protecting themselves against potential lawsuits. They fear implication in malpractice, or may potentially lose thousands of dollars and their reputation on the basis of a spontaneous, merciful intervention. If the doctor were to set a broken leg, and the leg were not to heal properly or if additional complications set in, the risk of being sued is simply too high for the doctor to undertake uncontracted treatment. The doctors will refuse or be reluctant to intervene in such situations where they could be helpful, for fear of being sued by the patient or their families. This is not yet the norm in Europe, yet the alarm signals are already infesting psychotherapy. Many professionals are already practising consciously or unconsciously infected by this kind of collective cultural fear. This polarity can ultimately be as detrimental to our practice as carelessness or abuse of other kinds.

Some practitioners will privately admit that they have modified their practice in the last decade – taking fewer risks, fearing unjust collegial criticism for therapeutic 'errors' or being concerned about avoiding unfair client persecution for unethical conduct by trying to play absolutely by the rulebook without any space for misinterpretation – as if this were possible! However, the professional phenomenon of 'minding our backs' is well under way in psychotherapy training, supervision and peer support. For example, a respondent in one study reported that he now tapes all sessions with female clients to ensure against false accusations of impropriety. I believe this is deeply disturbing and, much as it may prevent some abuses, it may create others. An example of this is the phobia about touching. I am told that some US insurance companies will not insure a psychotherapist against malpractice suits if they touch their clients at all. Against this, I would like to posit the question posed by Woodmansey (1988), 'Might we be depriving our clients by not touching them?'. On the other hand, we might prevent the case in our research where the clinician believed that they were 'working through the transference' by giving the client a massage? Does the emergence of defensive psychotherapy exclusively lead to an improvement in practice or sometimes to a concomitant loss of spontaneity, novelty, experimentation and appropriate risk? Has it become more important to avoid error than to do whatever is thought necessary and important to help the patient, rather than to protect the therapist from criticisms or lawsuits?

Defensive medicine and defensive psychotherapy describe a personal concern of practitioners in the avoidance of being sued or taken to court, greater than involvement in procedures which may be more risky but potentially more beneficial. The very fear of a client's reality being 'proved' different from yours in a court of law, at an ethics hearing or in the amphitheatre of public opinion can prevent what I believe to be creative and imaginative in a natural altruistic response to provide whatever help we can, according to the best lights of our judgement and competence at the time. This is another version of professional bystanding – an avoidance of taking action in situations which may be cruel, unjust or dangerous to another person (Clarkson, 1996).

Why is this happening now?

Why, just as psychotherapy is really beginning to clean up its act, regularise its practice, standardise its supervision, research its outcomes and genuinely re-evaluate its assumptions regarding gender, race, sexual orientation and religion in terms of their countertransferential implications? Why are the public being encouraged, aided and abetted by sensationalist media to suspect and attack the very people who dedicate their lives to professions devised to help?

I am not for a minute suggesting that some accusations of therapist abuse are not valid and I affirm that such abuse should be eradicated, with the offenders being rehabilitated or prevented from practising. There is no doubt that many patients have been genuinely victimised by their therapists and analysts. However, in an increasing number of cases there is a flavour of witch-hunting and a feeling of dull powerlessness as innocuous words from the mouth or demeanour of the psychotherapist are twisted and distorted into expressions of abuse, disdain or neglect. The problem is that reality is a flexible notion and the differentiation between so-called objective and subjective realities (whether culturally conditioned or individually chosen) increasingly hard to differentiate.

We will have to come to terms, as we stagger into the postmodern era, with the hard-to-avoid evidence that there are many different realities, and different ways of experiencing them, and that people seem to want to keep exploring them, and that there is only a limited amount any society can do to ensure that its official reality is installed in the minds of most of its citizens most of the time (Anderson, 1990, p. 152). The task of the therapist is working with ' multiple realities'.

An enormous amount has been written on the issue of 'delayed memory' or 'recovered memory' in working therapeutically with adults who have been, believe, discover or doubt whether they had been abused – sexually and/or satanically – as children (Sinason, 1994). In my opinion, in thinking about whether or not an adult patient had been sexually abused as a child, what it is important is their perception or experience of having been abused, which may or may not be grounded in empirical, logically testable reality. This experience is no less real to the memory, the body or the emotions – all the levels of reality which constitute an individual's psychic life.

I am not saying that therefore 'it did not happen'. I am suggesting that the argument is spurious, the doubts could be relieved if the therapists believe – the psychic scars, the dreams, the experience of a client says 'it did happen'. And as far as they and their therapist are concerned, it did. We know that the brain cannot distinguish between a real and a vividly imagined experience. The question of whether it happened in a consensually verifiable objective way mandates only a small slice of reality – that which can be objectively proved in a court of law. Psychological reality –

the one we live by – is different. More importantly, adopting a positivistic approach to 'prove objectively whether something actually happened or not' disallows and diminishes other forms of experiences. These may be vitally relevant if not central – although perhaps 'unprovable' – to psychotherapy and psycho-physiological life.

For example, it may be even the experience of an abusive parent's fantasies intruding into the child's psychic reality. Clinically I have often found that the traumatising effects of witnessing violence to a sibling, a dog or a servant and the visceral empathic response may be physiologically indistinguishable from actually physically being the subject of the violent attack (Clarkson, 1988). Furthermore, a mother's look of murderous hatred while her hand stops seconds away from smashing her child's face into a hot stove, a father's lascivious fantasies while he mentally undresses and rapes his adolescent daughter – can we say that these are not abuse because 'it did not actually happen'. The bodies and lives in my consulting room say they did – in all the ways that matter. This is the realm of psychotherapeutic expertise, not that of jury or judge. Psychotherapists are not trained to assess the objective reality of events they have not witnessed nor act as society's lie detectors.

Transference aspects of the victim's vengeance

Acting out a unilateral reality construction can be negative, destructive or psychotic transference – it can certainly demolish the psychotherapy if not worked through in the process. The psychotherapist's need to help and to be persecuted may be as a result of their own unresolved difficulties or part of a projective identification or hypnotic induction eliciting reactive countertransference, further leading to unconscious participation in a catastrophic drama. This threatens to wreak havoc with the working alliance and can destroy the analysis on occasion. No psychotherapist is entirely immune to failure. Some may still say: 'this would never happen if there was a good relationship'. But – to some respected and competent colleagues who judged the relationship 'good enough' – it already has.

Reality consequences of the victim's vengeance

Displaced vengeance enacted in the therapy for psychic hurt as a child can be more destructive to the adult patient in the here-and-now than the original trauma. Abusive attacks on the psychotherapist, the therapist's family or their reputation is often more damaging to the patient than to the therapist. It is frequently followed by guilt and remorse. As a wise person (source unknown) once said: 'It is hard to forgive others the evil we have done them'. The abuse of others leave scars on the soul sometimes worse that that of being the victim of abuse. When therapists protect themselves from undue persecution judiciously and compassionately, they are protecting the best interests of their clients. The prevention of psychotherapist abuse is not the same as avoiding the negative transference or denying real grounds for criticism or complaint.

Given the interpenetrability of our intersubjective worlds and the effects such as projective identification and hypnotic induction, it may be in many cases impossible if not irrelevant to discuss whether something actually happened in the sense that a court of law, a judge, jury or police office or, for that matter a biomedical scientist, may establish the judicial veracity of any particular claim. Yet, many modern psychotherapists are invited by clients to corroborate or witness past or current abuses as matters of fact, not fantasy. This may lead to a confusion of tasks for psychotherapy. Miller's (1985) position is that the victim is always reporting accurately; that the therapist has to believe that it actually occurred and be willing to act as advocate, sometimes even with the real family members. Did the abuse actually occur, and is it important for the psychotherapist to believe that it actually did happen? Psychotherapists are asked to vouch for the truth of events and to judge reality which would not be accepted in court as a reliable. Whether they are willing to do this, how and in which kinds of court – a family therapy session behind a one-way mirror, or a legal arena where battles are fought on another kind of grand scale – makes enormous and incalculable demands on the care and maintenance of a working alliance with someone who has been abused. And, who has not been abused in some way?

Victims attack rescuers

It is common knowledge that rescue workers going into disaster areas such as earthquakes need to have protection, often even carrying arms. Teachers of lifesavers usually warn them that drowning people may attack them – and they do. For example, the following account is from a young man who rescued his girlfriend from drowning at the beach.

> I remembered that when I did a life-saving course at school, there was a section on panic . . . Lots of people drown in relatively safe conditions, because panic makes them lose their minds. Also, I vaguely remember that there are things you are supposed to do when people panic. But only vaguely. Anyway, there's not much you can do because they hit you.

As he tried to rescue his girlfriend from the sea:

> She hit me. I tried to grab hold of her; she hit me again. I grabbed her arm, and we were both pushed towards the beach, and sucked back out again. I remember looking up at a wall of water above me . . . Then Lotta was on her hands and knees on the beach . . . Weakly, I stood up. I just wanted to laugh and laugh. Later, Lotta tried to explain why she wanted to hurt me, and it seemed to make sense, what with the panic, the fear, the scrambled, doomy thoughts. But at the time, it was a terrible shock. She stood up, turned round, and punched me in the face. I went right down, my nose bleeding. She

walked a few paces and sat down, weeping. We said nothing to each other. Afterwards, I told her it was lucky I hadn't been wearing my spare glasses. She nearly hit me again. (Leith, 1994, p. 12)

Entering certain concentration camps, the liberating officials apparently needed to wear flak jackets in case of attack by the victims, the very people they had come to save. Ambulance drivers in London have recently been issued with flak jackets; as they are often the first to arrive at the scene of an accident or violent attack, they are highly likely to be attacked by victims in shock (Middleton, 1994). In some tribal societies people actually say to those who are trying to damage them: 'Why do you hate me? I have never tried to help you.' There is a lesson here for psychotherapists. An attack may not be targeted to you or anything you have done – it may be simply because you arrived, ready to help, on the scene of the accident. It is not always all your fault. The responsibility for working with this aspect of the human soul where we meet it, is however not to be abrogated.

What a queer twist this is in the human psyche; and how vividly this is enacted in psychotherapy. Psychotherapists are attacked because they offer help. The microcosm of the consulting room reflects the macrocosm of society. There seems to be more and more enchantment with the idea of punishing rescuers (or putative rescuers) for the failures and abuses of God, parents, societies, organisations, governments and assorted others. These are the ones who, by virtue of their distance, cannot be attacked with the same amount of vengeance and vindictiveness as the person who comes towards you to save your life or simply to create a space with the intention of helping or alleviating distress. As Klein (1984) pointed out: 'The capacity to give and preserve life is felt as the greatest gift and therefore creativeness becomes the deepest cause for envy' (p. 202).

Therapist abuse as displaced vengeance

Much has been spoken and written about psychotherapist abuse of clients, but not so much about client abuse of therapists (Haeger, 1993). There are deliberate invasions of a psychotherapist's privacy; for example, where a client holds vigil outside the therapist's house having followed his car home, writing threatening letters to his children or his employer or attacking his property such as breaking into his car or his house.

There are many cases of sexual harassment and false accusations of unethical conduct. Often when the psychotherapist refuses a sexual advance, the ethics case rests on the psychotherapists having to prove that they did not seduce the client. Having participated in consultations to several other institutions I have empathically learned how psychotherapeutic institutions are vulnerable to attacks by disappointed staff or ex-trainees in a collective climate which may or may not favour the alleged victim. This must of course be differentiated from the scapegoating of courageous whistleblowers (see Clarkson, 1996). Then there are the deliberate lies, or delicate but telling omissions or envious gestures pregnant with intentions, which (without flaunting professional etiquette) can assassinate a previous therapist – now a colleague's reputation – for competitive advancement in the field.

I have come to believe that important limitations of our codes of ethics and professional practice concern the safeguarding of the psychotherapists' rights to privacy, respect, freedom from malicious or disclaimed invasion or attack. Perhaps this needs to be dealt with much more explicitly and meaningfully in training and supervision.

Whether as rescuers or as helpers, patients will or may attack; and, if not, we can wonder why not? It is important for our sanity to remember that sometimes it takes only one to tango. Let us consider the possibility that one party in a dispute may sometimes be entirely innocent – even if he or she is the one with perceived power such as Christ or Rumi. The working alliance is potentially under threat not only from individual resistance or externalisation of a bad object attack, it is also an effect of large and pervasive cultural collective pressures which permeate and infect all helping relationships.

For many adults who have been abused as children, the psychotherapist provides the first legitimate target who will sit still and not retaliate. It is a dynamic similar to the phenomenon of lateral violence that so puzzled commentators on the South African situation during apartheid. (So often black South Africans attacked other black people, not those who were guilty of actually oppressing them.) It can lead to victimisation of or abuse of the psychotherapist, when children are threatened, houses burgled and professional reputations ruined through malicious and untrue gossip. It is a psychological opportunity for the victim to strike back at some parent stand-in or substitute for the other authority figures who let them down in the past and who may forever remain psychologically out of reach. Of course, an unchannelled expression of rage, revenge and despair can destroy the working alliance. However, when the patient or client actually succeeds in causing damage of whatever kind to the psychotherapist, it is my belief that it is ultimately damaging to the client themselves. To wreak on others the shadow from which we have suffered must ultimately erode the fabric of our human responsiveness and interconnectedness – our visceral empathy with other human organisms who have the same propensity for violence, compassion and understanding as ourselves.

References

Anderson, W.T. (1990) Reality Isn't What it Used to Be. San Francisco, CA: Harper & Row.

Clarkson, P. (1988) Ego state dilemmas of abused children. Transactional Analysis Journal, 18(2), 85–93.

Clarkson, P. (1996) The Bystander. London: Whurr.

Garrett, T. (1994) Sexual contact between psychotherapists and their patients. In P. Clarkson and M. Pokorny (eds), The Handbook of Psychotherapy, pp. 431–50. London: Routledge.

Haeger, B. (1993). Personal communication.

Klein, M. (1984) Envy, Gratitude and Other Works. London: Hogarth Press and Institute for Psychoanalysis (first published 1957)

Leith, W. (1994) The day my girlfriend nearly drowned. Night and Day: The Mail on Sunday Review (London), p. 12.

Mahrer, A.R. (1985) Psychotherapeutic Change: An Alternative Approach to Meaning and Measurement. New York: Norton.

Middleton, A. (1994) London ambulance workers may be issued with bullet-proof jackets. Big Issue, 67, p. 7, 22–8 February.

Miller, A. (1985) Thou Shalt not be Aware: Society's Betrayal of the Child (trans. H. Hannum and H. Hannum), London: Pluto Press.

Sinason, V. (1994) Treating Survivors of Satanist Abuse. London: Routledge.

Thompson, A. (1990) Guide to Ethical Practice in Psychotherapy. New York: Wiley.

Watkins, J.G. (1954) Trance and transference. Journal of Clinical and Experimental Hypnosis, 2, 284–90.

Weldon, F. (1994) Affliction. London: Harper Collins.

Woodmansey, A.C. (1988) Are psychotherapists out of touch? British Journal of Psychotherapy, 5, 57–65.

ITEM 6
'Asking the Client's Permission' to do a Case Study

PETRŪSKA CLARKSON

This paper is written in response to several incidents, enquiries and development initiatives in the training, supervision and professional practice aspects of counselling psychology and psychotherapy. It is specifically concerned with the writing of case studies and the use of case material for supervision, examination, qualification, accreditation, audit and reaccreditation procedures. (This paper does not concern publication in professional journals or in books or monographs of any kind. At the time of writing the BPS are working on new guidelines for using client material in published sources.)

The issue of concern is the situation where a practising counsellor, psychotherapist or psychologist requests 'permission' of one client to use him or her for the case study which the practitioner intends to submit as part of the requirements for qualification – by examination or accreditation process. The worst case scenario is where a practitioner would ask a client for such permission while they were still seeing the client.

When a practitioner explains to a client that a condition of their work together and an aspect of the confidentiality they will keep includes the sharing of case material with the supervisor or colleagues, it is usually true to say that this supervision process is primarily in service of the client to improve the quality of practice of the practitioner on their behalf.

However, when the case study is being done solely for the purposes of the practitioner's examination, the benefit to the client may be secondary. That is, even though the client may receive more attention than other clients (which may or may not be beneficial), it is the advancement of the practitioner's career which is also in the balance – perhaps more.

Some examples

In some cases where permission has been asked, clients have reacted in ways that were quite destructive of the therapy. Of course, this may have been affected by the way in which the therapists asked permission to do the case study. However, my assumption is that the therapists would have been conscientious, careful, in supervision, and well meaning – but perhaps without sufficient forethought. What may be required is a fuller clinical and ethical understanding of the implications of the effects of such requests, mid-stream or towards the end of the client's therapy. Three fictional examples will illustrate some of the issues.

- In one case the practitioner had written the case study with the client's permission. They had agreed about what would be written, and the client had access to the documents and the opportunity to input from his perspective. It so happened that this client was a recovering alcoholic. As the trainee's examination date approached, the client went on a total and incapacitating binge. The client was never to return to therapy (as far as we know). There may be many reasons for this, not least the practitioner's anxiety about the approaching examination – or some variant of projective identification.

  However, it left the trainee in a position of going into the exam feeling demoralised and as if their work of four years with the client had come to naught. (We may not agree that this is an accurate assessment, but this is how the trainee felt in submitting this case study just before the exam.)

- Another example concerns a trainee who did a case study with the client's permission. After several months it became clear to both the trainee and the supervisors that the client's case was not suitable to take to the examination. Another client had to be found and the permission of this client sought. Did the trainee tell the first 'chosen' client that he was no longer the subject of the trainee's case study for examination? We can speculate about why the supervisor thought this case was not 'suitable' for submission for examination. Other clients of this therapist found out that two people had been 'chosen' for case studies. It became a matter for gossip and concern throughout the person's practice and the training institute concerned.

- A trainee, believing that he was doing the right thing, asked his client's permission to use her for his case study. She granted the permission enthusiastically. She welcomed the attention initially, and experienced it as a 'very special privilege'. However, within weeks it emerged that part of her history of sexual abuse involved her father's voyeurism. It soon became clear to the trainee that this had been a harmful interruption of the working alliance. He decided to choose another client for the case study, telling the first client that none of her experience would be used in any way except for the ordinary case supervision by his regular supervisor.

Some of the issues involved

Some examples of the issues that we need to think about in training supervisors and trainees in the light of such possibilities are considered in this section.

Transference

A client or patient may 'give permission' to please the practitioner in the way that he or she used to please a parent, comply with parental seduction, feel coerced in terms of threat to the love in the relationship, and so on and so forth. The client may want to help or hurt the clinician by destroying the goodness of the therapy or minimising the work accomplished together. The possibility that a client and therapist can agree such a permission before the end of the therapy without transferential implications is probably illusory. Toward the end of therapy, but before termination, is perhaps an even more delicate time. The client may be re-experiencing many of the pains and problems that first brought him or her to seek help, may be racked by envy or desires to make reparation. Feelings of love, hate and fears of separation may perhaps be more vivid than at any other time.

At worst this kind of concentration or expectation can precipitate, if not bring about, crises such as suicide – 'I could never live up to their expectations of me', a relapse into alcoholism, crime, psychosis or even acting out of a hatred or remorse in attacks on other people.

Countertransference

The therapist may be selecting this one particular patient because of proactive or reactive countertransference. In the first instance this patient may be selected as case study material because of the clinician's own unresolved past issues – for example, choosing someone who will disappoint him or her, or choosing someone who will reluctantly comply and then exhort some form of revenge or retaliation for 'having to give' to someone who already has so much and so on. The examples are as multifarious as human relationships.

In 'reactive countertransference', the clinician may, for example, respond emotionally or in terms of behaviour to the hypnotic induction of the patient to select the client as 'the only child' or 'the favourite child', the 'child with most promise', the 'most interesting (often the sickest) child'. Again the possible examples of such projective identifications multiply into infinity.

Psychotherapy is perhaps complex enough in terms of these possible vectors of transference and countertransference types not to exacerbate the relationship into the complications attendant upon asking the client to be 'the one client who gets to be used as a case study'.

Even if the practitioner does not accept (or centralise) the transference/countertransference dimension of the therapeutic relationship, there are other aspects to consider.

Fairness to others

Why should some clients be privileged (or punished) by having a case study done about him or her and not the other clients? What makes this selected person(s) special, and what are the consequences or rewards in doing that? Is it because he or she is particularly 'good' or particularly 'bad' or particularly 'ordinary'? (Whatever these words are chosen to mean.) Does it follow that the other clients do not have case studies done about them and if not, why not?

Professionalism requires case studies on everybody?

If a case study is one of the recognised and primary (but not necessarily the only or the best) ways of conceptualising our professional practice, are other clients not being deprived of something that should be their right? It may be that every client deserves to have a case study done about him or her. Perhaps the selection for audit or exam might even be done randomly – in order to ensure that all clients are given the appropriate concentration of theoretical thought, supervision and practitioner reflection.

If only one client is truly studied in depth, can it be said that the clinician has developed competence in dealing with a range of people and a variety of issues? What can we learn from an exam which is only based on one in-depth case study? So often the client chosen reflects in the parallel process dynamics of the clinician – by paying attention to these, might others be neglected? – only to accompany the practitioner for the rest of their professional career.

There are obviously many more such issues which space precludes me even mentioning. It is hoped that these issues have at least raised or reminded us of some of the directions for supervision or self-questioning on this important and very complex matter. Perhaps this will start the discussion. In the meantime here follows some ideas for suggested practice:

Suggested practice

Guidelines for the beginning practitioner

You need to be clear with your clients right from the beginning that anything they share with you will be taken to supervision and/or used for developmental and/or professional qualification, audit or re-accreditation procedures. It is the expectation that in all these situations the use of client material will be restricted to a small number of experienced senior professionals in the discipline who are bound by the same ethical rules as the practitioners whom they are examining, in terms of respect and confidentiality. A case study should not be published or made available to others outside of this definition without the express permission of the client.

An understanding and agreement like this could obviate the use of special (individually sought) permissions for unpublished case studies later.

Guidelines for trainees

These guidelines are intended for trainees already in practice before they write their case study for examination and who have not yet clarified this issue with their client.

It is necessary to clarify with all clients that they understand the limits of confidentiality without drawing them into the therapist's professional struggles or aspirations. In this case, some trainee practitioners have availed themselves in an annual practice 'hygiene' or quality maintenance procedure, which is to update people who are working with them on current conditions regarding fees, breaks, etc. This annual opportunity can be used to clarify the contract with clients, verbally or in writing, so that they understand that supervision, accreditation and re-accreditation procedures will apply to all clients within their practice. (This does not include the case where the client may refuse to be supervised – for whatever reasons they may request this or a practitioner may comply with such a request.)

Guidelines for audit or re-accreditation for qualified practitioners

In such cases, I think practitioners can follow a similar procedure to that suggested for trainees with opportunities for clients to discuss the implications. Every counsellor, psychologist, clinic, institute or university department will probably already have their own verbal or written version of such a working agreement, unsigned or signed by both parties.

Caveats

It is recommended that any discussion of the storage, access and use of client material be clarified, not only for the duration of the clinician's practice, but also what will happen to this material if a clinician should not be available, become ill or die. For a discussion of this see Traynor and Clarkson (1992).

Summary

In summary, a practitioner working ethically informs a client that a condition of their work together is that case material will be shared with a supervisor and/or colleagues, all of whom will be bound by the same ethics of confidentiality and respect for the client.

Good practice means treating all clients equally at the start. This means making it clear to all clients before even a contract is agreed that anything they share with you will be taken to supervision and used for developmental and professional examinations, qualifications, audit or re-accreditation procedures. This will ensure that every client starts from the same baseline and any differences in their response are then available for use in the therapy.

Reference

Traynor, B. and Clarkson, P. (1992) What happens if a psychotherapist dies? Counselling, 3(1), 23–4.

CHAPTER 7
When Rules Are Not Enough: The Spirit of the Law in Ethical Codes

PETRŪSKA CLARKSON AND LESLEY MURDIN

> [Weigert] (1970) points to certain generic characteristics of all professional rhetorics. They include a rhetoric of affiliation by which the profession aligns itself with higher status groups and distances itself from lower status groups; a rhetoric of special expertise that includes claims to valid theories and distinctive methods; a rhetoric of public service that simultaneously plays down careerist motives; a rhetoric of social passage that identifies and justifies credentialing requirements; a rhetoric of self-policing that defends against 'interference' from others; and a delegitimizing rhetoric of the rhetoric of outsiders, including 'pseudo-professions', 'charlatans', 'popularizers', and 'cranks' (Simons, 1986). Each of these genres, moreover, includes predictable lines of argument, topoi and stylistic characteristics. One recurring feature, for example, is that they are not labeled rhetorics at all. (Simons, 1989, p. 111)

Why do we need codes of ethics? In some ways the answer is self evident. The psychotherapy organisations, the United Kingdom Council Psychotherapy (UKCP) and the British Association for Counselling (BAC) are experiencing a great increase in the number of complaints that they are receiving both from clients and from trainees. There must be professional accountability if there is a profession at all. For the safety of clients and trainees, and for the benefit of practitioners, we need to think about what are the limits of safe and ethical practice. This we are doing. BAC has agreed codes of ethics and practice for counselling skills users, counsellors, supervisors and trainers. Complaints and appeals procedures have been drawn up and modified in the painful learning process that goes on as we learn how best to protect the public and ourselves.

We all acknowledge that we need these codes. Usually they provide an adequate basis for day-to-day good enough behaviour. The trouble is that as soon as a question arises with any degree of complexity, it is likely that two elements of the code will conflict or that the issue is not yet covered at all. Both the BAC and the UKCP Ethics Committees receive requests for help, advice and clarification precisely because the codes do not cover points of conflict. For example: if a counsellor thinks that a client is suicidal but has been asked by the client not to discuss him or her outside the therapy – with a GP or anyone else, at what point does the therapist decide to go against the client's wishes? (See Bond, 1993.) Clearly, this is just one of the many areas where the two ethical imperatives of confidentiality and the right of the client to make choices might conflict with the counsellor's own ethical imperatives about the value of life.

Conflicting demands

Sometimes a counsellor finds him- or herself trying to adhere to the codes of different organisations and finds that they make conflicting demands. The BAC requires all counsellors to be in supervision for the whole of their working lives. The LTKCP Guidelines require only that practitioners maintain their competence. This leaves us with either a difference between the provisions of counselling and psychotherapy or an ethical question to be answered by each individual: am I or is anyone sufficiently self-aware to practise without supervision or consultation?

Other areas of great difficulty arise frequently in training and supervision where the therapist has conflicting demands arising from the interests of the client and those of the trainee or supervisee. A dilemma of this sort may arise if we try to be open to training people with physical disabilities as counsellors. It is fair and just to allow a blind person the option of training if he or she is suitable, but is it fair to the clients to allocate them to a blind counsellor? A client might find it very difficult to object to having a blind counsellor, or to express negative feelings to the counsellor in the way that he or she might need to. Thus an action of fairness and justice on the one hand could perhaps be construed by some as an unfairness or injustice. Similarly, we work with members of ethnic minorities and, in order to do so, we might ask of them what they need? How can we speak to you, what are we doing wrong? To which the reply may well be: 'It is not my job to teach about being African, or West Indian. *You* find out.'

No code of ethics can deal adequately with such two-edged dilemmas: that is why we need to look more closely at the principles on which the profession is founded and from which it originates.

When we encounter a conflict or an area that the code does not cover adequately, the temptation is to say, 'Oh dear, we need to cover that point', and rush off to write a new clause. This can lead to a rule-bound profession in which spontaneity and creativity are ruled out. We begin to practise defensively so that the primary value is protection. There is something to be said for protection, both of the counsellor and of the client, but perhaps there are ways in which we can help ourselves and our clients to perceive the profession with its necessary protective and defensive structures differently.

Human communication implies value judgement

We hardly ever perceive a stimulus without the colouring of good or bad, better or worse, pleasurable or unpleasurable, more or less beautiful, more or less important. Just look at a sharp corner or a rounded one – which did you prefer? Perhaps you cannot say which or why. No one has satisfactorily explained the beauty of the serpentine line or wherein lies the charm of a beautiful face. Yet, to be human is to make value judgements. Some kind of selection according to constantly changing criteria enables the central nervous system to prioritise the attention paid to incoming stimuli. Whenever any one stimulus becomes figure, another becomes ground and is thus less attended to than the first. We all recognise the experience of the client who adjusts the material to suit the interests of the counsellor.

In humanistic and existential therapies there has always been an open and espoused position about the importance of values and their exploration in counselling and psychotherapy. A tradition which began with Moreno working in the parks of Vienna with latchkey children and prostitutes has continued through the radical psychiatry movement of the 1960s and has continued through involvement with, for example, Eastern European problems today. Many counsellors are also interested in social values and responsibility. Samuels (1993) shows that there is reason for counsellors also to be interested in politics and the values of our relationships within society and culture.

Clearly, we all have values in every sphere of thinking, feeling and sensing. Our duty is to be aware of what they are and to make them explicit and conscious, not imposing them on clients without knowing that we are doing so. Few of us would berate, preach to or exploit clients overtly, and yet we cannot avoid revealing our own values through every aspect of ourselves and our surroundings. The pictures or blank walls of our consulting rooms, for example, might say a great deal. Freud's taste in filling the space of his room with statues and figures certainly showed what he valued.

Is there ever value-free counselling?

You can try to be class-deaf or colour-blind. You can deny or overemphasise the differences between you and your client. You can speak about your views on homosexuality or claim to be neutral. But however hard you try not to, you will reveal that you do in fact value one end of each spectrum more than the other. There would certainly be differing views in the different models that we practise about the extent to which we would openly reveal our views to the client, but we need to open debates within ourselves and in the profession as a whole so that we can examine the ways in which we are tempted to indoctrinate. There is not space in this chapter to consider the ways in which we select and emphasise what we find valuable in order to help the client to whatever we think is the good life. Even the apparently value-free models which emphasise acceptance and non-judgement are loading value on to such concepts as autonomy, spontaneity, communication.

What we would most like to emphasise here is that there is a language that each counsellor speaks and teaches to his or her clients. The counsellor, we hope, learns to speak something of the client's language. Oppressed nations learn the language of the conqueror but the conquerors rarely learn the language of the slaves. This is not necessarily a bad thing. In the case of the Norman conquest, for example, the imposition of French had a very beneficial effect in immensely extending the range and subtlety of our language. It is possible that, where the Normans imported a new invention or concept, like 'roasting' or 'pleasure', we acquired a new word to convey it. Nevertheless, the language remained basically English. Counsellors have some choice over the extent to which they speak the client's language, but the choices made will alter the balance of power.

When one culture encounters another, there is a great range of possibilities along the continuum from agreed co-operation to coercion (D'Ardennes and Mahtani, 1993). When can it be said that a person has given informed consent? A person *in extremis* from anxiety or despair comes along and is so relieved by whatever the counsellor offers, whether that is speech or silence, helpful or unhelpful intervention. Is the client able to give informed consent? Most of us are aware of this difficulty. We might try, as the codes of ethics prescribe, to state the terms of what we are offering, and to disclose 'where appropriate' the method of treatment to be used. We might have certain self-protective measures that we use, such as the disclaimer, 'I don't have a magic wand.' This may sometimes need to be said, but the principle to be met is that we should try to give clients as much of a flavour of what they can expect as possible through the experience of the first session, not just through automatic disclaimers. There are two kinds of defensive practice that counsellors can operate. They may decline to take on anyone who is difficult, rejecting them as borderline or over-dependent or inclined to act out. On the other hand, there are those who will take on almost anyone who comes along and then practise defensively, making the minimal moves and playing safe at every point. There are times when that might be clinically indicated and times when it may simply be cowardice.

In any relationship there will be a continuum leading from uninvolved objectivity towards the overt exercise of power and influence. The analytic stance may be construed as uninvolvement or bystanding, particularly by those who see it from the outside. On the other hand, we need to be aware that there is a defensiveness about non-involvement at times. We can examine our neutrality for traces of avoidance. Accepting the *status quo* may at times mean favouring the aggressor or the dominant power. Codes of ethics do not have much to say about the obligation to search one's conscience over issues of power.

Non-involvement is not only a matter of leaving power where it has already accumulated. It may also be necessary to decide whether or not to offer help or support to a client beyond the usual constraints of the therapeutic framework. A relationship allows for needs to develop that have never been met before. Regression implies the expression of vast and painful need. The temptation for the counsellor to try to meet needs is in the headlines when it involves sexual contact, which is always wrong. Again, however, there is a continuum of fantasies and needs both in the counsellor and in the client, and it is just as likely that we could deny ordinary human help or concern in the name of professionalism and the maintenance of boundaries.

There is an argument that we should offer only the kind of help for which we are trained and that the client must go to find other sorts of help elsewhere. For some, the best kind of help may be the maintenance of boundaries. For others, there may also be an argument for making boundaries flexible in the interests of a client. We are all likely to have to face the question of whether or not to visit a client at home or in hospital when the client is ill or dying. Codes of ethics at such points as these leave us only with the barest essentials. We work for the client's best interest as we see it and we follow the oath of Hippocrates: 'In every house where I come I will enter only for the good of my patients, keeping myself far from all intentional evil-doing and all seduction and especially from the pleasures of love with women or with men be they free or slaves.'

We would like to consider here the possibility that the values implied by the practice of counselling lead to certain particular needs and, inevitably, to certain dangers. By considering what they are, we may be able to help each other and ourselves to practise less fearfully and also to make appropriate ethical principles central to all our training and subsequent practice. Are there any basic values to which we can all subscribe, in spite of our different models and methodologies?

Relationship: the basic assumption

Counselling and psychotherapy are both disciplines which emerged on the one hand from religion and philosophy and on the other from scientific observation and practice. Academics have tried to think through issues of good and evil: in laboratories some scientists try to circumvent such values and pursue objective reality. Although values are acknowledged to be a major element in therapy, as Clarkson (1995a) points out, perhaps more often by the humanistic practitioners and theorists, it is impossible to imagine the operation of any kind of therapy without an acknowledgement of the value of relationship. No psychotherapy can begin until two human beings make contact. Even if, in the future, we manage to devise computer programs that can do effective psychotherapy by interaction with a machine, nevertheless, there will have been someone to program the machine and to think and feel for the experience of the recipient. Even though some forms of therapy place more emphasis on internal than on external relating, nevertheless, we would argue that the purpose of therapy is to work with relationship, however brief and task-oriented it might be, to help people to relate to themselves and to others. From this one basic value, that it is worthwhile to relate to others or another, comes all our need for ethical codes, all our need to restrain our own impulses and all the complexity of the process of therapy.

So we come to temptation. Counsellors cannot avoid entanglement with the most profound of human emotions, as they engage in the therapeutic relationship. 'Who', as Macbeth said. 'can be wise, amazed, temperate and furious, loyal and neutral in a moment? No man.' And yet that is what is required of counsellors. The dangers are obvious and the temptations to enjoy and finger with the good feelings, the excitement, the idealisations are obvious. Sometimes counsellors can convince themselves that self-gratification is in the client's interests. He or she needs to be shown that he or she is still capable of inspiring love, sexual desire, etc. A safeguard when a therapist is tempted by these emotions is to think of how he or she would describe and explain the words and actions to colleagues. How would all this fit with the rationale by which that counsellor works, and how would others both of the same and of different theoretical persuasions view this? Could it truly be said to be non-exploitative and the best that could be done at the time and under the circumstances?

Codes of ethics explicitly state that the counsellor must relate to his or her client only as a therapist and that other sorts of relationships with clients are prohibited. There are very good reasons for this. We have a much-heightened awareness as therapists of the ways in which the more powerful person in a relationship can harm and damage the other. Sexual abuse of children is now the currency of pop psychology as well as the concept on which Freud based his understanding of psychoanalysis through studying hysteria. We know that the therapist can damage a client by exploiting him or her. There is little evidence that partnerships and marriages based originally on a therapeutic relationship work well. A study of such relationships would be a useful piece of research.

As Clarkson points out (1995b), there are many areas of dual or multiple relationship where the counsellor cannot avoid having other sorts of connections with clients. How do we judge the ethics then? As soon as a counsellor takes on a role with any public connections at all, such as working for a national professional organisation, which may lead to being quoted or interviewed in the media, he or she has a potential dual role. Does that mean that we should all refrain from writing, teaching, publishing, talking in public, amateur dramatics, singing in a choir? Clearly this would be absurd. We cannot turn ourselves into enclosed orders of monks and nuns. Instead, each individual needs to think about how his or her life and lifestyle might affect current or potential clients and what difference it makes to his or her effectiveness as a counsellor and most particularly to the power balance in the counselling. The therapeutic relationship involves at least two people and, as we know, the client may be abused, but it is also possible that the therapist may be abused by the client.

Who protects the counsellor?

So far, we have talked about the ethical issues that underlie codes of ethics and practice, in order to consider at more depth why we should, or should not, behave in certain ways. Most codes assume that their purpose is to protect clients from the wrongdoing of counsellors. That is certainly their major function and they are needed for that purpose. We might also consider the need of therapists for some protection and help. Transference theory teaches us that clients will see us in illusional, and, at times, delusional ways as the need arises for them. Depending on the model that we practise we will be more or less inclined to encourage and develop the transference, but few people would deny that it exists. Clients may well bring complaints against therapists out of the extremes of pain and anger endured in the transference. Yet transference, as we know, attaches itself usually to some hook in the therapist's personality or behaviour in the present. Therapists are at risk from the client who sees a formal complaint as a means of dealing with the pain that transference experience brings and will be convinced that the experience is completely real in the present, and is based entirely on the therapist's actual shortcomings.

There are many aspects of the therapeutic relationship that lend themselves particularly to the 'victim's revenge' (Clarkson, 1995c). Sometimes, the therapist is induced to make the mistake that produces the scenario the client needs to repeat. It is possible to forget to give basic information, to be sadistic with fees, holiday dates, absence, etc. If we do act in these ways, to the extent that it is unethical or unprofessional, then I suppose we have to accept the process of a complaint. On the other hand, the Psychoanalytic Section of UKCP has been trying to think whether organisations could make allowance for the possibility of delusional transference in codes of ethics and practice and in complaints procedures.

For example, a complaint might be made against a therapist who has suggested that a client should work towards an ending. The therapist might think that it is in the client's best interest for all sorts of reasons to go to someone else or to stop altogether (see Murdin, 1994). Yet the client might feel that the suggestion is the same as an abandonment in the past and be consumed with rage and a desire for revenge. If this is so, we might say that the time is not yet right for an ending. But what if the relationship is not working well or the therapist has his or her own personal reasons for needing to stop? Most of the difficulties that we encounter can be dealt with by the therapist within the relationship and very often within the transference that exists. Sometimes, however, there is what seems to be an unmanageable breakdown. The result is most often that the client simply leaves and either carries the scar permanently or goes to another therapist who may be able to help to stop the repetition of the damaging pattern.

Making the therapeutic relationship a priority

We would like to suggest that the profession as a whole might be helped if we were able to help each other more with therapeutic relationships that have run into difficulties. Since our work is about relationship, the first consideration when there are questions of ethics must be the maintenance and usefulness of the therapeutic relationship. Would we be able to offer to clients and ourselves some sort of consultancy, rather like marriage guidance, where a senior member of the profession would see both the therapist and the client and discover whether anything could be done to help the relationship to get back to work? At the moment, the investigative stage of hearing a complaint may have that effect. If the client feels that his or her side of the story is heard, the effect may be to introduce the second parent into what is often felt to be the terrifying mother–child dyad where father is nowhere to be seen. If father can be brought in symbolically, the third person may well be able to avoid reaching the stage of a formal complaint which implies that the relationship has broken down already. The teaching profession might have something to offer us from its experience. Since the Children Act of 1989, teachers have been subject to many complaints from children and parents, sometimes with little or no evidence in support, and have usually been suspended at least. New guidelines are now taking into account that teachers also need protection, justice and a method for reinstatement (*Times Educational Supplement*, February 1995).

Practical benefit might come to all of us if we were able to consider that help might be available if we needed it without our having to think we were admitting failure. In the same way, clients might be better helped if they felt and knew that their therapists had the possibility of bringing in an independent but professional third person. We might also then be able to create an atmosphere of attempting to help and improve what is difficult rather than the sense of dread and isolation that currently surrounds the possibility of a complaint. Such is the anxiety about complaints that there is a tendency to scapegoat the ones who are complained against in order to preserve the rest of us as whole and virtuous. We need to try wherever possible to work with the difficulties that arise, to educate and provide care rather than to police and punish. We have the task of working to evolve more fruitful and creative relationships while maintaining all the necessary safeguards against human frailty.

References

d'Ardennes. P. and Mahtani, M. (1993) Transcultural Counselling in Action. London: Sage.

BAC (1992) Code of Ethics and Practice for Counsellors. Rugby: British Association for Counselling.

Bond, T. (1993) Standards and Ethics for Counselling in Action. London: Sage.

Clarkson, P. (1995a) Values in counselling and psychotherapy. In The Therapeutic Relationship. London: Whurr.

Clarkson, P. (1995b) In recognition of dual relationships. In The Therapeutic Relationship. London: Whurr.

Clarkson, P. (1995c) Vengeance of the victim. In The Therapeutic Relationship. London: Whurr.

Holmes, J. and Lindley, R. (1991) The Values of Psychotherapy. Oxford: OUP.

Murdin, L. (1994) Time to go: Therapist-induced endings in psychotherapy. British Journal of Psychotherapy, 10(3), 355–60.

Samuels, A. (1993) The Political Psyche. London: Routledge.

Simons, H. W. (1986) Persuasions: Understanding, Practice, and Analysis (revised edn) New York: Random House.

Simons, H. W. (1989) Distinguishing the rhetorical from the real: the case of psychotherapeutic placebos. In H. W. Simons (ed.) Rhetoric in the Human Sciences, pp. 109–18. London: Sage.

UKCP (1993) Guidelines for Codes of Ethics and Practice for Member Organisations. London: United Kingdom Council for Psychotherapy.

Weigert, A. (1970) The immoral rhetoric of scientific sociology. American Sociologist, 5, 111–19.

ITEM 7
Professional Practices and Ethical Guidelines for Administrative/Ancillary Staff at Counselling and Psychotherapy Practices, Institutes and Colleges

PETRŪSKA CLARKSON

As far as I know there are not many codes of ethics for administrative and ancillary staff in these settings, even though the professional staff are very thoroughly bound to their code. I would like to offer this as an example to other bodies and thus share my experience in this area. Some points are covered but not all, and I would welcome feedback and comments. I see this as the beginning of a dialogue on the subject of ethical guidelines in administrative settings.

Confidentiality

Working at a large training institute which runs an assessment and referral service means that many clients and trainees, trainers, supervisors and other professional staff may discuss matters which are confidential or within their strict code of ethics, usually outside of your hearing. Sometimes, however, through your presence at meetings or recordings of workshops or written communications between patients, clients, staff trainees, ethics committees etc., you will be exposed to and handle confidential material that is governed by professionally strict rules of non-disclosure. In this sense you are most similar to legal or medical secretaries and will be expected to adhere scrupulously to the same code of ethics as the professional staff insofar as it affects your functioning alongside and in support of them and the people they serve.

Security of written information

Confidentiality of name, address and other significant details of all clients and trainees must be protected under all circumstances. This

122

includes whether or not a particular person has contacted any of the institute staff or not, and whether or not they are in counselling or psychotherapy. The appointments book must be kept safe under lock and key and the cover name of the book should be coded.

All client or trainee information must be kept secure in locked files. Specific members of staff should be named as being responsible for ensuring that security procedures are maintained and that no one can have access to these files who is not also bound by the BAC, ITAA, GPTI and BPS codes of ethics (or any one of these) in addition to the institute code. Please ensure that anyone who teaches or supervises at the institute is a member and/or agrees in a written contract or letter of employment (whether short- or long-term) to adhere to the code of ethics and professional practice.

A coding or password system will protect all confidential letters etc. which are on computer or disc and appropriate security – including lodging duplicate keys at the bank or solicitors – may be required for sensitive material. Remember that administrative support staff may go off sick or be unavailable in emergencies, and access to information at all times for professional staff is equally important as keeping it secure. Please ensure that the institute is at no time in breach of the Data Protection Act and take all necessary steps and advice wherever you are unsure.

Security of spoken information

All information about the institute/centre/college, its staff, clients and meetings is to be kept confidential to the institute and not used without permission in outside conversations or communications. The privacy of the clients and staff, the decision-making processes and business plans are the mutual concern of everyone and need to be protected. Where there may be exceptions, please check this first with your head of department or the principal beforehand.

Conversations about people

Conversations about people should be restricted to necessary confidential discussions and in appropriate spaces – i.e. with doors closed. This also applies to telephone conversations or arguments that may need to be conducted in privacy. Your co-operation in helping everyone to keep to such boundaries will be appreciated. Sometimes trainees and others may need to be reminded that all discussions of clients must be conducted in a non-trivialising way within supervision, training or meetings and not as part of social conversation – even in break times. Kitchen or caretaking staff are sometimes unnoticed during enthusiastic discussions, and they too need protection from the burden of undue information. Clients or trainees may also be in the refectory or the passages, and due care and respect for all is usually preserved when an awareness of the delicacy of our work and the open nature of a learning institute is maintained. It is in the nature of working outside a padded cell that people in a training and psychotherapy institute may sometimes accidentally overhear things which are private. Such unusual occurrences are of course also to be treated with the utmost respect and privacy, and never to be referred to or discussed by outside parties.

Conversations about counselling and training

It is unprofessional to engage in conversations about the nature of psychotherapy or counselling, its related training and entry requirements, to read references, or to select or confirm people on courses without the explicit, preferably written, instruction of the trainers and or head of department concerned or head of school (as appropriate), or to discuss details of accreditation and validation procedures, etc. which are not within your limits of competency. These are the province of the professional staff who both have the information (or resources) and the skills to deal with such questions, decisions or discussions. Always encourage enquirers or trainees and supervisees to write directly to the heads of department and/or the head of school on professional matters or to make appointments with them for such discussions, rather than attempt to be helpful outside of your legitimate brief.

Code of ethics and grievance procedure of the organisation

All staff should familiarise themselves with at least the institute code of ethics and the BAC code of ethics for counsellors, trainers and supervisors. There are also grievance procedures for dealing with ethics and professional guidelines and appeals procedures for dealing with trainees' concerns about examinations or assessment.

Handling complaints

Whenever you become aware of concerns about professional staff in terms of these guidelines, it is your duty to speak to them directly in the first instance to seek clarification of a matter that you may have misunderstood or may have been an oversight on their part. If you feel that your concern has not appropriately been responded to, then you should approach the administration manager, and the relevant head of department to follow the matter through. A written record of this meeting should be lodged with the principal, conserving the rules of confidentiality as far as the professional and administrative or ancillary staff members are concerned.

When people make complaints about the management, facilities, training, trainers or supervisors, please direct them to discuss problems directly with the people concerned rather than secretly in your presence. Offer help if they are unsure how to proceed. There is usually an under-used suggestion box which is eagerly opened and frequently successful in implementing suggestions where feasible and realistic. If there are complaints about the administration or yourself, please ask the person who is complaining to be specific, and if possible to put it in writing with suggestions for improvement. In consultation with the administrative manager, the head of the department concerned and the principal, make the necessary adjustments as soon as possible, apologise where appropriate and solicit the help of the professional staff concerned in preventing recurrences or adapting procedures in more efficient ways in future. Many errors of system and procedure can be prevented by review of existing ways and creative problem-solving between all the parties affected by the problem. There is an old saying, 'Those who are not part of the solution are part of the problem'. That applies to everyone. Refer people to the solution team structures as well when there are concerns which need revision, improvements or changes. Welcome appreciation and encouragement and give it so that more of these nourishing elements can circulate throughout the system.

Relationship with colleagues

It is part of most professional codes of conduct to treat colleagues with respect and courtesy. Even when disagreeing with them it is vital that you use the management structures, each other and/or facilitators to resolve differences openly and cleanly. It is equally important that you respect yourselves and do not accept disrespectful treatment from professional colleagues toward you or your colleagues. Please ask for help in communicating clearly when you cannot or should not disclose confidential information or when you need to refuse something to someone, and in learning how to be assertive in ensuring that your work is smooth, efficient and well-supported by the professional staff.

It is important to demonstrate that everyone values and respects each other – clients, trainers and other staff and colleagues – whatever their race, gender, religious beliefs or sexual orientation may be.

Dealing with emergencies

All staff, including the caretaker and housekeeper, should have special training in first aid, fire prevention and the management of physical, psychological and other emergencies of the kind that can occur within a counselling establishment. If someone is distressed or in need of help in a public part of the building, please help them to a private room (you will know which are free) and call the help of a professional staff member. It is your duty to ensure that you are adequately equipped for supporting this kind of professional work and to help others who are new to it. In the rare cases where you are exposed to painful or disturbing material through your work (e.g. case notes or ethics enquiries), you should contact the director of clinical services or the principal who will arrange suitable counselling.

Feedback

It is good professional practice constantly to review and improve systems, procedures and habits and in this spirit also additions and improvements to this chapter would be welcomed.

CHAPTER 8
Collegial Working Relationships – Ethics, Research and Good Practice

PETRŪSKA CLARKSON AND GEOFF LINDSAY

> To ignore an ethical violation is an ethical violation in itself . . . (Bernard and Jara, 1995, p. 67)

PART I: SOME RESEARCH FINDINGS

- What should you do if you hear that a colleague as a result of some 'impairment' is too mentally or physically unfit or incompetent (in your judgement) to work effectively with clients on a temporary or a permanent basis?
- What should you do if a client tells you confidentially that he was one of several boys who had been sexually abused by a counsellor, but despite knowing that he had the right to complain, he did not want any complaint made?
- What should you do if a colleague tells you that an eminent colleague has been expelled from their organisation's lists because he made a complaint and that therefore clients and supervisees are no longer to be referred to him?

These are only three examples of the kinds of dilemmas about collegial conduct many of us face or may face in our professional lives. (Some answers to these dilemmas are embedded in this chapter. You could check them again at the end to see if your view has changed.) That ethical dilemmas are complex and interwoven in our sociolegal cultural context is taken for granted. The list of references of the work of others and our own covers much ground which cannot be discussed in any one book or chapter. Here we wish to focus on only one aspect which has a way – notwithstanding all efforts to circumscribe it – of permeating all of our ethics codes, moral awareness and standards of practice anyway – namely our working relationship with our colleagues.

All professional ethics codes contain items regarding collegial working relationships and most have procedures for dealing with breaches of such principles of ethical practice (BAC, 1992; BPS, 1995; UKCP, 1995–6). Yet as Friedson (1970) pointed out:

a code of ethics has not necessary relationship to the actual behaviour of members of the occupation. . . . In this sense a code of ethics may be seen as one of many methods an occupation may use to induce general belief in the ethicity of its members, without necessarily bearing directly on individual ethicality. (p. 187)

It remains one of the most fraught areas of our professional theory and practice of ethics and calls into question complex foundational moral questions of integrity and responsibility towards the professional organisations one belongs to, the clients' or students' interests we claim to be protecting and one's own survival issues as a professional with a livelihood to make in these professions.

This chapter briefly reviews in a preliminary way some early findings taken from research into ethics in terms of collegial working relationships, offering some guidance from the literature and from experience as reminders of good practice. Quotations from respondents in this and other stages of the study are used to highlight qualitative aspects of these ethical concerns. (We have not used any quotations we were requested not to use.)

Background to this analysis of ethical dilemmas concerning collegial conduct

As explained in Chapter One, following on North American (Pope and Vetter, 1992) and British research studies (Lindsay and Colley, 1995) of ethical dilemmas of psychologists, a joint survey was undertaken into the ethical dilemmas as experienced by a random sample of 1000 UKCP psychotherapists as described in the first chapter of this book. This sample was posted a simple survey form with pre-paid reply envelopes and asked for a response to the following question: 'Describe in a few words, or more detail, an incident that you or a colleague have faced in the past year or two that was ethically troubling to you.' This was a replication of the previous North American and BPS research designs. This preliminary report highlights only some findings.

Of the UKCP psychotherapists who replied, 73.2% reported experiencing ethical dilemmas, 22.1% reported that they had experienced no dilemmas and 4.7% wrote that they were unable to comment for various reasons. In the opinion of the researchers such a high proportion of practitioners grappling with ethical dilemmas indicates a serious commitment to engaging with such issues in our professions. Since we believe that there is hardly any clinical or supervisory event at all without its ethical – or moral – dimensions, we would hope that, in time, with increased education and professional awareness, the figure reporting no dilemmas will rise to 100%. This research and this chapter are an attempt to increase appreciation and exploration of this dimension of our work in all its guises.

The most frequently reported troubling ethical dilemmas for UKCP psychotherapists included in the first Clarkson and Lindsay survey (1997) were: confidentiality (29.2%), followed by colleagues' conduct (13.5%), then dual relationships (11.8%), then sexual issues (8%), then academic training issues (5.6%) and then by issues of competence (4.9%). Other issues were proportionally somewhat less significant.

The fact that colleagues' conduct emerged as the second highest source of ethical dilemmas if all mentions were aggregated for UK psychotherapists seemed to warrant much further and deeper investigation. A detailed secondary analysis of all respondents' comments specifically mentioning colleagues' conduct was thus made to facilitate such consideration. Since this is a qualitative study, it is not suggested that these results are necessarily representative of the profession of psychotherapy – or counselling for that matter – but merely a starting point for exploration and discussion. (The BAC does not differentiate between counselling and psychotherapy and, although we do not know how many responding UKCP members in this survey are also BAC members, counselling was frequently mentioned. We are thus assuming – until further research may prove otherwise – that for the purposes of education, exploration and practice improvement the issues regarding ethics for counsellors and psychotherapists are substantially the same.)

So the overall theme is our working alliances or working relationships with our colleagues. Paraphrasing the definition in *The Therapeutic Relationship* (Clarkson, 1995), a working alliance or relationship is defined as: 'that part of a colleague–colleague relationship which enables them to work together even when either of them experiences some desires to the contrary'. As professionals we are required to work together – for the benefit of our clients, our students and members of the public – also for the sake of profession as long as we are members of these professions. There are many times when we have to work effectively together with people with whom we disagree or don't like or with whom we may not want to be 'close friends'.

As long as people remain members of the same professions, they are highly likely to serve on committees or research projects together; they may be involved with different members of the same family or with students from the same organisation; and they will hopefully be joined in the common purpose of competent and ethical service to clients, students, colleagues and members of the public – notwithstanding their own personal foibles, preferences, rivalries or fears. Therefore members of the professions are required to maintain such working relationships in order to fulfil the items of code regarding not bringing the profession into disrepute.

Professions exist on the public trust (MacDonald, 1995), so that particularly in such circumstances the good of the students, the clients and the public will prevail and that mutually effective working relationships will be developed, maintained and secured. When a surgeon and an anaesthetist engage in professional rivalry over a patient, the life of the patient may be endangered. In psychotherapy the stakes are no less high – sometimes a life, sometimes sanity and frequently professional careers. The maintenance of effective working relationships – particularly when there are conflicting desires or potential difficulties – is thus of the greatest and most crucial value to the profession of psychotherapy in its claim to be protecting and serving the interests of the public. Some respondents in our study also argued that there was not sufficient guidance about collegial relationships:

This shows up a general lack in the profession of laid down criteria/ethical code guidance for collegial relationships within our organisations and procedures for the breach of them.

We thought, however, that the guidance did in fact exist in the relevant codes (see later), but that it was not frequently taught or implemented. Many responses indicated ignorance or confusion. Qualitative interviews with complainants (and those complained against) about the procedures in which they participated appear to bear this out.

The situation is often exacerbated from the outset with professional bodies often being very defensive and reacting in a hostile way to enquiries regarding complaints. Sometimes they may be shrouded in mystery and it is difficult to get hold of the basic necessary information, such as the code of ethics or the complaints procedures. Failure to readily give clear information at the outset can contribute significantly to considerable feelings of mistrust (Clarkson and Lindsay, 1999).

It has been suggested (e.g. Bernard and Jara, 1995) that a primary reason for the comparative neglect of teaching and education about responsible collegial behaviour is that all kinds of 'unwritten protection laws' have proliferated along with fear – justifiable or not – of the destructive consequences of becoming responsibly involved. Some of our respondents had experienced this:

The organisation was furious when we made the complaint . . . a colleague lost her job without due notice.

Fear of such official kinds of retribution held people back from making complaints. Several respondents expressed regret of some kind for not acting appropriately in cases where they had grave cause for concern:

Sadly this seemed to me to indicate some confirmation of my own fears and I regret that I did not take more strong action at the time they were still seeing me.

Quotes from respondents are in italics. Quotes used in this chapter are largely verbatim except where changed for sense or the protection of identifying details.

Others were reasonably clear about personal responsibility for choices along the continuum from bystanding to responsible involvement: it's the problem of being aware that:

> some other practitioner is working with what I see as an incompetence that is culpable and damaging. I may understand well why but since I'm not being approached by them for supervision, I feel uncomfortably powerless but when it's close to home and I feel obliged to act then ultimately it is to be about recognising abuse and not tolerating it.

Research results: the types of ethical dilemmas concerning collegial conduct

Eighty-one specific ethical dilemmas (with two coded in two instances) regarding collegial conduct were mentioned in this part of the research project and a category analysis revealed the following results in terms of rank order for type of reported dilemma. The 83 code items break down as shown in Table 8.1.

Table 8.1: Analysis of ethical dilemmas

Type of dilemma	Number of responses
Serious concerns about colleagues' competence	29
Sexual misconduct with clients or students	19
Attacks by colleagues on professional reputation	8
Boundary breaks	7
Financial exploitation of clients and students	7
General misconduct	4
Issues to do with moral competence including lying about qualifications	4
Issues to do with discrimination of various kinds	2
Issues to do with the abuse of power over clients or students or members	2
Mismanagement of colleague's death – effect on clients (see Item 9 in this book, pp. 168–72)	1

Here follows a brief discussion with examples on the most frequent of these issues for more general consideration. It is envisaged that any one of these types of dilemmas could benefit from a paper, a chapter or even one or more books written about them. Hopefully this initial attempt will encourage colleagues to join us in the endeavour of finding more information and more questions about these very complex dimensions of being a responsible professional living and working with integrity in the confusing, uncertain and rapidly changing world of our current time. Of course this is not a spurious demand for perfection, but a serious call to accountability and responsibility. We know only too well, as Bauman (1993) puts it:

What the postmodern mind is aware of is that there are problems in human and social life with no good solutions, twisted trajectories that cannot be straightened up, ambivalences that are more than linguistic blunders yelling to be corrected, doubts which cannot be legislated out of existence, moral agonies which no reason-dictated recipes can soothe, let alone cure. (p. 245)

Serious concerns about colleagues' competence

This was the largest sub-category including concerns about both trainee and qualified colleagues. Due to the open-endedness of our question, it is not possible to quantify this properly, given the fact that some North American studies found that 50% of psychotherapists have admitted to practising while incompetent (Pope, Tabachnik and Keith-Spiegel, 1995), one can see why this is such a serious issue.

The dilemma for the supervisor is how to help the supervisee admit that she needs to actively challenge her client and at the same time to contain the supervision group split between collusion and alarm, it feels as if some speedy action is advised, intervention rather than exploration, as the client's welfare and that of others is at stake.

The issue of client welfare should of course be of overriding concern and the very foundation of claims to being a profession. The dilemmas reported in this study often concerned how to deal with or how to inform the organisation and prevent or stop the abuse while not breaking codes of confidentiality. These were often interpreted to mean that 'nothing can be done'. This leaves members of the public at risk of abusive and damaging professionals while other members of the profession know of such abuse, but feel they cannot act. If this is the case, the profession cannot regulate itself, and its claims to the public to have viable ethics codes which are enforced is devoid of truth.

I am afraid that she [supervisee] might eventually be a very damaging counsellor, but I don't seem able to let anybody know this, even in the vaguest of terms, because I have no contact with her course tutors.

If a training institution's course tutors have not had contact with course supervisors something is seriously wrong. It seems to us that the published rules of professional and ethical conduct requiring confrontation of a colleague when in doubt, well covers these issues of competency. It appears that the differentiation often made between trainee and qualified colleagues is spurious in these cases. Alternatively, it may be misunderstood because where the psychotherapist or counsellor suspect abuse or damage as a result of competency issues, both the client and the practitioner can best be served by some direct, personal and compassionate intervention.

Some professionals reported difficulties about the source of their information:

> This confidentiality was shared with me in my role as a therapist but it also overlapped the boundaries of my responsibility as a trainer and supervisor and also the organisation whose code of ethics I adhere to.

Only after respectful discussion with the colleague concerned (always on the assumption that one may be wrong), can one make a reasonable professional estimate of risk to clients. If such a discussion with the colleague does not resolve the issue satisfactorily (e.g. with a clarification, explanation or commitment to get help of a particular kind) then it is usually an ethical requirement that client welfare take precedence over protecting the confidentiality of the practitioner. Then either the supervisor, training organisation or relevant professional organisation needs to be appropriately involved and then only with those breaches of confidence strictly necessary to deal ethically with the case.

Sexual misconduct with clients or students

The second largest group of responses about collegial conduct concerned sexual misconduct with clients or students. A practitioner expressed 'grave concern' about a sexually abusing colleague who is still practising sexual misconduct – the client won't complain and the practitioner has

> not checked whether this organisation takes third party complaints.

The disruptive effect of sexual relationships between trainers and students was another cause for distress in our sample (as in other studies).

> Issue for the organisation in terms of interpreting ethics – and unreconciled conflicts between organisation and wider community.

Attacks by colleagues on professional reputation

> I found that what I had heard seriously damaged my confidence in my colleague's integrity as a psychotherapist. Yet there seemed to be no appropriate place to take my concerns, especially as the source of my information was so informal.

The BPS differentiates between disagreeing with views or methods or opinions as different from attacks on the person or the professional reputation of a colleague. 'For instance, two counsellors engaged in a heated public debate would not fall into this category [of undermining public confidence in counselling] unless either party became personally abusive and defamed the other or violence resulted' (Bond, 1993, p. 148). That gives considerable leeway for responsible collegial conduct.

Boundary issues

A supervisee was breaking an ethical code in continuing to counsel a client with whom she was in another relationship. Had I withdrawn supervision or initiated the complaints procedures, she would have continued to counsel the client unsupervised. My decision was to continue to address the unethical behaviour in a challenging way – but also in the interests of client safety – to continue the supervision.

General discussion

Although the research question was phrased in a very open way, not asking for this kind of information at all, it was also possible to make an indicative sub-analysis of responses in terms of what kind of action was considered or taken. These results, so spontaneously mentioned, are definitely not to be generalised, but again provide fruitful food for thought. They may also indicate the depth and quality of the respondents' appreciation of and engagement with the complexity of the problem raised by the ethical dilemma in each instance. Another study could research this in much more depth. So, just because no action or reflection or outcome was mentioned in a particular response, we cannot assume that much more thoughtful consideration and a definite outcome did not actually follow in cases where these were not included in responses.

The injunction to do no harm [non-malificence] can be construed to include the mandate not to remain passively acquiescent when fellow professionals are violating ethical principles and standards of practice (Pope et al., 1995, p. 78).

Several respondents specifically mentioned not filing ethics complaints, some feeling that others (such as a boss) should have done 'something'. This is compared with one fourth (plus 9.3%) of respondents in a North American study who have actually filed an ethics complaint against a colleague. If only some 10% of colleagues were willing to act on information about other colleagues' violation of ethics codes, that means that 90% of ethical violations against clients, colleagues and members of the public are possibly unconfronted and perhaps continuing.

Some highlights from the results

In 19 instances taking action was considered, but not taken. One respondent wrote:

Moral problem: Where does my responsibility lie? With him or my patient so as not to be provoked into being the expected punishing father or to the world who will probably meet an angry therapist with deeply unreached power issues?

Another example:

Do I have sufficient grounds to 'interfere' in some long-term relationships he is engaged in with clients? (junior colleagues)

and

I chose to stay with my patient and actually did not signal my profound anger at what I consider a deeply immoral action on his part. And of course he still left therapy.

In 21 instances some form of action was reported. For example:

After discussion with my supervisor I took the necessary step to report him

and

Although I felt it might have implications at a clinical level for my clients, I went ahead and pursued a formal complaint against the individual and member organisation. I'm glad I did and in the end it has helped my clinical work rather than hindered it.

Some reflected on short-term discomfort weighed up against long-term negative consequences:

The supervisee is very upset, and I feel guilty – but I would have felt guilty had I kept quiet.

Several respondents reported difficulties even when complaints procedures were implemented, for example:

Many areas of this therapist's practice concerned me and my female members of the panel – his advertising, failure to contact GP, seek supervision, etc. We could not examine the emergent factors because that (apparently) did not form part of her complaint.

Several comments concerned the institutions' capacity to deal appropriately with ethical concerns, for example:

It has been an enormously empowering learning curve for both of us. It leaves us in great doubt about the ability of institutions to manage counselling courses. Their philosophical, management and financial ethos is at great odds with that of the therapeutic world.

North American studies also found respondents who were worried about 'diploma mills' (termed 'a crisis' by one UK respondent) 'but many had concerns about programs accepting students 'with marginal ethics and competence who were so identified in graduate school and no one did anything about it' (Pope and Vetter, 1992, p. 54). From some of our other research, particularly into organisational issues, the training institution's pressure to make money from 'bums on seats' and to save money by employing staff with inadequate qualifications and experience is a source of concern for the ethical welfare of the profession and the public which it professes to serve. Lindsay and Colley (1995) also found evidence of 'professional gagging'.

In only one case in this particular study was there a sense of precipitate action, and in no case where reporting was considered was there a sense of impulsive or malicious making of 'improper complaints', i.e. a breach of the rules stating, 'Psychologists do not file or encourage the filing of ethics complaints that are frivolous and are intended to harm the respondent rather than to protect the public' (APA, 1992, code 8.07).

There were seven specific reports of not having taken action as if the respondents felt that appropriate action was precluded by other items of ethics codes. As we have shown, we don't necessarily agree that this is a proper understanding of the ethics codes. However, a respondent's understanding gives us an insight:

> *The training system demanded that his therapy remain confidential; and if my supervisee had not found a way of conveying to the training committee her reservations, I would have felt compelled to contact them myself. (Competence issue) It concerns a junior colleague, but the problem seems to be the training committee's perceived rules which prevented proper access.*

Popper (1992) contrasted

> the attitude of the old professional ethics leads us to cover up our mistakes, to keep them secret and to forget them as soon as possible. . . . the new basic principle is that in order to learn to avoid making mistakes, we must learn from our mistakes. To cover up mistakes is therefore, the greatest intellectual sin . . . since we must learn from our mistakes, we must also learn to accept, indeed gratefully, when others draw out attention to our mistakes . . . (p. 202)

Other points of interest

Some respondents mentioned the valuable role of self-doubt and reflection:

> *This is not to say that I haven't myself been in difficult situations, confused and emotionally upset. But at least then I knew that something was problematic and could hold on to myself and try not to act before the fog had cleared.*

and some others the uses of countertransference reactions in understanding the psychodynamics of ethical conflicts:

> *I was overcome with rage, about the whole position she is in, and I think this reflects the unhealthy, incestuous and abusive aspects of her domestic situation.*

The purpose of the codes is to clarify what is acceptable practice and what is not.

> If an organization possesses the awesome power to remove a practitioner from its register, with all the consequences that this will have on his or her life and livelihood, it should feel a compulsion to provide for that person a template against which to measure his or her conduct and practice. (Palmer Barnes, 1998, p. 8)

It was thus interesting to read of some concerns for violators and the effect of sanctions such as exclusion from the profession on their livelihood:

> *I am not questioning the unethical nature of his action but would be interested in there being some thought about the ethics of depriving someone in their 50s of their livelihood for one such misdemeanour. I wonder if there is any possibility of a programme of 'rehabilitation' (including therapy and supervision) for such offenders.*

Psychotherapist impairment due to psychological dysfunctioning 'is not often remedied through either educative or disciplinary actions, but may succumb to psychotherapy and other rehabilitative efforts. . . . Generally such programs are staffed by professional colleagues who volunteer to work for little or no fee on a limited basis' (Thompson, 1990, p. 137).

We also believe that it is important to separate the ways in which we deal with misconduct from difficulties due to health problems such as dementia.

> The willingness to monitor and correct unethical and incompetent behaviour by colleagues is difficult to instil or to encourage. Yet without such willingness the entire structure collapses. (Thompson, 1990, p. 133)

A good working relationship between colleagues is fundamentally based on a shared care for clients, other colleagues (including particularly clients, students and supervisees) and members of the public. To this end disagreements of policy, values, theory and practice should be made explicit within an atmosphere of mutual respect for the persons involved so that difficulties can be addressed, mediated and resolved through ongoing dialogue and co-operation with or without the assistance of dispute facilitators or mediators. Where there is reason to believe that a colleague (whether novice, peer or senior) is contravening an ethics code item, the principles of a good working alliance requires that such hearsay or suspicions be checked with the practitioner in question (or the person who reports this be encouraged to deal with it directly, personally and privately in the first instance).

The colleague may have been misunderstood or misreported, or may even welcome the opportunity to correct either a misperception or a misconduct. (This is the 'do as you would be done by' rule.) When appropriate, a concerned third party should offer to act as a mediator or refer the client (or gossiping colleague) to an impartial mediator or specially appointed dispute resolution or ethics consultant. It should not be assumed that bad intent is always the motivation – often it is lack of education and even lack of intellectual ability to understand the complexities of ethical consequences and moral choices in our world.

If this is not successful, it is the practitioner's ethical duty to report it, particularly in cases where detriment to others, self or the profession is concerned. Such reporting needs to be done with strict confidentiality, ensuring as far as possible psychological safety for all concerned. If complainants are penalised, this demonstrates by example that complaints will not be welcomed and is more likely to encourage abuse and drive concerns underground.

It is thus our moral and ethical responsibility to each other and to our clients, students and members of the public to take action with proper confidentiality preserved, after appropriate and timely consultation and without malice, but yet a professional may be wrong, deliberately or accidentally falsely informed, misled or simply making a mistake. These additional concerns may prevent professionals from acting appropriately. The code items usually specify words like 'where there is reason to suspect', 'where there is ground to believe', etc.; the codes do not require that the complaint be proved true or valid before it is formally made. It does imply a requirement to make an informed professional judgement about the seriousness of the charge and the urgency of confronting the colleague or calling for an investigation. It is important for colleagues seeking such redress of harm to clients or colleagues, for example, to be aware that if they have taken proper consultation to avoid malice or breaches of confidentiality, they may still be wrong about such assessment of probabilities without incurring the risk of being sued for defamation. In normal circumstances libel, slander and defamation tort would apply, but in professional circumstances there is – usually – the defence of qualified privilege which extends precisely this protection to responsible professionals for taking such risks – since it is actually their ethical duty to do so.

PART II: COLLEGIAL DUTY AS A PRINCIPLE OF SELF-REGULATION (SHAM, SHAMBLES OR SHARED RESPONSIBILITY?)

The effectiveness of these [professional ethics] codes depends on four main factors: (1) the benefit that members perceive in retaining their membership; (2) the effectiveness of the association in communicating the code and a sense of its importance to its members; (3) the willingness of members to monitor the behaviour of fellow members and to apply the sanctions when appropriate; and (4) the efforts by the profession to educate the public as to what constitutes competent and ethical behaviour by its members and to support any legitimate complaints about such behaviour by members. (Thompson, 1990, p. 130)

As counsellors, psychologists and psychotherapists we are primarily engaged in the work of alleviating human suffering and facilitating desired development. Most of us work with words ('the talking cure') within different kinds of therapeutic relationship towards these goals. We aspire to professionalism which leads to us publishing claims to the public that we are legitimate practitioners of our science/arts and that those of us who exploit or damage the public's trust will be subject at first to confrontation and if necessary to sanctions – at worst expulsion from membership of the profession. Those who do not belong to the profession usually represented in the relevant register are commonly suspected of being 'quacks' or otherwise dishonest or incompetent. Most frequently a profession undertakes the duty of protection of the public by writing and implementing a code of ethics – the equivalent of a professional legal system which codifies appropriate and unethical conduct for members of that profession. (Employment law of course exists for handling disputes and grievances of employees.) All members of a profession at least subscribe to its ethics code and agree to abide by its rules or submit to its sanctions.

So far, so good. If members of the public who receive services from a member of one of the professional organisations such as BAC, UKCP, BCP or BPS feel that their practitioner has contravened the ethics code of that profession, they can usually choose to discuss their dissatisfaction with the practitioner (and sometimes a facilitator), or they have the option of taking the complaint up with the relevant professional body through the published ethics procedures. Whether this is effective depends on many factors but particularly on:

- whether clients know and understand the codes and standards of ethics and complaints procedures in our professions
- whether clients or students generally feel that they can effectively discuss their feelings about possible ethics violations with the practitioner concerned
- whether the complaints procedures are effective, just and fair
- whether the client can manage, or can get help in negotiating them.

The basic questions

Do our clients/students know and understand the standards and codes of ethics and complaints procedures?

There are anecdotes of insurance companies who recommend that practitioners do not display their ethics codes in their consulting rooms – in case this should act as 'provocation' to making complaints. Do we as counsellors and other professionals in this field even know and under-stand our codes of ethics? Marzillier (1999) reported his realisation in 1992 'that clinical psychologists as a group had virtually no exposure to training in ethics and that was a serious deficiency both for ourselves and our clients'. Partly to explore this, we are conducting research on ethical dilemmas as our colleagues have experienced them.

Do clients/students generally feel that they can effectively discuss their feelings about possible ethics violations with their practitioners while they are still in therapy/training?

Other researchers have found that clients and students who, for example, do not object to (or may even desire) sexual contact at the time *subsequently* feel that the contact with a therapist or educator was coersive. Pope (1989) reported that 'While 80% viewed such advances as ethically inappropriate at the time they occurred, 95% now [at the time of the study] viewed those advances as ethically inappropriate' (p. 171).

Are our complaints procedures confidential, reasonably swift, fair and justly processed by unbiased investigators and adjudicators?

From my interviews with complainants and those complained against, as well as other data available from the Prevention of Professional Abuse Network (POPAN), the answer is an overwhelming 'no'. Participants are often left even more traumatised by the process. The adjective frequently used is 'appalling'. The fact that the UKCP's ethics and complaints procedures has recently had to be taken to judicial review further causes the deepest concern. (An application for judicial review is successful when the High Court has to order a body with responsibility to members of the public to follow their own procedures!) Judicial review is the legal answer to the question: 'Who judges the judges?'

The knowledge of legal process and/or resources to apply for judicial review in the case of a mismanaged or unfair complaints process would usually be prohibitive to many clients and students. Many professionals involved with ethics procedures furthermore lack the expertise, experi-ence and competence to conduct complaints to proper standards (Collis, 1998). In other cases it is process itself that is experienced as inadequate, for example:

> *The case was dismissed for lack of hard evidence. I was quite convinced, however, of malpractice.*

Are clients or students assisted in confidence and without fear of retribution or sanctions in making complaints and negotiating official ethics complaints procedures?

From her UK experience Palmer Barnes (1998) writes:

> What must always be borne in mind is the bravery involved in making a complaint. It is much easier to close down on a bad experience. Pathologising the patient or colleague who has made a complaint is all too easy, and unfortunately it happens all too frequently. Instead of being perceived as a souce of fear or panic, complaints could be taken as an opportunity for learning in its broadest sense. (p. 113)

There is definitely a lack of research on how complainants and complained against experience our professional processes. As part of our ongoing research project we would welcome anyone who would like to confidentially explore further their experiences in this regard.

But ask yourself – how many students of counselling or psychotherapy courses do you know who have made successful formal ethics complaints against their organisational tutors or supervisors or directors and still went on to successfully complete their qualifications? Or should we assume that all staff of training and professional organisations are ethically and professionally perfect? History indicates that this is unlikely. So do our daily newspapers. Research (Bersoff, 1995) adduces, for example, the 'crisis' of 'diploma mills' along with serious concerns about incompetent and unsuitable students being allowed to qualify (p. 54). Similar concerns also showed up repeatedly in our research.

These are some of the reasons why it is a requirement of professional organisations to report suspected unprofessional conduct by colleagues – usually after attempting to resolve the issue informally. The fact is that

> Many, if not most of the ethical violations by professionals come to the attention of fellow professionals when clients [or students] seek them out, sometimes to remedy the wrong that was committed, but more often because their original problem was not satisfactorily resolved. The clients[or students] may not even be aware that they were mistreated because they lack the requisite knowledge of professional standards [or accurate information]. Their current therapists can choose to ignore the matter, actively persuade the clients [or students] that no real wrong or harm was done, pursue the matter themselves (normally with the client's permission), or support their client's efforts to do so. Which course of action is chosen is crucial in the aggregate, in determining the effectiveness of the profession's self-policing. (Thompson, 1990, p. 133)

Can we believe that most professionals will take the course of action which is likely to make them unpopular with their colleagues, appear 'unsupportive' or even cause damage to their reputation and income? As anyone knows who has offered to act as witness to a car accident, the time and stress and cost of appearing in the legal process on another's behalf (e.g. in court) has little benefit and much stress and inconvenience. For counsellors and psychotherapists their reputation or even their livelihood may be put at risk. It has been suggested (e.g. Bernard and Jara, 1995) that a primary reason for the comparative neglect of teaching and education about responsible and ethical collegial behaviour is that all kinds of 'unwritten protection laws' have proliferated along with fear – justifiable or not – of the destructive consequences of becoming responsibly involved. One might even be accused as not having good working relationships if one challenges or makes complaints about the unethical conduct of colleagues. Some of our respondents had also experienced various personally and professionally damaging attempts to exclude or punish them.

Of course, any good respectful collegial relationship actually mandates the exchange of challenges as well as support and the engagement in mutual regulation as well as mutual affirmation.

The ethical duty to confront or report colleagues

The need to act appropriately by confronting and/or reporting colleagues when there is reason to suspect misconduct is enshrined in our codes of ethics. BAC, BCP, BPS and UKCP all publish this undertaking to the profession and the public, thus fostering the legitimate expectation that professionals are ethically obliged to act in cases where they have reason to be concerned about their colleagues' unethical behaviour. As we have seen, clients are most likely to be disadvantaged by such practitioners' unethical conduct. Clients are also usually least informed and least resourced in acting on their own behalf in such situations. If the professionals – who are most likely to hear about abuses from clients and students – abrogate their responsibilities to and for each other, these claims become flagrant misrepresentations to the public and professional self-regulation descends to an empty sham.

Collusion has been raised as a possible concern by Ingrid Lunt in her President's Column in the *Psychologist* about a case which has become a *cause célèbre*. A senior psychologist had been found to have behaved inappropriately and in a sexual manner with his therapeutic clients. Although subsequently disputed by Slade's colleagues, Lunt raises, in addition to other concerns, the issue of whistle blowing:

> . . . why did not his colleagues initiate action early on when they realised what was happening, particularly as Peter Slade had been removed from the Register for two years for a previous case of professional misconduct. (Lunt, 1999, p. 59)

The *Ethical Guidelines* of the UKCP state:

> 2.11 (ii) Psychotherapists are required to take appropriate action in accordance with Clause 5.8 [initiate the relevant complaints procedure] with regard to the behaviour of a colleague which may be detrimental to the profession, to colleagues or to trainees. (UKCP, 1995–6, p. 1)

The relevant item from the BAC *Code of Ethics* (1992) reads as follows:

B. 2.4.2 If a counsellor suspects misconduct by another counsellor which cannot be resolved or remedied after discussion with the counsellor concerned, they should implement the Complaints Procedure, doing so without breaches of confidentiality other than those necessary for investigating the complaint (see B.9). (p. 4)

Example items from the BPS *Professional Practice Guidelines* (1995):

Psychologists shall conduct themselves in their professional activities in a way that does not damage the interest of the recipients of their services or participants in their research and does not inappropriately undermine public confidence in their ability or that of other psychologists and members of other professions to carry our their professional duties. . . 5.3 not exploit any relationship of influence or trust which exists between colleagues, those under their tuition, or those in receipt of their services to further the gratification of their personal desires;. . . and 5.10 bring allegations of misconduct by a professional colleague to the attention of those charged with the responsibility to investigate them, doing so without malice and with no breaches of confidentiality other than those necessary to the proper investigatory processes and when the subject of allegations themselves, they shall take all reasonable steps to assist those charged with responsibility to investigate them. (p. 453)

Not acting in cases of concern about colleagues' conduct is therefore in itself a breach of ethics. 'This is a matter of their personal accountability as professionals; if they do not act they will be equally guilty of misconduct by not taking action' (Palmer Barnes, 1998, p. 64). No one in our study so far even mentioned any of these specific ethical code items which oblige all professionals to act in cases where they have reason to suspect misconduct. It may, of course, be possible that every professional knows these and acts on it so automatically that it is taken for granted.

On the other hand, it may be that there is in practice a collusion which privileges a closing of ranks with our friends and colleagues against the interests of the public – or as one of our respondents put it:

the greatest [ethical] dilemma is whether or not to remain belonging to UKCP and ensure my status is safe, for future (e.g. legislation), whilst at the same time believing it is creating a false position and status for its members (of safety and effectiveness) in the eyes of the public, that they generally don't deserve (based on any objective evidence) and are in fact simply creating a closed shop under the banner of protecting the public. PS. This is true of many of my colleagues.

Szasz (1999) has also challenged us at the 1997 University's Psychotherapy Association Conference with the question of whether professional psychotherapy organisations don't really exist in order to protect the professionals from the public. Yet this 'duty to report' is a fundamental undertaking published for the public in most of our ethics codes. In this way we lead members of the public to believe that professionals would intervene with their own colleagues – on behalf of both our clients and our profession – in cases where there were grounds for thinking that a collegial situation needed investigation or correction or regulation. Thompson from the USA puts it like this:

> The desire for power and identity [of professional associations] may or may not be accompanied by a strong desire to serve the public and to do so in more effective ways, even though the profession espouses such goals. The immediate, often tangible, benefits of protecting and enhancing one's prestige and one's political and economic status may often be more powerful incentives than those of good service to the public. Should the two conflict, or appear to conflict, the latter is apt to give way. (1990, p. 129)

Several of the respondents in our research made comments such as the following:

> *I have difficulty reconciling . . . my own moral standards with that of the organisation I'm involved in with at any given time and my need. . . to earn a living . . . I feel that the counselling and supervision network is quite a small network . . . therefore in order to pay myself OK I need to be on reasonable terms with most people who might . . refer clients to me.*

Palmer Barnes (1998) acknowledges that: 'Whistleblowers are unusual in therapeutic organizations and agencies, but in the future there may need to be more if high standards and ethical practice are to be maintained' (p. 64). These issues should be seen in the light of the fact that concerns about colleagues' ethical conduct emerged as the second highest aggregated source of ethical dilemmas mentioned in the first phase of our study. Only confidentiality caused more concern to UKCP psychotherapists than dilemmas about the ethical conduct of colleagues.

Yet it is known that: 'This kind of difficulty can be very painful because the practitioners often know each other as colleagues or friends. It is often only after considerable heart-searching that such complaints are expressed' (Palmer Barnes, 1998, p. 62). Is bystanding collegial misconduct not more comfortable and definitely safer? (See Clarkson, 1996, Chapter 8.) There are so many benefits from claiming professional status while avoiding the responsibilities or accountability – not least maintaining falsely good working relationships with colleagues who may refer clients, supervisees or teaching contracts. Given such extremely negative consequences of dealing with collegial misconduct the reluctance of professionals to act ethically in this respect is very understandable, but very worrying at the same time.

To illustrate, here follows in rank order the kinds of ethical dilemmas about collegial conduct which we found in just this phase of the study:

1. Serious concerns about colleagues' competence, for example:

Am I right in thinking there's nothing I can do?

2. Sexual misconduct of colleagues with clients or students. For example:

A practitioner expressed 'grave concern' about a sexually abusing colleague who is still practising sexual misconduct, but since the client won't complain has decided there is nothing he can do.

3. Attacks by colleagues on professional reputation by slandering or pathologising them if they raised uncomfortable issues, caused much concern.

Boundary breaks and financial exploitation of clients and students, for example, ranked joint fourth; general misconduct (unspecified); and issues to do with moral competence, including lying about qualifications, ranked joint fifth. Issues to do with discrimination of various kinds and issues to do with the abuse of power over clients or students or members ranked joint sixth and the effect on clients of the mismanagement of a colleague's death ranked last in this sort.

From our research some other reasons emerged that throw some light on what the current situation is as well as implications for might be done to improve it.

Perceived conflicts between ethics code items

Apart from explicitly self-protective agendas which prevented professionals from acting on their concerns about suspected collegial misconduct, we found cases where respondents felt that appropriate action was precluded by other items of ethics codes.

> *The training system demanded that his therapy remain confidential; and if my supervisee had not found a way of conveying her reservations to the training committee, I would have felt compelled to contact them myself. (Competence issue) It concerns a junior colleague, but the problem seems to be the training committee's perceived rules which prevented proper access.*

Perceived lack of adequate information about complaints processes

We were concerned that respondents may not take action, even to establish what the possibilities are, even though all our ethics codes require that where there is reasonable grounds for doubt, confrontation and reporting should happen. Without this willingness, abuses will continue and perhaps proliferate as professionals experience a kind of protectionism born of ignorance or fear of retaliation at the expense of the people we are supposed to serve. It is worth repeating for emphasis what Thompson (1990) and others have pointed out:

> The willingness to monitor and correct unethical and incompetent behaviour by colleagues is difficult to instil or to encourage. Yet without such willingness the entire structure collapses. (p. 133)

Ignorance of ethics codes and the duty to report

In some cases it was clear that respondents are working without adequate knowledge or training of ethics codes and processes as far as their practice is concerned.

> *Do I have a moral duty to tell the client's training organisation that the client really needed several years of analysis to resolve this problem, before being ready to take on his own casework? (concerns peer colleagues as well)*

Some respondents appeared to the under the impression that collegial misconduct was not an ethical issue, but only a moral one:

> *Such a dilemma challenges my trust in myself. It is as I see it a moral, not an ethical matter. I won't collude with therapists and counsellors' bad practice on the grounds of professional 'ethics'. Ultimately my commitment has to be to my supervisee, not to my colleagues' egos.*

No use of consultants/facilitators

There was no mention among our respondents at all of informal attempts to resolve dilemmas with colleagues, in contrast to the APA's (1992) guidance:

> When psychologists believe that there may have been an ethical violation by another psychologist, they attempt to resolve the issue by bringing it to the attention of that individual if an informal resolution appears appropriate and the intervention does not violate any confidentiality rights that maybe involved. (code 8.04)

Nor was there any evidence of attempts at mediation or use of consultants or third parties to resolve issues. Stone (1983) recommended referral of a client (who has been victimised by a colleague) to consult a third party, an 'administrator' to reduce the dual role conflict of being both client's advocate and client's therapist. If the consultation goes ahead, the consultant assumes the responsibility of working with the client in proceeding with any legitimate complaint.

Sometimes concern for welfare of client took precedence, sometimes concern for the colleague's welfare did

> The purpose of the codes is to clarify to what is acceptable practice and what is not. If an organization possesses the awesome power to remove a practitioner from its register, with all the consequences that will have on his or her life and livelihood, it should feel a compulsion to provide for that person a template against which to measure his or her conduct and practice. (Palmer Barnes, 1998, p.8)

Constructive suggestions

Several respondents reported making constructive suggestions for improved practice based on their experiences, but we do not know whether these suggestions were taken up. We also believe that it is important to separate the ways in which we deal with misconduct from difficulties due to health problems such as dementia from disciplinary issues.

There are certainly grounds to conclude from this and our other studies that there is a great deal of room for improvement in practitioners' understanding and appreciation of the role of ethics and our shared responsibility towards our colleagues in the profession.

Education and mediation need to supplement genuine regulation. Gawthop and Uhleman (1992), for example, showed that the recognition of ethical dilemmas and the ability to resolve them improves with training. Many of the studies done indicate that the teaching of ethics by osmosis, 'add-ons' or the compliant introjection of 'rules' or group 'norms', without ongoing critical reflection or constant grappling with the complexities of ethical and moral decisions, is not enough. In addition, philosophical training is essential since some research and wise opinion have indicated that the intellectual ability to deal effectively with complexity is a pre-requisite for dealing intelligently, compassionately and competently with ethical issues (e.g. Pope and Vetter, 1992; Pope et al., 1995).

How can we foster such abilities and moral courage in training and supervision? We would suggest that a 'learning by enquiry' research-minded attitude to ethics and professional practice is more likely to keep us all questing and questioning than to lead to 'conformist obedience', cavalier carelessness or professional collusion.

> . . . good enough reason to make training in standards and ethics a formal part of every counselling course. There will be gains to clients in a greater sense of personal safety. Counsellors will also benefit because a sound understanding of standards and ethics is something which can unite counsellors from many different orientations. (Bond, 1993, p. 208)

In conclusion

Of course the very fact of participation in this study demonstrates a willingness on the part of our respondent colleagues (21% of a sample of 1000) to think about, reflect on and do something to enhance the ethical understanding and practice of our professions. It also shows good and effective collegial relationship manifesting as an enacted value of deep and serious concern about own and others' conduct and the principles of our professions.

Finally, as researchers and professional colleagues of our respondents we were very touched by the respondents who expressed appreciation for our work. This included addressing us by name, 'I hope this helps', suggestions for improved practice, 'Thank you' and 'I appreciate your efforts in doing something about this very delicate and painful as well as important issue.'

We in turn heartily thank all our respondents who have helped in the research so far, trusting that future generations will benefit from our joint efforts.

We would like to end on a quote from Hannah Arendt (1964) who demanded that

> human beings be capable of telling right from wrong even when all they have to guide them is their own judgment, which, moreover, happens to be completely at odds with what they must regard as the unanimous opinion of all these around them. . . . These few who were still able to tell right from wrong went really only by their own judgments [during the Holocaust], and they did so freely; there were no rules to be abided by . . . because no rules existed for the unprecedented (pp. 294, 295)

We may yet face many unprecedented events and currents in the ethics and morals of our professional worlds of psychotherapy.

Anyone reading this who would like to be confidentially interviewed about their experience of ethical dilemmas or their experience of complaints procedures, ethics investigations or any restated issues should contact Petrūska, who is continuing with the qualitative interviews of anyone who has been involved in

informal or formal complaints procedures. In this way concerns about our professional ethics can be considered, communicated, addressed and perhaps improved without the painful personalisation and fear or experience of retaliation that is sometimes the result of responsible involvement according to our ethical duties. In this way the principle of beneficence can also be served.

Address

POPAN (The Prevention of Professional Abuse Network) 1 Wyvil Close, 10 Wyvil Road, London SW8 2TG. Tel. 020 7622 6334.

References

APA (1992) Ethical principles of psychologists and code of conduct. American Psychologist, 47, 1597–611.

Arendt, H. (1964) Eichmann in Jerusalem: A Report on the Banality of Evil. New York: Viking Press.

BAC (1992) Code of ethics and practice for counsellors/counselling skills/trainers/supervision of counsellors (4 leaflets). Leicester: British Association for Counselling.

Bauman, Z. (1993) Postmodern Ethics. Oxford: Blackwell.

Bernard, J. L. and Jara, C. S. (1995) The failure of clinical psychology graduate students to apply understood ethical principles. In D. N. Bersoff, Ethical Conflicts in Psychology, pp. 67–71, Washington, DC: American Psychological Association.

Bersoff, D. N. (1995) Ethical Conflicts in Psychology. Washington, DC: American Psychological Association.

Bond, T. (1993) Standards and Ethics for Counselling in Action, London: Sage.

BPS (1995) Division of Clinical Psychology, Professional Practice Guidelines. Leicester: British Psychological Society.

Clarkson, P. (1995) The Therapeutic Relationship. London: Whurr.

Clarkson, P. (1996) The Bystander. London: Whurr.

Clarkson, P. and Lindsay, G. (1997) Secrets, sex and money: ethical dilemmas of psychologists and psychotherapists. Poster displayed at British Psychological Society Division of Counselling Psychology Annual Conference, 30 May–1 June, Stratford-upon-Avon.

Clarkson, P. and Lindsay, G. (1999) Collegial duty as a principle of self-regulation (Sham, shambles or shared responsibility), submitted to Counselling.

Collis, W., (1998) 'Judge over your shoulder'. Judicial Review: Balancing the scales. Revised May. The Treasury Solicitor's Department in conjunction with the Cabinet Office (OPSS) Department Divison.

Friedson, E. (1970) The Profession of Medicine. New York: Dodd, Mead.

Gawthop, J. C. and Uhleman, M. R. (1992) Effects of the problem-solving approach to ethics training. Professional Psychology: Research and Practice, 23(1): 38–42.

Lindsay, G. and Clarkson, P. (1999) Ethical dilemmas of psychotherapists. The Psychologist, 12(3), 20–3.

Lindsay, G. and Colley A. (1995) Ethical dilemmas of members of the British Psychological Society, The Psychologist, 8, 448–53.

Lunt, I. (1999) President's column: disciplining psychologists. The Psychologist: Bulletin of the British Psychological Society, 12, 59.

Macdonald, K.M. (1995) The Sociology of the Professions. London: Sage.

Marzillier, J. (1999) Training of clinical psychologists in ethical issues. Clinical Psychology Forum, 123, 43–7.

Palmer Barnes, F. (1998) Complaints and Grievances in Psychotherapy – A Handbook of Ethical Practice, London: Routledge.

Pope, K.S. (1989) Teacher-student sexual intimacy. In G. O. Gabbard (ed.), Sexual Exploitation in Professional Relationships, pp. 163–76. Washington, DC: American Psychiatric Press.

Pope, K.S. and Vetter, V.A. (1992) Ethical dilemmas encountered by members of the American Psychological Association. American Psychologist, 47, 397–411.

Pope, K.S., Tabachnick, B.G. and Keith-Spiegel, P. (1995) Ethics of practice: the beliefs and behaviors of psychologists as therapists, in D. N. Bersoff, Ethical Conflicts in Psychology, pp. 72–84. Washington, DC: American Psychological Association.

Popper, K. (1992) In Search of a Better World. London: Routledge & Kegan Paul.

Stone, A.S. (1983) Sexual misconduct by psychiatrists: the ethical and clinical dilemma of confidentiality. American Journal of Psychiatry, 140(2), 195–7.

Szasz, T. (1999) Discretion as power: Language and money and status in the situation called psychotherapy. Universities Psychotherapy Association, Review No. 7: 1–14.

Thompson, A. (1990) Guide to Ethical Practice in Psychotherapy. Chichester: John Wiley.

UKCP (1995–6) Ethical Guidelines of the United Kingdom Council for Psychotherapy, in National Register of Psychotherapists.

Item 8
Libel, Slander and Defamation and their Derivatives in Professional Codes of Ethics

Petrŭska Clarkson and Vincent Keter

Shakespeare's Othello puts the case thus:

> Who steals my purse steals trash;
> 'tis something, nothing; ...
> But he that filches from me my good name
> Robs me of that which not enriches him,
> and makes me poor indeed. (*Othello* III.iii.157–160)

Every profession's ethical codes contain clauses (which may be differently phrased) which proscribe the disparagement of the reputation of colleagues – especially to trainees, supervisees and clients.

British Psychological Society

The BPS's Professional Practice Guidelines (BPS 1995a), under the heading 2.2 'Relationships with colleagues' require that:

> 2.2.1 Psychologists should adhere to high standards of behaviour towards members of their own and other professions, within an atmosphere of mutual respect. They should not publicly denigrate colleagues regarding their personal, professional or ethical conduct. (p. 16)

Other example items from the BPS Code of Conduct:

> Psychologists shall conduct themselves in their professional activities in a way that does not damage the interest of the recipients of their services or participants in their research and does not inappropriately undermine public confidence in their ability or that of other psychologists and members of other

150

professions to carry our their professional duties. . . . 5.3 not exploit any relationship of influence or trust which exists between colleagues, those under their tuition, or those in receipt of their services to further the gratification of their personal desires; . . . and 5.10 bring allegations of misconduct by a professional colleague to the attention of those charged with the responsibility to investigate them, doing so without malice and with no breaches of confidentiality other than those necessary to the proper investigatory processes and when the subject of allegations themselves, they shall take all reasonable steps to assist those charged with responsibility to investigate them. (BPS, 1995b, p. 453)

Gestalt Psychotherapy Training Institute

6.7 Responsibilities to GPTI Colleagues and Other Professional Groups
6.7.1 Members should conduct themselves in ways which promote public confidence in psychotherapy. Any reference made to or about Gestalt psychotherapists, practitioners in other fields of psychotherapy or members of other professions should be respectful.
6.7.2 If a Member is seriously concerned about the conduct of another Member, he or she should seek to discuss this with the person in question. If the matter cannot be resolved satisfactorily, then the Institute's Complaints Procedure should be implemented. (GPTI, May 1996)

Institute for Transactional Analysis in Britain

3. Members of the ITA shall, in their public statements, whether written or verbal, refrain from derogatory statements, inferences and/or innuendoes that disparage the standing qualifications or character of members, as well as other psychotherapeutic practitioners, bearing in mind their responsibility as representatives of ITA and of Transactional Analysis. (ITA statement of ethics, p. 1)

United Kingdom Council for Psychotherapy

The UKCP code states:

2.11 Detrimental Behaviour
2.11 (i) Psychotherapists are required to refrain from any behaviour that may be detrimental to the profession, to colleagues or to trainees.
2.11 (ii) Psychotherapists are required to take appropriate action in accordance with Clause 5.8 with regard to the behaviour of a colleague which may be detrimental to the profession, to colleagues or to trainees.(Ethical Guidelines of the UKCP, 1993, p. 1)

British Association for Counselling

The relevant item from the BAC Code of Ethics and Practice reads as follows:

B.2.4 To other Counsellors:
2.4.1 Counsellors should not conduct themselves in their counselling-related

activities in ways which undermine public confidence in either their role as a
counsellor or in the work of other counsellors.

2.4.2 If a counsellor suspects misconduct by another counsellor which
cannot be resolved or remedied after discussion with the counsellor
concerned, they should implement the Complaints Procedure, doing so
without breaches of confidentiality other than those necessary for investigating the complaint (see B9). (BAC, 1992, p. 4)

Qualified privilege

[Qualified privilege is] the defence that a statement cannot be made the
subject of an action for defamation because it was made on a privileged
occasion and was not made maliciously, for an improper motive. Qualified
privilege covers statements made fairly in situations in which there is a
legal or moral obligation to give the information and the person to whom
it is given has a corresponding duty or interest to receive it and when
someone is acting in defence of his own property or reputation. (Martin,
1997)

If any ethics procedure is not subject to qualified privilege, as it appears
that of at least one new university is, it mandates against any legitimate
complaint being fairly heard without the threat of defamation. Since
defamation actions are prohibitively expensive, it may again prevent all
those except the very rich from acting appropriately in the execution of
their moral and professional ethical duty.

The main consequence of the distinction between the two forms of action
[libel and slander] is that in libel the law presumes damage has been suffered
and the plaintiff is not required to prove any loss. In slander, however, the
plaintiff will have to satisfy the court that he or she has suffered financial
damage arising from the defamatory statement'. There are exceptions to this
rule which include slanderous statements which 'disparage a person in his or
her business, calling or profession'.
    In fact, it does not require any great amount of special knowledge or skill
to identify defamatory statements or acts. Most people know when a statement exposes someone to 'hatred, ridicule or contempt' or lowers him 'in
the estimation of right-thinking members of [a] society generally'. (Crone,
1991, pp. 2–4)

References

BAC (1992) Code of Ethics and Practice for Counsellors. Amended, AGM September
    1992. British Association for Counselling.
BPS (1995) Division of Clinical Psychology, Professional Practice Guidelines.
    Leicester: British Psychological Society.
Crone, T. (1991) Law and the Media, 2nd edn. Oxford: Butterworth-Heinemann.
Gestalt Psychotherapy Training Institute (1996) Code of Professional Practice.
    London: GPTI.

ITA Statement of Ethics.

Martin, E.A. (ed.) (1997) A Dictionary of Law, 4th edn. Oxford: Oxford University Press.

UKCP (1993) Ethical guidelines. In the UKCP National Register, p. xi. London: United Kingdom Council for Psychotherapy.

CHAPTER 9
The Ethical Dimensions of Supervision

LESLEY MURDIN AND PETRŪSKA CLARKSON

Theory and practice

Supervision as an ethical enterprise for carers is, we know, a multidimensional enterprise which requires both the exercise of considerable skill and also an awareness of the part played by ethics and values in all that we do. Psychotherapy has so far resisted attempts to see it and practise it as a science with a body of tested theory and a range of techniques agreed and practised by all. The Strasbourg Declaration of the European Association for Psychotherapy declares that psychotherapy is a scientific discipline governed by scientific method. We all position ourselves somewhere along the spectrum that leads from replicability and generalisable truths at one end to the art of responding to the individual and his or her unique self at the other end. Nevertheless, to ignore research findings from psychology, physics and mathematics seems to blindfold us unnecessarily and on the other hand, not to spend time considering the part played by the values on which a psychotherapist and supervisor might be basing their work would be equally disabling.

Supervision has its laws. The BAC was the first organisation to write a code of ethics and practice for supervisors (BAC, 1995) although the British Association for Psychoanalytic and Psychodynamic Supervision (BAPPS) has since produced its own code as well. These codes set out guidelines and requirements for attitudes and conduct in the practice of supervision. These work well for the majority of supervisory relationships most of the time, but sooner or later everyone comes across a conflict or an ambivalence where the code is not sufficient guidance.

Because the spirit of the law is as important as the letter, we also need to consider the values that underlie the work of the supervisor (Clarkson and Murdin, 1996). Since the work of psychotherapy supervision is in relationship and about relationship, any discussion of the ethical questions facing supervisors will have to take into account the complexities of all the relationships involved in supervision. We are always working in supervision with a role that may range between levels of responsibility depending on whether the work is with a trainee or an experienced colleague. The supervisor shifts into a different register but the exact positioning of a given piece of work may need careful thought.

There are legal and ethical considerations as well as the more personal ones of taste and inclination and very importantly the model of work being supervised which will inevitably affect the values underlying the supervision. For example, at its most obvious, the importance of working with countertransference may vary depending on the extent to which the model emphasises intra-psychic processes as distinct from inter-psychic. We may think of these aspects of the work in metaphorical terms as the depth at which it is carried out. In addition to the dimension of depth, we are also bound to be concerned with the topographical dimensions of the relationships involved

A map of supervision

Supervision involves an extremely complex interacting system. Figure 9.1 shows the basic subsystems which can be said to be present in any supervision. They all have their own values attached and their own ethical, moral and legal compulsions both conscious and unconscious.

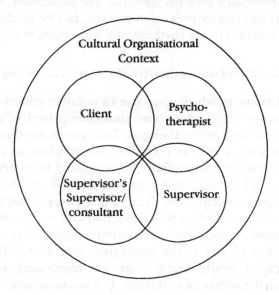

Figure 9.1: Overlapping supervisory systems (version of a diagram first published in Clarkson, 1998).

This map provides a way of diagrammatically locating where the supervisory dilemma is most concentrated, and therefore where the supervisor may most fruitfully focus attention. The discussion which follows takes the supervisor's vantage point.

The supervisor's relationship with the supervisee's client

The supervisor's primary concern should be with the welfare of the client. Our concern in this chapter is to look at the conflicts that might be implied by the supervisor's concern for the client having to meet the concern for and the actual contract with the supervisee.

Consider the following dilemma. A psychotherapist, Mrs P, is seeing a very angry client, Mrs C. The client makes great demands on the psychotherapist. She has suffered a great many losses in that both her parents died when she was small and she was brought up by a succession of aunts who passed her from one to another like a parcel. She now has two children of her own, aged three and five, and no partner present. She is tempted to hit the children and has been coming to counselling for several months in order to try to understand this violence in herself.

The psychotherapist finds this whole subject difficult to work with and has just decided to go on a two-week holiday because she is overtired. The supervisor knows that she is tired but also suspects that she is not dealing well with the resonances that this client's situation has with the psychotherapist's own background. The supervisor may well have no choice in this matter over what is done, but he or she does have a choice over whether to say anything, and how much to say.

The supervisor's relationship with the supervisee's psychotherapist

Another relationship which gives rise to possible ethical and technical difficulties is the relationship, often unacknowledged, of the supervisor with the supervisee's psychotherapist. This is a relationship that is potentially fraught with conflict or collusion. The conclusions that the supervisor draws about the psychotherapist are bound to be deductions from the supervisee's behaviour and responses and will tend to come to mind when there are problems. The thought that arises is that this blind spot should have been picked up by the psychotherapist. Questions about the psychotherapist's competence, motivation or insight may arise.

In the case of Mrs P, the supervisor might well hope that the psychotherapist would know what was happening and would be working with the source of avoidance. This is a reasonable hope, but Mrs P is likely to be avoiding in her own therapy as well as in her work. The supervisor then grows more and more angry with Mrs P's

psychotherapist and more and more inclined to intrude on the therapeutic work. In addition, the supervisee may sometimes talk about the
psychotherapist or the therapy. A supervisee may appropriately
mention that it is difficult to work with a client who is afraid of cancer
because he is going through his own fear of dying of cancer in his
therapy. This point of contact is helpful but there are other sorts of
overlap that may cause much more conscious or unconscious difficulty.
For example, Mrs P says, 'I decided to give the client a hug because that
is what my psychotherapist does.' Obviously this can be discussed in
relation to the client and the kind of work being offered. It may also
lead to judgement of the psychotherapist by the supervisor. If the
judgement is negative or dubious, it may lead to an unconscious
condemnation of the supervisee: how can this person do good work if
his therapy is dubious?

Therapy of the supervisee is also a fruitful ground for conflicts to
arise for the supervisee between the values of the supervisor and the
values of his or her psychotherapist. Usually, one would hope that these
values could be brought into the open and discussed. A supervisee may
say, 'I did what my psychotherapist would have done, but I know it's not
what you would do.' I have to find out first whether that is true first of all
and also decide how to deal with the possible conflict.

Often the conflict is over technique, and yet fundamental values may
reside in the choice of technique. Recently a psychotherapist was
expressing a conflict because her psychotherapist is very open and
willing to answer questions and make personal revelations. One way of
working usually implies interpreting rather than answering or reacting
immediately. With an area of technique such as the acceptability of
touch, the difference will be obvious and may be able to be addressed. It
does, of course, represent a difference of theory and inevitably, beneath
that, a difference of values. Not touching could imply an overvaluing of
the mind as opposed to the body. It could more constructively imply an
orientation which stresses the development of the capacity for thought
and reflection as opposed to gratification. In any case, a supervisee is
likely to be greatly influenced by what he or she has grown used to in
therapy. If the supervisor appears to disapprove of the psychotherapist,
that may cause damage just where the psychotherapist is most in need of
the possibility of useful work. Sometimes, however, the supervisee is
ashamed of what his or her psychotherapist does, wishes to treasure it in
secret and will not expose it to the potential harsh judgement of the
supervisor. This may or may not arise from a realistic assessment of what
the supervisor actually thinks. Often these areas of conflict remain
hidden unless a particularly difficult client brings them unavoidably to
the surface. Secrets that are felt to be guilty may arise and lead to
confused or ineffectual supervision.

The supervisor's relationship with the supervisor's consultant

The concept of supervising supervision is relatively new to psychotherapy although the BAC requires it for the supervision of counsellors and most supervision trainings would also require it. We would like to note here the way in which its increased relational complexity allows for greater resonance and complexity of values and ethical systems. At the most obvious level, the supervisor at the end of the chain has an ethical responsibility for what he or she knows is happening all the way down the line, but may have a primary duty to the immediate relationship with the supervisor presenting work. This is fine while all is going well, but may become difficult to manage when conflicts of values arise at any point in the complex structure.

The supervisor's relationship with society

The outside circle on the diagram is to represent the enclosing arms of the social and cultural context in which the supervision takes place. All supervision happens within cultural contexts of gender, ethnicity, ability, class and many other factors. In addition, supervision is always taking place within or on behalf of an agency or institution. Even when in independent private practice, psychotherapists and supervisors are still connected, at the very least, through the ethics codes of their professional societies. Many supervisors are paid for or funded by the NHS, a GP practice or a training body. Some are working within the context of a private company or a voluntary body such as a charity. Each of these will set its own ethical standards, and conflicts will arise from the choices of priorities and duties that must be made.

The supervision may take place in the context of a private practice where there is no responsible body other than the therapists' and supervisors' training organisations and registering bodies. These gaze with a watchful parental eye, increasingly so as complaints and media interest in our shortcomings force themselves on our attention. Whatever the institutional context, we are all limited and shaped by social and political assumptions and norms. The supervisor works within a society is undecided about the value of psychotherapy or counselling; that has no consensus about the importance of religion; that is still fighting over the meaning of political correctness and damage done by language.

Samuels (1993) has developed our understanding of the psychotherapist's relationship to the political psyche of his clients, and the supervisor might well consider the effect of his or her own political convictions on the work. In addition, the political and social context determines such questions as who can be seen for psychotherapy (see Appendix 1 in Clarkson, 1996). We will come back to the ethics of assessment later, but there is research which indicates the difficulty for ethnic minorities in reaching the therapy that might benefit them. We also know of the ethical problems involved in financial disenfranchisement of large numbers of people. Eurocentrism of both theory and technique is an issue which must be of concern to supervisors as well as to psychotherapists (Clarkson and Nippoda, 1997).

Conflicts in supervision

Having mapped out the territory in terms of depth and the overlapping circles of influence, we come now to look at some of the specific kinds of conflict that arise in supervision. The diagram in Figure 9.1 has one great advantage. It shows clear boundaries. These are of course metaphorical and illusory. In reality one of our areas of greatest difficulty but also of the most potential for growth and development is in drawing and shaping boundaries that are sufficiently firm to feel safe for the self, but sufficiently flexible to allow contact with another.

If we begin with the psychotherapist–supervisor relationship itself, we can see that much has been written on the main aspects of the supervisory relationship and the dangers of overemphasising one role at the expense of others. The supervisor must not become the friend, the psychotherapist or the teacher too much, not allowing any element of those roles to become dominant or the supervision itself will be contaminated. Each of these roles has its theoretical and technical problems and also each has an ethical dimension. To take the possibility of friendship with a supervisee first, some regard supervision as a refreshing change from the clearer more rigorous boundaries of therapy itself. With a supervisee one may ask ordinary social questions: 'How are you?' might be permissible, might be regarded as a necessary enquiry in order to assess how the work is likely to be done. This is a small example of the way in which the different tone of supervision may inhabit a grey area between therapy and something much closer to friendship, even when one is working with trainees. As the supervision proceeds along the spectrum to where one is working with colleagues who are themselves experienced therapists, the question of how much friendship is ethical becomes more and more difficult. Ethics cannot be divorced from a theoretical rationale, of course.

Ethical principles in the practice of psychotherapy are derived from various sources: the Judaeo-Christian tradition of ethical absolutes modified by Utilitarian principles of the greatest good of the greatest number. These principles themselves have to be filtered through the understanding of the instinctual wishes and impulses that we have derived from psychoanalysis and analytical psychology. We would be unlikely to say that something is wrong from an ethical point of view if it was clearly for the good of the client and psychotherapist and did not affect anyone else adversely. When it comes to friendship or social relationships between supervisor and psychotherapist, we have on the one hand the imperative that says something like 'love one another'. On the other hand, we have to see transference and parallel process and those may not show unless there is a fairly blank screen to reflect them. That is a theoretical reason to maintain a clear boundary. Other reasons deriving from ethical traditions would be similar to those governing other professions where it is not acceptable to provide professional services to friends or family. Judgement is clouded by emotional involvement and where unpleasant decisions must be made, a close emotional tie will make them more difficult if not impossible. It is difficult enough to disentangle the supervisor's countertransference response to the supervisee from that to the client's material, without adding in the complications of a close or social relationship to the supervisee. Looking at the close links between theory and ethics, we inevitably see the difficulty of making any judgements about colleagues and friends supervising each other.

Many experienced therapists form pairs or small groups for supervision and work together for many years so that they know each other very well. Clearly this is a very different kind of supervision from supervising trainees. It would be foolish to say that it is unethical or unhelpful. On the other hand, it requires some discipline to make it bite. The group or the pair presumably need to ask each other from time to time whether they are sufficiently critical and perceptive of each other's weaknesses. Guggenbühl-Craig (1971) comes to the conclusion that the only thing that will save us from identification with the archetype of the charlatan or the charismatic leader is the honest appraisal of friends.

Perhaps in supervision, therefore, there is room for friendship if it already exists and is used well. On the other hand, if it is introduced into a supervisory relationship to satisfy the therapist's erotic or narcissistic needs it is unethical and may well decrease the scope for useful parallel process or for necessary constructive criticism. Supervision often gives us trouble with our position in relation to the archetypes of the wise old man or woman, as well as the charlatan or leader. We all like to be admired, respected, as the experienced colleague or the teacher. Again, we would all agree that a supervisor may employ some teaching techniques and, particularly in training, supervision has some responsibility to pass on ideas, theoretical knowledge, reading, etc. and to try to bring out the best from supervises.

On the other hand, the supervisor needs to resist the temptation to enjoy the teaching function too much. The supervision can become a seminar in which there is a mutual enjoyment of intellectual discussion. Technically this would cease to be useful supervision because it would be unlikely to lead to helpful developments of the therapy for the client. Ethically it is problematic because the supervisor's task is to develop the psychotherapist as a psychotherapist in all respects. The supervisor may be modelling only one aspect of what a psychotherapist needs to be and, undoubtedly, parallel process working backwards may lead to a restricted functioning in the therapy. Since all supervisors must presumably themselves be therapists, there is always a pull towards becoming the psychotherapist of the supervisee. The boundary between the two is often difficult to see and to maintain but it needs constant vigilance. We have come across fairly dramatic crossings of this boundary.

Recently a supervisee came saying that she needed supervision because her previous supervisor had been so interested in her, and so uninterested in her clients, that they had both decided that she had better go to him for therapy and find another supervisor. This requires suspended judgement. What is coming across is a blurred boundary and a failure of the supervisory responsibility. This has to be held in suspension because it is only a second-hand account, as always. At least the nature of the relationship was understood and the important thing is always to make it conscious and clear to both parties.

The opposite tendency is revealed by a different example. A trainee had need of extra supervision and reported that his psychotherapist had offered to supervise some client work. This also would have been separate from the therapy time and would have been presumably clearly distinct to both people, but the ethical question remains: is it possible to be in this literal way both psychotherapist and supervisor? The answer seems to be that if the work is psychodynamic at all, and transference and countertransference are used, two relationships at once would be confusing to say the least. It is also important to note that to conduct a therapy relationship and a supervisory relationship at the same time with the same person contravenes the BAC Code of Ethics for supervisors (1995, B 1.6). Boundaries are important in individual relationships; they are, if anything, even more contentious within organisations or institutions carrying out counselling or psychotherapy.

Conflicts over boundaries are bound to arise if there is any overlapping of supervision and line management. A line manager is unlikely to be able to maintain the boundary between the needs of the organisation and the needs of the client. Confidentiality is also likely to be difficult to maintain. Managers need to manage waiting lists and throughput and will want to know the reasons why certain clients need more time. A supervisor is often the person who has to hold the difficult interface between the pressures of time and money on the one hand and an assessment of the benefit that may be possible on the other. This is an unenviable place to be. Psychiatrists are often unwilling to leave therapists and supervisors to go at their own pace and may, because of the pressures that they themselves are under, seek to know more of the detail of the therapy than is appropriate.

Training organisations provide some of the most difficult boundary problems in that they demand assessment of trainees. The supervisor's assessment is often the most important element in a training and carries the most weight. Assessing trainees is a skilled and demanding job, but is something that most supervisors have to pick up either from their own internalised experience or from other experience such as teaching. There are profound ethical questions involved.

A frequent conflict is between the need or wish to give the dubious trainee time to develop and the question of whether he or she is actually depriving clients of a better experience with another psychotherapist. This is inevitably a difficult question to answer as it brings us up against the inevitable lack of direct knowledge of the client. Nevertheless, a trainee may show the same difficulties with a number of clients, as long as the training requires that a number of clients must be seen. If the lack of progress and helpfulness shows itself in several cases, the supervisor may well have grounds to draw the boundary and say that this person is not good enough at the work to continue.

Useful questions that tend to bring out the essentials are:

- Is the trainee able to give this client the opportunity to develop further?
- When it is a question of qualification?
- Would you refer patients to this person?

The issues raised by assessment are, of course, numerous. Much of the responsibility will be held by the training organisation concerned, but supervisors will still have their own consciences and their own professional responsibility.

The supervisor's responsibility

One of the major ethical problems for supervisors is to determine the extent and the limits of the supervisor's responsibility. We envisage the responsibility of the supervisor to lie in four main areas:

- for assessment and management of the client
- for competence and ethical/professional behaviour of the psychotherapist
- to the organisation that employs or sponsors the therapy, society at large
- to the profession as a whole.

Within these four main spheres, there is a great deal of room for debate about how far the supervisor can and should be responsible. There is, of course, a difference between the supervisor of a trainee or of an employee within an organisation where there is a clear contractual responsibility, and the supervisor of a qualified and experienced psychotherapist. We could simply say that the contract between supervisor and psychotherapist must make clear the extent and limits of responsibility. This is important and there should be some sort of contract and understanding, but whenever a difficulty arises, there is likely to be a problem in interpreting the contract and deciding just what the supervisor will do and say. In the first areas, for example, the supervisor will presumably hear about the assessment of clients.

Trainees may not have freedom of choice about whom they see and may not be doing the actual assessments. More experienced therapists, on the other hand, are probably assessing their own clients and deciding whether or not to see a difficult client. This is precisely the sort of case that is most likely to be brought to the supervisor.

The following is an example of the kind of case where the supervisor may feel responsible for what happens and will have to decide whether in fact he or she does has any responsibility beyond facilitating the supervisee.

> A fairly experienced, qualified psychotherapist brought an assessment to discuss. The client was a man of 43 subject to fits of rage at work and at home. He said that he wants to be a better husband and father. He had been to Relate for a few sessions and says that he found it quite helpful because 'it got my wife off my back for a while'. Recently he had begun to hit his wife again.
>
> The history was problematic. He had very little memory of it but had been told by his brother that he was neglected by his mother who preferred the older daughter and found boys a problem. The father had left home when the client was 2 or 3. He remembered best the years from 16 to 20 when he went round with a football gang. He had been convicted of four offences involving violence but none so serious that he was given a custodial sentence. He was fined and cautioned.
>
> He settled down after he got married to a strong woman , but he says that he finds it difficult to be what she wants him to be and particularly to talk to her. She has urged him to come for therapy. The psychotherapist is deeply ambivalent. She is a woman of about 55 and not easily frightened. She says that she was struck by this patient's red hair and the fact that he never made eye contact. She says, 'I can't make out whether he is just not used to being open or whether there is really something for me to be frightened about.' There are indications that he is motivated to work but also questions about what kind of transference might be created with an older woman. In a bright and somewhat dismissive way, the psychotherapist brushes the problems to one side and says 'Well, I'll take him on. I think it'll be all right and I think he has potential to use this kind of work.'

The supervisor may see it as his or her job simply to support the psychotherapist or perhaps to go more deeply into the ambivalence. How far does the responsibility both for the client and the psychotherapist go? If the supervisor's countertransference experience of the client is negative and disturbing, would it be right to refuse to ask the psychotherapist not to take the client or even to refuse to supervise him? What if the supervisor is very doubtful that a particular client can make use of psychoanalytic work at all?

In this case, the psychotherapist confessed to having omitted to make any sort of trial interpretation or to have forgotten the outcome of whatever was said. Not only does assessment raise questions about the responsibility of the supervisor; there are many ongoing matters of management and technique that we all face frequently. Clients who are suicidal, potentially psychotic, severely regressed or physically ill all raise difficult questions and can put enormous strain on the supervisor's trust of the psychotherapist. The temptation may well be to take too much responsibility and tell the psychotherapist what to do. This may be the safest policy, but is it supervision?

On the other hand, there is an unresolved question about the supervisor's legal responsibility. As far as the law is concerned in the UK at the moment, there is no definitive answer as supervisor involvement in, for example, a tort of negligence or a criminal offence has not been tested. Legal opinion, however, is that a supervisor could be an accessory. It behoves us therefore to take reasonable care for the well being, not only of the client but of others who may potentially be harmed.

Supervisors, like other citizens, may well find themselves with knowledge that is difficult or dangerous either to use or to suppress. Clearly, a satisfactory supervisory relationship will allow these sorts of questions to be worked through so that the resulting practice will be the consensus of both supervisor and psychotherapist. As long as this is the case, ethical codes and codes of practice will simply be part of the background and will inform but not need to dominate practice. Under the pressure of a stressful or difficult problem, however, the consensus may break down. The psychotherapist may do or fail to do what the supervisor thinks is essential. What does the supervisor do if the psychotherapist fails, for example, to get the client to speak to the GP or to deal satisfactorily with possible child abuse? As in the therapeutic relationship, the first priority is to have the client or psychotherapist to deal with the problem him or herself, but if that does not or cannot happen, then the supervisor may have to take responsibility and require certain action.

Organisational contexts

Taking responsibility may be helped if the work is being done within an organisation. A supervisor may then be able to discuss the difficulty with a legitimate source of authority such as the head of a clinic or service, and two people may then share the decision that needs to be made. On the other hand, organisations may require that supervisors take responsibility for such matters as reducing waiting lists, limiting the amount of time that any given client may have in therapy.

Overt or covert racism and prejudice may influence the availability and quality of client care and supervision. Working with supervisees and clients from a different ethnic or cultural background raises questions of awareness, personal values and discriminatory practice for the supervisor (BAC 1995, B.1.9). Such differences may range from gender to sexual practices to class. Arguments can be heard that mixed race supervisory relationships are inadvisable on the grounds that there is always a cultural power imbalance or on the theoretical issue that psychoanalytic theory is inherently eurocentric. Whatever the supervisor's views, he or she may need to be aware of the range of opinions and the need for addressing issues of difference very seriously (López, 1997).

The financial difficulties of the organisation will also impact on supervision either indirectly through client input or directly in, for example, limiting the amount of supervision available so that too many clients must be covered in too little time. Where supervision is in any way affected by managerial issues such as training opportunities, promotion, resource allocation, status or any other such factor of threat or reward, quality client supervision may become impossibly compromised in terms of authenticity, honesty and risk.

Organisational support may make some supervisory decisions easier or at least inevitable, but the supervisor will still be left with some of the most difficult problems. When a psychotherapist is ill, or becomes incompetent, in some cases, only a supervisor may know of practice that is unsafe or inadequate. On the other hand, when therapists are incompetent, they are likely to avoid supervisors altogether or hide the nature of the work that is being done.

Professional responsibility

One of the most difficult areas for many supervisors is to insist on detailed accounts of work with clients so that there is some chance of judging what the practice is like. Even if you are fairly sure that you are hearing the detail of what is going on, there is no easy way of judging where work that you do not like or do not approve of has become so bad as to be incompetent or unethical. A supervisor may have to judge whether it is better to continue supervising someone in the hope of improving the practice or whether he or she can no longer be associated with the work that is being done. If that point is reached, the supervisor may have to report the psychotherapist to a professional body and that is one of the most difficult things for anyone to do.

Under the heading of responsibility to colleagues and profession, supervisors must obviously consider whether a therapist's practice is likely to bring the profession into disrepute. Is it fair to land supervisors with this kind of guardianship role? Many of us have non-judgmental tendencies and have chosen this profession out of a desire to be neither a powerful participant nor totally a bystander (Clarkson, 1996). Often we find it contrary to both inclination and training to take responsibility for another. We still have to ask ourselves whether we can take on the role of supervisor if we are not prepared to take some responsibility. An example of this sort of difficulty has come to our notice. A psychotherapist has been hospitalised for mental illness but has recovered sufficiently to be discharged. The psychotherapist wishes to see his clients as soon as possible. The supervisor is the only person who is in a position to say whether or not the psychotherapist is fit to practise. A more common experience is bereavement, where the psychotherapist is obviously not functioning as well as usual – but where exactly do we draw the line and say that he or she must not work, especially as in many cases work is providing a form of therapy for the psychotherapist?

Most supervisors will sooner or later come across a problem with a supervisee that is not solved within the normal supervisory process. The avenues of discussion have been tried and suggested improvements or changes have been ignored. What happens then? According to recent research (Lindsay and Clarkson, 1999) the second ranking source of dilemmas for UKCP psychotherapists was colleagues' conduct. This indicates that supervisors are likely to come across conduct in supervisees which they cannot condone. The codes of conduct would require that the supervisor either makes a complaint against the psychotherapist to the relevant professional body or at least transfers him or her to another supervisor. This does not often happen in practice. We could all see reasons for this. Supervisees are a part of a practice and there are economic and conservative motives to keep the same person and hope that there will be some improvement.

Rationalising may also go on along the lines that the person needs time to improve, or is perhaps not quite as much at fault as may have appeared. Fundamentally, we are reluctant to invoke a disciplinary procedure or make any sort of complaint against a colleague. A supervisor understands only too well that a complaint would have to be well substantiated and the process would be time consuming and disturbing. We can certainly hope that the occasions on which there would be any question of such action would be rare, but perhaps supervisors need to be willing to accept that they do have a responsibility to the profession when they cannot find any way of amending a therapist's work.

References

BAC (1995) Code of Ethics for Supervisors. Rugby: British Association for Counselling.

Clarkson, P. (1996) The Bystander, London: Whurr.

Clarkson, P. (1997) Supervision in counselling, psychotherapy and health: An intervention priority sequencing model. European Journal for Counselling, Psychotherapy and Health, 1(2), 195–212.

Clarkson, P. and Murdin, L. (1996) When rules are not enough: the letter and spirit of the law. Counselling, 7,(1), 31–5.

Clarkson, P. and Nippoda, Y. (1997) Cross-cultural issues in counselling psychology practice: a qualitative study of one multicultural training organisation. In P. Clarkson (ed.) Counselling Psychology: Integrating Theory, Research and Supervised Practice, pp. 95–118. London: Routledge.

Guggenbühl-Craig, A. (1971) Power in the Helping Professions. Dallas, TX: Spring Publications.

Lindsay, G. and Clarkson, P. (1999) Ethical dilemmas of psychotherapists. The Psychotherapist, 12, 3: 20–3.

López, S.R. (1997) Cultural competence in psychotherapy: a guide for clinicians and their supervisors. In C.E. Watkins Jr (ed.), Handbook of Psychotherapy Supervision, pp.570–88. New York: Wiley.

Samuels, A. (1993) The Political Psyche. London: Routledge.

ITEM 9
What Happens if A Psychotherapist Dies?

BARBARA TRAYNOR AND PETRŪSKA CLARKSON

The role of the psychotherapeutic executor

This chapter is intended for counsellors and psychotherapists, and concerns the ethics and practicalities involved in appointing a psychotherapeutic executor in the event of death, illness or becoming incompetent to practise. It explores our responsibilities towards ourselves and our clients in these circumstances. The original idea came from Petrūska Clarkson and is included in the Code of Professional Practice of Metanoia Psychotherapy Training Institute (1990).

The guidelines and examples given here are not prescriptive. One possible option is offered, which has been found effective. The authors hope to engender discussion in an important and neglected area.

We have examined the Code of Ethics and Practice for Counsellors of the BAC (BAC, 1990), the ITAA Statement of Ethics (ITAA, 1989) and the Code of Ethics of the GPTI in the UK (GPTI, 1990). We think the ideas we express are implicit in the above codes but believe they should be made explicit.

There are four types of psychotherapist/client endings:

- client's planned termination
- client's unplanned termination
- psychotherapist's planned termination
- psychotherapist's unplanned termination.

Ideally we can take time to discuss and prepare for termination, preferably when both client and psychotherapist are agreed. As psychotherapists, we sometimes have to deal with clients who terminate suddenly, or when we consider the time is not right in view of the presenting problems. When we are responsible for the termination, for example for a pregnancy or a move, we can plan withdrawal. However, although much is written about the first three types of ending, less is written about unplanned termination by the psychotherapist and that is the focus of this chapter.

The implications of our long-term responsibilities to our clients are complex. They may ask, 'What happens to me if anything happens to you?' A more suspicious client maybe concerned about what happens to their notes. I (Barbara Traynor) have found that they are relieved that I have considered this eventuality, thereby acknowledging that I have a commitment to them that extends beyond the immediate.

Most psychotherapy books or texts assume that the practitioner is always alive and well. But psychotherapy is a profession practised by a large number of older people. There are few young psychotherapists, and often people work beyond the statutory retirement age. It is therefore essential to plan for how the client is to deal with termination if for some reason the psychotherapist is no longer available.

In the event of the psychotherapist's unplanned termination of contract, there is a caretaking responsibility. Clients are precious human beings who entrust themselves to our care and may be in various stages of vulnerability. They confide in us, and their records and psychological processes should be safeguarded. It is appropriate professional practice to take responsibility for the client in these circumstances, and to ensure that arrangements are made that are mindful of their continuing psychological journey and which protect confidentiality.

In a group practice, fellow psychotherapists can provide support, arrange referrals, etc., but we suggest that, no matter how small the practice, all counsellors and psychotherapists should write a 'letter of direction' to accompany their current legal will which includes instructions for the termination of their practice and appropriate care for clients, and inform their executors of the contents.

The appropriateness of informing the client about this arrangement, and whether or not it is discussed, depends upon the individual client. For example, someone whose parents died when they were young may have problems making a therapeutic alliance. If they are concentrating on early issues, it may be important to bring this into focus. Another client might ask directly about it. Equally, if you have any reason to believe that a client has deep-rooted or out-of-awareness fears about the death of another person, it might be appropriate to discuss the issue. The act of making a will has to do with facing up to one's own death and dispensability. It is particularly important for psychotherapists to do this so that they can help clients to deal with issues of death, dying and mortality. In order to be able to leave, I need to ensure my affairs are in order. By bringing this into focus for the client, the therapist is, amongst other things, modelling self-support.

It would be preferable to choose as psychotherapeutic executor a fellow practitioner, someone who is not so close as to be emotionally bereft at one's loss but close enough to be familiar with one's way of working and sympathetic to the idiosyncrasies of the filing system. There is a considerable amount of work involved in the execution of these duties so it is important that a proviso for the psychotherapeutic executor to claim expenses for the estate is written into the letter of direction.

Practicalities

Outlined below are some of the issues I (Barbara Traynor) have covered.

- Instructions to ensure that my psychotherapeutic executor and the two executors of my estate will contact each other.
- Instructions about gaining access to my flat, study and records.
- Information about where my files are kept. My practice file contains names, addresses, phone numbers and GP details of my current clients. At the front of the file I have written a detailed explanation of the key. I have used coloured stickers to denote who is in my various groups, who is in training in what discipline (e.g. gestalt, transactional analysis or counselling) and who is seeing me for supervision. In this way I have ensured that clients can be referred appropriately.
- Some clients have given me personal letters and material to 'hold' for them. These are kept separately and clearly marked as the clients may wish to reclaim their property.
- In order to ensure confidentiality, when a client leaves my practice I go through their notes, removing their names and material which will obviously identify them. I keep their notes in a plastic numbered envelope. A card index system is kept separately, so that I may relocate their notes should they return to my practice.
- Instructions to the executor to destroy all past and current client notes and references. I give details of where my tapes are stored and instructions to wipe them all and retain them for use in the executor's practice.

Instructions as to disposal of photocopied material, articles, journals, books on child development, health, philosophy, psychology, psychotherapy and notes from workshops I have attended. Instructions to keep any books, notes, stationery for the executor's practice as she deems useful. Otherwise to offer them for sale as a charitable contribution to training bursaries.

- Instructions to send my accounts, petty cash receipts, vouchers, etc., to my accountant for auditing; I give details of where they are filed. An outlined procedure for the aftercare of my clients includes:

- contacting all clients as soon as possible
- arranging for a facilitator to take my groups and, where appropriate, to do bereavement work
- arranging for a facilitator to see individual clients and continue in bereavement process with them until they have either transferred or terminated, so that the transition can be dealt with appropriately.

Ethics

The BAC stresses the counsellor's responsibility for maintaining confidentiality includes personal information 'which may result in identification of the client' (BAC, 1990, B4.2, p. 7). The GPTI's code of ethics states that 'All exchanges between client and Gestalt psychotherapist must be regarded as confidential' (GPTI, 1990, 2, p. 5). The BAC requires that the counsellor 'Should not counsel when their functioning is impaired due to personal or emotional difficulties, illness, disability, alcohol, drugs or for any other reason' (1990, 2,2,18, p. 5). GPTI states that 'The welfare of the individual client must be the therapist's first concern' (1990, 1, p.5). The ITAA (1989) combines a relevant statement on confidentiality and professional responsibility:

> However, certain professional responsibilities continue beyond the termination of the contract. They include, but are not limited to, the following: (a) maintenance of agreed-upon confidentiality; (b) avoidance of any exploitation of the former relationship; (c) provision for any needed follow-up care. (8, p. 78)

They further state that:

> If members of the ITAA become aware that personal conflicts or medical problems might interfere with their ability to carry out a contractual relationship, they must either terminate the contract in a professionally responsible manner, or ensure that the client has the full information needed to make a decision about remaining in the contractual relationship. (11, 78)

Although none of these ethical codes deals specifically with the issue of the psychotherapist's unplanned termination, it seems to us that this article reflects the spirit of their humanistic existential philosophy and follows good counselling and psychotherapy practice.

We look forward with interest to hearing the opinions of our colleagues.

Discussion issues

- What would happen to your clients if something happened to you, which precluded you working or making any necessary arrangements?

- How do you imagine individual clients would react if you were to die?
- If you were to die without having left adequate provision for clients to be contacted and referred appropriately, might this present a specific negative repetitive experience for any of your clients?
- It has been said that record keeping from a liability perspective is a compilation of evidence of the adequacy of care a patient has received. Do your records reflect the quality of your work and would this be evident to a reader?

References

BAC (1990) Code of Ethics and Practice for Counsellors. Rugby: British Association for Counselling.

GPTI (1990) Code of Ethics. London: Gestalt Psychotherapy Training Institute.

ITAA (1989) Statement of Ethics. San Francisco: International Transactional Analysis Association.

Metanoia Psychotherapy Training Institute (1990) Code of Ethics and Professional Practice. London: Metanoia Psychotherapy Training Institute .

Chapter 10
Ethical Dilemmas in Supervision, Training and Organisational Contexts

Petrūska Clarkson and Geoff Lindsay

> The greatest dilemma is whether or not to remain belonging to UKCP and
> ensure my status is safe, for future (e.g. legislation), whilst at the same time
> believing it is creating a false position and status for its members (of safety and
> effectiveness) in the eyes of the public, that they generally don't deserve based
> on any objective evidence and are in fact simply creating a closed shop under
> the banner of protecting the public. (Anonymous quotation from research)

PART 1: SUPERVISION AND SUPERVISION OF SUPERVISION

Ethics and professional practice are important elements in any training
and professional developmental path of a psychotherapist or supervisor,
trainer or organisational leader. Arguably, they are the most important.

Supervision and supervision of supervision

The ethical and moral dimension of supervision embraces issues of
professional practice and of ethics as these relate to the trainee or student
in his or her relationships with clients, the public, training organisations
and with professional peers. Supervision is here defined as 'a contractually explicit conversation between two or more professionals with the
purpose of educating, monitoring, and developing service to
patient(s)/clients(s)' (Clarkson, 1998, p. ix). A spectrum of issues –
encompassing confidentiality with clients, how to deal with advertising a
practice, and difficulties in dealing with a professional colleague – may at
times take priority as the focus of supervision. According to the accreditation procedures of the British Association for Counselling (BAC), for
example, the supervisor is required to ensure that the professional in
supervision both knows and implements the Professional Practices
Guidelines and the Code of Ethics of their relevant organisations.

In short, the supervisor has *accountability* which concerns the unavoidable obligation to take cognisance of others – particularly third parties such as the organisation, the profession or the children – this is ethically (if not always managerially) inescapable. The supervisor also has *responsibility*, which I see here as the way in which supervision can be on one's own cognisance – it is autonomously chosen, one is response-able, free to engage in an essentially equal collegial partnership. Thirdly, the supervisor is concerned with *potentiality* – that which concerns nurturing the aspiration to that which is desirable for oneself, others and the world. It has to do with the needs of our capacities to fulfil our own potential and contribute significantly to the lives of others and our planer.

Often it is the supervisee who specifies what he or she wants of a particular supervision session – the supervisory contract. They will generally bring to supervision problem areas or interesting issues, sometimes requiring urgent attention. However, the supervisor's judgement may also determine the selection of a particular focus in the supervision for trainee or experienced supervisors.

If a psychotherapist is overlooking an ethical issue, the supervisor cannot hesitate too long to draw attention to the *ethics and professional practice* dimensions of the work – even if this is not in the 'contract'. Our professional responsibilities require us to act in this way – the sanity or lives of others may be at stake. It is also the compassionate and wise course of action. Veterans as well as trainees may consistently avoid certain areas in supervision. For example, one trainee consistently avoided focusing on the actual interventions he was making with a client (the microscopic look at his work), although quite ready to discuss assessment, therapeutic strategies, direction and theory.

Culture

Problematical issues of culture and organisational context suffuse every supervisory relationship, yet 'to date, the influence of organisational variables on supervision has rarely been studied, and the role of cultural diversity has not been studied at all' (Brown and Landrum Brown, 1995, p. 284). This probably does not indicate that such issues do not exist, merely that they are still invisible – or at least not mentioned.

In the training and organisational graze on the first Clarkson and Lindsay UKCP sample (1997) there were only four specific examples of dilemmas concerning culture – all of them painful and including the patronising by colleagues of a black Jamaican who was assumed to be less self-confident (and therefore not capable of handling peer criticism) because of living in a predominantly white European society – perhaps 'because of an unconscious sense of insecurity and superiority on the part of the white group members'.

In research conducted in cross-cultural issues (Clarkson and Nippoda, 1998) we found that some 22% of respondents – even in a genuinely multicultural training organisation – experienced negative effects of racial, ethnic and cultural factors on their counselling and psychotherapy. (See Clarkson and Nippoda, 1998 for further details and discussion of this theme.)

There was also one report in our research of a trainee being refused training on the grounds of being 'disabled'. Collusive ignorance or avoidance of these issues can be profound and habitual and will also usually take priority over any other consideration, such as what the supervisee wants from a particular session. Most supervisors will often be concerned to reduce potential harm and to deal urgently with the practice issue involved for the welfare of all involved.

From nearly 30 years' experience I have come to believe that there is hardly any supervisory issue that does not bring in its wake at least general, if not specific ethical considerations or problems. Each one of these brings an opportunity for growth in understanding and appreciation for the complexity of being human. Exploring these with trainee and experienced supervisors as well as trainees enriches the process of psychotherapy supervision and training and contextualises it within a much vaster enterprise of the alleviation of suffering and the facilitation of beneficial development, not only for the individual, but also for our multicultural society as a whole.

Ellis and Ladany's (1997) impressive integrative methodological review of more than 2000 sources on the subject of psychotherapy supervision investigated six sets of inferences:

- inferences about the supervisory relationship
- inferences entailing matching in supervision
- inferences regarding supervisee development
- inferences relating to supervisee evaluation
- inferences about client outcome
- inferences about supervisees – new measures.

The bad news is that their conclusions are, as they write:

> sobering . . . we essentially concluded that these theories and the central premises thereof remain untested . . . simplistic and incomplete, partially accurate and partially inaccurate. (pp. 497, 493)

Their findings in terms of developmental approaches to supervision are also

> disheartening . . . beleaguered by unpleasantly conspicuous conceptual and methodological problems . . . largely uninterpretable . . . no tentative inferences from the data to the models seem justifiable . . . the use of practicum level as a proxy for experience level is ill-advised'. (p. 483)

They also question the very notion of supervisee development. Indeed, they suggest that there may be a more potent underlying construct such as cognitive development or cognitive complexity (Blocher, 1983; Holloway, 1987; Ellis, 1988). Neufeldt et al. (1997) also conclude their chapter that, given the current state of affairs, 'whether specific supervision strategies are more effective than others in provoking therapist development cannot be known' (p. 520). Edward Watkins, the editor of the *Handbook of Psychotherapy Supervision* (1997), even doubts whether psychotherapy-based approaches to supervision actually exist.

Knapp and VandeCreek (1997), in addressing legal issues in supervision, recommend:

- more thorough teaching of ethics
- formal teaching and supervision of supervision skills
- an enacted concern for the psychological health of all trainees across the spectrum from noticeable problems to the enhancement of personal and professional fulfilment.

There is in our fields a growing conviction (although not particularly any evidence) that psychotherapy supervision is important, not only for training, but also as part of our continuing development, whether for the duration of our professional lives, or intermittent and periodic periods of supervision – and for the supervision of and/or consultancy to practising and experienced supervisors for as long as we are engaged in this work.

Unfortunately research into the effectiveness of supervision has but little to say conclusively except:

> There are few practical implications of the research reviewed here. The research suggests that the quality of the supervisory relationship is paramount to successful supervision (Ellis and Ladany, 1997, p. 495)

and

> Whatever the view taken, however, the supervisor–supervisee relationship appears to be necessary ingredient to the making, doing, and being of the supervision process itself and seemingly facilitates or potentiates whatever takes place within that process. (p. 4)

This seems to support our conviction that relationship is the matrix not only of professional development, but also of ethical behaviour.

There is little if any research on ethical dilemmas specifically involving supervision – in the Pope and Vetter (1992) studies it emerged as one category amongst all the others. As part of our ongoing international research project, building on and replicating the methodology of previous studies here and in the USA (e.g. Pope and Vetter, 1992; Lindsay and Colley, 1995; Clarkson and Lindsay, 1997), we therefore wanted to focus on ethical dilemmas as they emerge in supervision. We therefore adapted the question for qualitative analysis to read: 'please describe in a few words, any ethical dilemmas which you or a colleague have experienced regarding supervision in the last year or so.'

There has been, as far as we are aware, no intentional comparison of ethical dilemmas in supervision between the different disciplines of counselling, counselling psychology and psychotherapy. Experience and previous research leads to the expectation that commonalities will outweigh differences. Since at the time there were only 258 counselling psychologists in the UK, we mailed all of those as well as a randomly selected sample of 258 UKCP psychotherapists and 258 BAC counsellors to make proper comparison.

One of our objectives of this ongoing study included the exploration of the kind of ethical dilemmas concerning supervision experienced in these disciplines, their relevant importance and the extent and significance of differences, if any. (Some respondents to this set of questionnaires included their names and offered to be interviewed confidentially in more detail about their dilemmas. In subsequent questionnaires such confidential opportunities were offered and the resulting interviews are currently being aggregated in a discourse analytic study of people who have been involved in ethical dilemmas and procedures.)

There were no significant differences between these three disciplines (counselling, counselling psychology and psychotherapy) to be observed from our data at this level of analysis. Neither were there any significant differences when types of ethical dilemma were compared.

Since this is work in progress, I would like to highlight some themes of interest emerging from a qualitative analysis of the discourse used in the responses (aggregated across disciplines) and share my own impressionistic subjective responses to these from my own experience as practitioner, teacher and supervisor.

Table 10.1: Comparison of responses relating to ethical dilemmas in supervision

	No. of responses	No. reporting no dilemma
BPS Counselling Psychology Division	60 (23.3%)[a]	11 (18.3%)[b]
BAC	58 (22.5%)	10 (17.2%)
UKCP	43 (16.7%)	8 (18.6%)

[a]The number of supervisors sampled from each organisation was 258, and percentages in this column relate to that figure.
[b]The percentage of respondents who indicated 'no dilemma'.
Note: No dilemma includes no comment.
Source: *Psychotherapy*, Rome, June.

No dilemmas?

Firstly, there is our surprise and shock even that there are qualified practitioners – *almost one-fifth* of our respondents – who claim that they have not encountered ethical dilemmas in supervision in the last couple of years. Since supervision often involves at the very least three people, and often many more, it is likely that ethical dilemmas are likely to proliferate in supervision. As discussed earlier, it is my deeply held conviction that every action or non-action of a psychotherapist contains moral and ethical implications. To counteract the notion that 'ethics' or 'cultural issues' are to be 'add-ons' to the curriculum, my students and I explore all our professional work as a matter of course for explicit, implicit or potential ethical and cultural concerns and possibilities, as much to discover those which are embedded in our work as to develop professional reflexes attuned to these too frequently ignored and neglected dimensions of human relationships.

Is it possible that respondents did not understand the meaning of the word 'dilemma' which is usually understood as something like 'a position of doubt or perplexity'?

Dilemma is equally usually understood to mean something 'concerning thought or reflection between several alternatives'. Thus an ethical dilemma would be something that caused a practitioner to question their own or their colleagues' practice. I want to believe that such semantic misunderstanding is the only reason some professionally qualified colleagues would write for example: (details changed):

> *I have worked in a psychiatric hospital for 12 years, as a residential thera-pist working with physically, emotionally and sexually abused children for 10 years and as a counsellor in private practice for 7 years. I have never encountered an ethical dilemma.*

Never?

Another response with the wording (but not the sense) again somewhat changed:

> *I have not had to face any serious ethical dilemmas. One situation caused me anxiety but the agency took responsibility . . . this was about a man who disclosed that he was a contract killer who had killed eight people.*

Another example tells clearly how supervisees sometimes need the moral and emotional sensitivities of their supervisors before they naturally begin to think and work in ethically attuned ways.

> *A psychotherapy student was critical of her training organisation because of inadequate training. In passing she mentioned how one of her very well known teachers had used tape-recordings of clients as demonstration material without the clients' knowledge or consent for this to be shown to*

others. . . . My dilemma was whether to demand his name and report this or whether to say to the student that such conduct was totally unethical and leave her to take it up. Although she was a reasonably competent student, it was not until I explained my outrage that she even thought about the betrayal of the confidentiality that his behaviour represented!

Appreciation of ethical complexities

Contrasted with this is the large number of colleagues who thought well and deep, not only about obviously ethical, but also about moral and cultural issues, usually discussing their concerns with supervisors and/or colleagues often until some satisfactory resolution had been achieved. Some stories were truly inspirational showing how practitioners grapple with their professional reputation (for example, being shown to be complicit in fraud), their compassion for their clients (a fragile client with vulnerable children), their loyalty to the organisation paying for the employee counselling (under false pretences), the secrecy and shame in the countertransference which were all worked through in supervision to a result which was practically, clinically, professionally and legally appropriate.

Practitioners' reports of dilemmas sometimes ended with multiple questions, for example:

This was to do with a previous supervisee of mine having visited an ex-patient of his. A sexual encounter was reported as having taken place. This information was given to me in confidence by a current patient of mine who had been told this in confidence by the ex-patient who was a friend. My dilemmas – truth, fiction or mixture? – interpret as transference – approach the ex-trainee? – if true, what action if any? – how to safeguard the boundaries of the current therapy with me? – and how to understand the information?

My supervisee informed me that her previous partner had fallen in love with a young patient and was pursuing the relationship. We agreed in the first instance that she would share with him the guidelines on ethics of his professional body and warn him of the seriousness of the situation for his future career even though she saw him as potentially suicidal and capable of taking violent revenge on my supervisee. My dilemma concerns how to handle the confidentiality aspects and whether to propose an investigation.

Table 10.2 shows a comparison of ethical dilemmas in supervision between the three professional groups sampled (BPS, UKCP and BAC).

Fear

Among our respondents there were several expressions of fear of legal consequences; for example, someone who:

only recorded female clients to prove there had been no impropriety and that professional boundaries had been maintained if they alleged otherwise.

Table 10.2: comparison of dilemmas in supervision

	BPS[a]	BAC	UKCP
Confidentiality	13	19	15
Research			
Questionable intervention	1		
Colleagues' conduct	11	16	9
School psychology			1
Sexual issues	7	5	7
Assessment	1	1	1
Organisational	7	5	5
Dual relationships	7	11	4
Payment matters	8	2	2
Academic/training	4	6	1
Competence	4	2	5
Supervision	1	3	
Forensic	7		7
Ethics codes/committees		1	1
Publishing			
Advertising			
Medical issues			
Ethnicity		2	1
Treatment records	2		1
Helping the financially stricken			
Termination		3	
Miscellaneous		1	
Moral issues	8	2	1

[a]Division of Counselling Psychology

This is an example of what has been called 'defensive psychotherapy' (see Chapter 6). Furthermore

> *a trainee with whom I was working reported in my estimation abusive behaviour with a practice client. Issues of proof, action and my vulnerability to legal action by the trainee was discussed in supervision.*

Matters of appearing in court as witness for or against clients and the fact that records needed to be shown are also of concern to practitioners.

Others reported fear that if they made complaints about legitimate issues they would be 'black-balled' by the organisation or that they would be punished in other ways such as exclusion, as in the case of a manager not inviting a staff member to meetings any more because she had made a complaint:

> *what I'm trying to do is to give the students a positive learning experience and I feel that because of [such] aspects beyond my control, I have not been able to do that.*

Several mentions were made of how small the counselling, psychotherapy and supervision network is and the importance of

staying on reasonable terms with people who might send clients to me

or

the fear of losing my job if I made the complaint . . . so I did not, but I still don't feel good about it.

In this latter case the supervisors consulted advised the potential complainant not to pursue the legitimate concerns

since 'getting the qualification is the most important thing plus earning a living'

Individual and organisational financial concerns

The role of financial concerns was in contrast actually quite wide and worrying, for example:

and that particular institution has a . . . financial problem, so it's desperately trying to increase its income . . . and its student numbers.

A patient was clearly finished with therapy at . . . the place where I work and supervise. She had completed all treatment goals and was ready to terminate. The Clinical Manager balked at my suggestion of discharge because of financial reasons – 'the client's insurance company was not pressing for discharge, hence we should continue to treat as long as the insurance money keeps coming in'. In my opinion, totally unethical as well as reprehensible. Not only was I unsupported by my own supervisor, but now I was also forced to lie to the student working with the client 'to continue treatment' when in reality treatment was only creating more income for the institution.

In terms of dual relationships, there were several instances of supervisors being managers or in some way involved with promotion, determining pay scales and in one case even advising the organisation concerned on how to make his supervisee redundant – resulting in the supervisee losing her livelihood!

In a number of cases there is evidence that organisations are unwilling or unable to deal with such issues and that people who raise such uncomfortable issues are penalised:

They [the organisation] are lashing out but we feel we have acted ethically and professionally always keeping the students' interest in heart and mind. It leaves us in great doubt about the ability of certain organisations to manage counselling courses. Their philosophical, management and financial ethos is at great odds with that of the therapeutic world.

Competency of people in training and supervision

*the other thing is, because I like working there and because I'd like to have a
bit more work there in future, if one of 28 students fail in my group, what
does it say about me?*

This issue is taken up in part 2 of this chapter.

Recovered memory

*Colleague was faced with the problem of a client who had recalled child-
hood sexual abuse by a family member who is currently employed in a care
capacity looking after children. The client does not wish to go public or
confront the abuser and my colleague now faces the issue of breaking a
confidence gained from knowledge of his client, taking no action (as his
client wishes) and possibly putting others at risk. There is no corroboration
of the allegation made by the client.*

PART 2: ETHICAL ISSUES CONCERNING
TRAINING/ORGANISATIONS
PETRŪSKA CLARKSON

First of all, it seems that the relationship within a group of teachers forming
the staff of an institute is akin to that in a good marriage. The members will all
be separate individuals, perhaps with a variety of orientations, different styles
and views of their own, all of which will provide a rich resource of knowledge
and skill upon which the students can draw, and by which the staff can
continue to learn from each other. We will expect strong tensions within
these relationships, arising from these differences, but members will be
prepared to continue to communicate, constantly negotiating compromises
and resolving conflicts, each accepting that it is normal and healthy for us to
want our own way, but also knowing that it is not usually good for us to get it
all the time, since we can see ourselves more clearly through the reflections
provided by others, and can therefore grow, learn and develop in skill only by
accepting some measure of painful, confrontation and challenge. (Skynner,
1989, p. 204)

There is little if any research into ethical dilemmas which concern
training or organisational issues.(It is largely absent in most texts.)
Although the data for the study of training and organisational influences
on the practice of ethics is still in a preliminary stage of analysis, certain
trends are indicative of concerns which deserve inclusion in this book at
this stage. The first sub-analysis done simply grazed the first Clarkson
and Lindsay (1997) data (respondents' ethical dilemmas) for instances
where training and organisational issues were specifically raised in the
dilemmas. (It will be remembered that for the first Clarkson and Lindsay
(1997; see also Lindsay and Clarkson, 1999) study we replicated the USA

Pope and Vetter study (1992) and used their categories and scoring system where training and academic issues emerged as the fifth largest category.)

As we know (Denzin and Lincoln, 1994), qualitative data does not necessarily lend itself to the kind of statistical precision that quantitative studies can accomplish. It is more concerned with the quality of the phenomenon researched – metaphorical literacy rather than numeracy. The fact that people responded in their own words to our invitation to describe an ethical dilemma that they or a colleague had encountered may, for example, not indicate that training or organisational issues were involved in the dilemmas, whereas there were such issues involved. Our respondents may or may not have found it necessary to mention this even if it were since neither 'training', nor 'organisation' nor 'supervision' was mentioned in our research question to the first 253 respondents who then reported ethical dilemmas. (As a result of our findings, subsequent questionnaires in our ongoing research programme have specifically investigated these dimensions.)

Therefore the fact that some 68 items of the original responses (approximately 26% – more than a quarter of the sampled responses) specifically included spontaneous mentions of training and/or organisational/professional issues is considered extremely significant and a serious cause for concern. This finding may reflect the lack of training, research or literature on such matters as well as the comparative youth of many training organisations in the UK – the UKCP is some 10 years old. As an organisation, the BCP is younger. The BPS, for example, has many more decades of experience of grappling with such dilemmas formally and structurally as well as ethically. Yet training and organisational issues interpenetrate all psychotherapy activities. They often determine who gets help, from whom, of what kind, under what kind of conditions and whether or not complaints will be heard, understood or retraumatising for the people involved.

Here I will only indicate a few highlights of our explorations for the sake of opening debate, questioning and discussion of this dimension of our collegial relationships. These naturally relate to our duties to protect our clients, the public, our colleagues and ourselves – as well as the fair name of our profession.

Colleagues on training courses judged to be unsuitable, dangerous, incompetent, etc. in relation to their work with patients

The most serious and recurrent theme appears to be the ethics and competence of colleagues in training who are seeing patients.

If we subtract the 7 incidents concerning professional colleagues who appear from the responses to be already qualified, but whose ethical behaviour is causing concern, there is still a worrying 34 of the 61 (55% of items in this sample) that report concerns about training and organisational issues regarding the incompetence, misconduct and unsuitability of counsellors/psychotherapists in training with various training organisations. That is, more than 50% of psychotherapists' concerns about ethical dilemmas are to do with junior colleagues who, for some reason or other, are not considered fit to practice by qualified practitioners. Yet they are currently seeing clients – presumably with the agreement of their training organisations. Some examples from respondents follow:

I'm afraid that she might eventually be a very damaging counsellor, but I don't seem able to let anybody know this, even in the vaguest of terms, because I have no contact with her course tutors. Am I right in thinking there's nothing I can do?

A trainee therapist – just beginning – comes to me for personal therapy. The trainee is deeply narcissistic, unable/unwilling to work on quite severe intra/interpersonal difficulties and leaves therapy after two sessions. I was in a difficult dilemma about conveying to the training body any of my doubts regarding the trainee's suitability and the fact that the required therapy had not been completed etc. Bound by confidentiality, I did not, trusting that problems would be addressed in supervision and training, but I felt uncertain about the thoroughness of the training body's selection procedure of new trainees.

I experienced a peer and colleague fellow supervisor/therapist ethical dilemma about whether to convey to the NHS psychotherapy department in question my concerns regarding her inadequate supervision and lack of experience of 'acting out' patients. She presented difficulties in containing personality-disordered patients in terms of external environment issues to the responsible consultants, and wanted to include me in her concerns. I found it very tricky to separate my own position from hers and to decide whether to convey information about her.

Having knowledge about individuals applying for training which could affect their acceptance on a course. A trainee with whom I was working for two years as a therapist sought permission from her supervisor to begin working with practice clients. Because of undealt-with issues in her own process, I did not think it appropriate for her to begin counselling. She broke with me, found a new counsellor and was given permission within two sessions to begin working.

Students on training courses no longer have to obtain permission to begin working with practice clients from their own psychotherapists. S. came to me at the beginning of her third year in a four-year course which requires her to be in therapy throughout. She had already left one therapist because he enraged her and didn't give her the support she needed, and so was no better than her parent had been. Her fifth session with me was spent entirely in a rage; she ranted for a full 50 minutes calling me, for instance, a stupid bitch who was as inconsistent and cruel as her mother had been. She cancelled the next appointment, taking the opportunity of ranting on the phone. Later, she phoned to terminate the therapy. During the same period, she changed her general practitioner for being insufficiently courteous.

Clearly she can't at present deal with her enormous transference problems. (She knows what transference is, but insisted that this wasn't anything to with it.) My dilemma is that her course tutors invite no feedback from her therapist(s), and she seems to be doing well enough on her course to qualify successfully. She already works as a voluntary counsellor for several agencies.

I became convinced that a trainee therapist I was supervising was being very ineptly handled by her therapist, who obviously could not cope with her. Usually I can manage this with tactful suggestions to the supervisee. In this case I knew the therapist in the training context; things had reached a really desperate ('gruesome-twosome') state. I advised her to stop working with him; I then met with him to clarify what I had done. He had of course been angered by my intervention, but he didn't take the opportunity to ask me for any 'supervision' on what was going wrong. There was nothing more I could do. In the end the outcome, for the supervisee, was beneficial, for she was stronger than he.

Such a dilemma challenges my trust in myself. It is as I see it a moral, not an ethical matter. I won't collude with therapist and counsellors' bad practice on the grounds of professional 'ethics'; ultimately my commitment has to be to my supervisee, not to my colleagues' egos.

Cultural issues and issues of difference

Nadirshaw (1992) found that:

there is increasing concern amongst [ethnic] groups about the lack of available, accessible, adequate, appropriate and relevant services to black people. The concern is ever greater in black and ethnic communities as they remain at the receiving end of little or no services. That includes psychotherapy and counselling services. (p. 257)

If matters of difference and culture are not part and parcel of all training curricula, it is possible that individual practitioners (perhaps with a preponderance of middle-class white women?) may not develop discriminating sensitivities to these issues. It is likely that the more experienced psychotherapists become, the more they would be seeing other psychotherapists who are in training and supervision and the less likely it is that they would be working with seriously disturbed financially disadvantaged clients who may have difficulty with English and punctuality, appreciating analytic neutrality or 'non-directiveness' and the importance of keeping (or cancelling in advance) all appointments.

The absence of black or differently abled people in the management structures of many psychotherapy organisations attests to the problems many people experience in finding role models or a sense of being welcomed – apart from a liberal kind of tokenism. Lip service attempts only too often founder on the rocks of academic requirements that are not suited to cultural pluralism or cannot tolerate genuinely Afrocentric world-views (Ani, 1994), which Eurocentric theories usually simply exclude. For further discussion of research which Nippoda and I have conducted (Clarkson and Nippoda, 1998) and for further discussion of some moral issues concerning these issues please refer to *The Bystander* (Clarkson, 1996) and Racial and Cultural Issues in Psychotherapy (Clarkson, in press).

Organisational management of colleague's death

A colleague of mine, who I knew to be in analytical psychotherapy, let me know her analyst had cancelled two appointments and then 'not been there' when she went for her sessions. My good friend after five weeks was notified (by a member of the analyst's family) that 'she had died'.

I was aware of my colleague's anxiety – being in the dark . . . I then realised her psychoanalyst was the one who had been found dead in suspicious circumstances. My colleague was asking me what to do for further news. I encouraged her to approach the organisation she'd 'got' her therapist from. I maintained supportive listening to my colleague, who did ring the organisation. Eventually, after about three months she was told she could have an interview to 'talk' about this death, and discuss continuing her analysis. My colleague has not so far been approached for this interview, though she tells me she will do something when she feels more settled. The ethical dilemma which I feel I contained (as a colleague to protect her) is uncomfortable and feels deceptive. So, is this a boundary problem? or, as I think, an ethical one? Also, I'd suggest 1) All therapists keep lists accessible of names and addresses of patients; 2) the organisation provides quicker and more sympathetic back-up in death of therapist cases for patients (and also for colleagues).

My own experiences as colleague and supervisor in the early 1970s led me to formulate recommendations to implement appropriate procedures to deal with such eventualities for all psychotherapists. Traynor and Clarkson (1992, and reprinted in as Item 9 in this volume) recommended the inclusion of these guidelines in all ethical codes. It is gratifying to see this item appearing more in our professions' publications whether the source is acknowledged or not. (See Item 6 and also Chapter 11 in this regard.)

The organisation of professions

In recent years there has been increasing concern about the large number of students going on training courses of one kind or another hoping to make a first or second career or supplement their existing income. In a climate of economic uncertainty and pressure from the UKCP for example on training organisations to prove themselves financially viable *ad infinitum*, there are inevitable pressures to get 'bums on seats'. According to our respondents and from other anecdotal evidence this often results in the sacrifice of quality for quantity.

In the UK the General Medical Council and the British Psychological Society respectively hold the Registers for the professions of medical doctors and psychologists of acceptable standard from whichever university they have trained in medicine or psychology. Of course some institutions will close for financial or other reasons, but the central body will continue to exists as long as these professions exist. The codes of ethics and disciplinary procedures are held and implemented centrally by the profession for the profession as a whole.

Unfortunately organisations such as the UKCP and BCP are constituted by an amalgam of training organisations and some smaller professional organisations . So 'votes' or delegates are represented by these institutional bodies – instead of a democratic process involving all the members whatever their historical training body or university. Unlike the GMC or the BPS, the UKCP and BCP at the moment more resemble trade associations. Such conflicts are of course evidenced by most of their organisational members independently 'staying in business' – rather than necessarily protecting the good of the public by acting concertedly to safeguard both the rights and the responsibilities of professions.

Ineffectiveness of complaints procedures

The notion that ethics codes can be impartially and independently administered or heard by employees of the organisation – particularly organisations which are naturally concerned about their reputation and income – is patently false by all the standards of natural justice. It is an increasingly voiced opinion that the federal type of organisation represents a confusing conflict of interests – particularly if we take into account that these organisations have public duties. (Such conflicts are of course evidenced by the successful application (1999) to have the conduct the UKCP Complaints procedures judicially reviewed in the UK High Court: see Chapter 13.)

Organisations such as the Prevention of Professional Abuse Network (POPAN) as well as formal and informal interviews with people who have experienced these complaints procedures almost uniformly express dissatisfaction with the complaints processes as currently practised in the UK. The book by Palmer Barnes (1998), describing the procedures and practices of complaints and ethics matters, only serves to highlight the sad discrepancy between good practice and actual practice. Furthermore, the complaints panels themselves are often unable to act, as in the example below. How many of these situations are there?

In the last year I have been a member of an adjudication panel dealing with a complaint from a patient. I was concerned that we could only deal with the issues that actually conflicted with the code of ethics: there seems to be no place for dealing with standards – i.e. seeing both husband and wife in individual therapy, seeing patients in a social setting, asking for fees in lieu of one month's notice. None of these issues contravenes the code, but I and my colleagues felt that they show a lamentable lack of high standards of work.

Questions regarding the validity of training psychotherapists at all . . .

As someone who has founded several professional organisations and trained several hundred counsellors, psychologists and psychothera- pists, I would like to draw attention to the following information through the device of quoting Corney (1997, pp. 14–15) directly and at length as follows:

> Critics of psychotherapy such as Szasz (1988) and Eysenck (1966) suggest that therapy is not ultimately distinct from relationships like friendship and that therapy brings about an improvement in the same way as talking to a good friend.
> McLennan (1991) compared students who received informal help from academic staff, friends and family members with those who received formal counselling from professionals. Those receiving formal help reported their experience as more private and more 'impactful', but not necessarily more effective. McLennan speculated that even minimal training for informal helpers might close the gap perceived between formal and informal helpers.
> Most people agree that the kinds of skills which form the basis of counselling training [or psychotherapy] are not wholly distinguishable from the kinds of skills used by health professionals. These include attentive listening, accurate understanding, an ability to understand the viewpoint of another person and an ability to engage emotionally with others.
> Research studies have compared the outcomes of counselling provided by trained and untrained counsellors. Their findings suggest that the value or impact of training is overestimated. Durlak (1979) undertook a box score analysis of 42 studies and found that paraprofessionals achieve results which were equal or significantly better than those obtained by professionals. Hattie and colleagues (1984) reanalysed 39 of these studies using a meta-analysis and found the same results. Berman and Norton (1985) disagreed with the categorisation of some of the studies and reanalysed the data omitting some problematic studies. Nevertheless, they found that professionals and paraprofessionals were generally quite effective. Training gives the counsellor or therapist a theory, technique and status but it is unclear whether it makes them more effective in helping people.
> Those involved in training (be they trainers or trainees) may find this evidence difficult to accept. Trainers indicate that they can observe the differ- ences in their trainees throughout their training, as their trainees learn to offer subtler, more accurate and more consistently helpful responses in their work (Feltham, 1995).

I happen to agree with Feltham. However, I hardly need point out the obvious fact that psycho-practice (counselling, psychoanalysis and psychotherapy) has become a multi-million pound industry and training schools and training courses are often financially dependent on finding and maintaining adequate student numbers for training in these fields. Students enter training schools or institutions often making enormous investments for energy, personal therapy and money in qualifying for these professions. They frequently complain about their training organisations 'moving the goal posts' after they had begun training. Complaints, and sometimes even simple questioning, can result in scapegoating or various forms of bureaucratic sabotage – not to mention effects on their academic grades or professional opportunities. Students, as is evident from the analyses of collegial relationships in Chapter 8 and elsewhere, naturally have investments in protecting themselves, their colleagues and the training organisations on which they are dependent for social, professional and often financial reasons (e.g. referrals, assignments of research funds, funding for conferences etc. etc.). And – after having made such expensive and long-term investments (perhaps £30,000 or more) will these professionally trained therapists work with those who are usually most in need – those who precisely cannot afford their professional services? The evidence from black and working-class colleagues shows the contrary.

> To know how to question means to know how to wait, even a whole lifetime. But an age which regards as real only what goes fast and can be clutched with both hands looks on questioning as 'remote from reality' and as something that does not pay, whose benefits cannot be numbered. But the essential is not a number; the essential is the right time, i.e. *the right moment, and the right perseverance.* (Heidegger, 1987, p. 206, emphasis added).

References

Ani, M. (1994) Yurugu: An African-Centred Critique of European Cultural Thought and Behavior. Trenton, NJ: Africa World Press.

Berman, J.S. and Norton, N.C. (1985) Does professional training make a therapist more effective? Psychological Bulletin, 98, 401–7.

Blocher, D.H. (1983) Toward a cognitive developmental approach to counseling supervision. The Counseling Psychologist, 11(1), 27–34.

Brown, M.T. and Landrum Brown, J. (1995) Counselor supervision: cross-cultural perspectives. In J. G. Ponterotto, J. M. Casas, L. A. Suzuki and C. M. Alexander (eds) Handbook of Multicultural Counseling. Thousand Oaks, CA: Sage.

Clarkson, P. (1996) The Bystander. London: Whurr.

Clarkson, P. (ed.) (1998) Supervision: Psychoanalytic and Jungian Perspectives. London: Whurr.

Clarkson, P. (ed.) (in press) Racial and Cultural Issues in Psychotherapy. London: Whurr.

Clarkson, P. and Lindsay, G. (1997) Secrets, Sex and Money: Ethical Dilemmas of Psychologists and Psychotherapists. Poster displayed at British Psychological Society Division of Counselling Psychology Annual Conference, 30 May–1 June 1997, Stratford-upon-Avon.

Clarkson, P. and Nippoda, Y. (1998) Cross-cultural issues in counselling psychology practice. In P. Clarkson (ed.) Counselling Psychology: Integrating Theory, Research and Supervised Practice, pp. 95–118. London: Routledge.

Corney, R. (1997) A Counsellor in Every General Practice? London: Greenwich University Press.

Denzin, N.K. and Lincoln, Y.S. (eds)(1994) Handbook of Qualitative Research. Thousand Oaks, CA: Sage.

Durlak, J.A. (1979) Comparative effectiveness of para-professional and professional helpers. Psychological Bulletin, 86, 80–92.

Ellis, M.V. (1988) The cognitive developmental approach to case presentation in clinical supervision: A reaction and extension. Counselor Education and Supervision, 30, 225–37.

Ellis, M.V. and Ladany, N. (1997) Inferences concerning supervisees and clients in clinical supervision: an integrative review. In C. E. Watkins, Jr. (ed.) Handbook of Psychotherapy Supervision, pp. 447–507. New York: Wiley.

Eysenck, H. J. (1966) The Effects of Psychotherapy. New York: International Science Press.

Feltham, C. (1995) What is Counselling? The Promise and Problem of the Talking Therapies. London: Sage.

Hattie, J.A., Sharpley, C.F. and Rogers, J.H. (1984) Comparative effectiveness of professional and paraprofessional helpers. Psychological Bulletin, 95, 534–41.

Heidegger, M. (1987) An Introduction to Metaphysics. New Haven, CT: Yale University Press. First published 1959.

Holloway, E. L. (1987) Developmental models of supervision: Is it development? Professional Psychology Research and Practice, 18, 209–16.

Knapp, S. and VandeCreek, L. (1997) Ethical and legal aspects of clinical supervision. In C. E. Watkins, Jr. (ed.) Handbook of Psychotherapy Supervision, pp. 589–99. New York: Wiley.

Lindsay, G. and Clarkson, P. (1999) Ethical dilemmas of psychotherapists. Psychologist 12, 182–5.

Lindsay, G. and Colley, A. (1995) Ethical dilemmas of members of the Society. Psychologist 8: 448–51.

McLennan, J. (1991) Formal and informal counselling help: students' experiences. British Journal of Guidance and Counselling, 19(2), 149–59.

Nadirshaw, Z. (1992) Theory and practice: brief report – therapeutic practice in multi-racial Britain. Counselling Psychology Quarterly, 5(3), 257–61.

Neufeldt, S.A., Beutler, L.E. and Banchero, R. (1997) Research on supervisor variables in psychotherapy supervision. In C. E. Watkins, Jr. (ed.) Handbook of Psychotherapy Supervision, pp. 508–24. New York: Wiley.

Palmer Barnes, F. (1998) Complaints and Grievances in Psychotherapy: A Handbook of Ethical Practice. London: Routledge.

Pope, K.S. and Vetter, V.A. (1992) Ethical dilemmas encountered by members of the American Psychological Association. American Psychologist, 47, 397–411.

Skynner, R. (1989) Institutes and how to survive them. In. J.R. Schlapobersky (ed.) Mental Health Training and Consultation. London: Routledge.

Szasz, T. (1988) The Myth of Psychotherapy. Syracuse, NY: Syracuse University Press.

Traynor, B. and Clarkson, P. (1992) What happens if a psychotherapist dies? Counselling, 3(1), 23–4.

Watkins, C.E. (1997) Some concluding thoughts about psychotherapy supervision. In C.E. Watkins, Jr. (ed.) Handbook of Psychotherapy Supervision, pp. 603–16. New York: Wiley.

ITEM 10
Seven Domains of Discourse in Exploring Ethical and Moral Dilemmas

I was thinking about finishing this book and omitting a philosophically epistemological perspective. Then it seemed to me that there was a possibility of conceiving of ethical relationships in psychotherapy as only a matter to do with oughts and shoulds which are either 'introjected' or 'integrated' from our professional or social cultures and 'ethics' codes – or rational concerns about facts and probabilities, for example, what a court is likely to decide or what kind of 'standard' or 'evidence' would be acceptable for the efficacy of a certain approach or certain intervention (or omission) to psychotherapy. This would be doing violence to what I think is an infinitely more complex process. Neither do I personally consider that 'common sense' or 'clinical intuition' takes us as far is we need to go in order to uphold our claims of 'ethicality' to the public or our aspiration of integrity to ourselves. We are talking about talk – discourse and how different rules and processes operate at different levels – or domains of discourse, how they can get conflated and confused and what we might be able to do about that so that not only our thinking, but also our living can be clearer and perhaps even 'truer' – in all the different senses of that notion.

Apparently most ethical decisions, including decisions to intervene on behalf of another, are made not after careful rational deliberation, but as instinctive responses under pressure. Nobody can really predict how they might behave *in extremis* and the Milgram (1963 and 1974) experiments (where white middle-class students were led to believe that they were voluntarily inflicting painful and then deadly electric shocks on volunteers in experiments) have shown us that we are all capable of the worst of evils for reasons ranging from fear of our lives (cannibalism or betrayal) to a simplistic and unquestioning compliance with perceived authority. Add to that the human tendency to abdicate responsibility to unbelievable degrees in a crowd or group (as is evidenced from the bystander experiments and historical examples) and I think we cannot leave ethical matters solely to the provinces of reason (the

discourse domain of rationality) or professionally accepted moral codes
(the domain of normative discourse).

There is, as we have noticed so far, also a domain of discourse which
is theoretical – where we tell each other stories, narratives, myths about
our experience, our explanations, our 'schools', our hypotheses. Of
course, as soon as a theory is proven (to our consensual reality in a
particular time and place) it becomes a fact or a statistical probability.
For example, is it a fact that humans are less likely to intervene on behalf
of another the greater the number of people in the crowd watching an
atrocity – even though numerically they could often overwhelm the
'perpetrators' – or at least enquire about the event at the time when
intervention still is possible (before the black man is lynched, the
questioning member expelled, the child murdered)? It is characteristic
of facts or statistically proven probabilities (whether 0.05 or 0.001) that
people of that culture and that time do agree about them if they can
investigate the evidence, the figures, the legal precedents, the statistical
tables or the research methodology.

There is little argument in the domain of facts. If a fetus is destroyed
in a particular manner, it invariably dies. So many Jews can be burnt in
ovens fuelled by so much coal. So much torture can be committed
before visible scars are left. So many people will die in a atom bomb blast
of so many megatons.

It is in the realm of the normative that arguments are endless – 'it is
good to be human with your clients' or 'it is essential never to disclose
anything about yourself to your patients'; 'it is better to take a full
psychological history' or 'it is essential to let the patient unfold their
own story'; 'you must diagnose the patient accurately and follow the
standardised treatment plan for that condition' or 'diagnosis is an
assault on a human being who should be met in their full existential
reality' and so on and so forth. There is little factual evidence for any of
these kind of statements – if there were, we would not be arguing about
them. They are preferences or ideologically influenced stories or the
normative values which we believe in and hold dear – the 'flag statements' of psychotherapy for which there is no factual backup. If there
were factual evidence for these mutually conflicting theories, we should
all be doing the proven 'right' thing – or be in violation of caring to our
best ability and knowledge for our patients.

This is analogous to a medical practitioner not prescribing antibiotics
for a potentially fatal pneumonia because he or she 'doesn't believe in
antibiotics' and would rather prescribe enemas because he or she
trained with the enema-giving training school (and still has shares in it),
and feels more 'comfortable' in giving enemas. There are very few facts
indeed in psychotherapy. If the situation were different, we would not
have 450 different approaches to psychotherapy/psychoanalysis,
constantly ambiguous research results (see Chapter 12 for review) and

endless claims of 'mine's better, longer, shorter, faster, deeper, cheaper, more exclusive (etc.) than yours'. When these kind of claims distinguish our discourse, we are not in the realm of facts, reason or probabilities, but in the discourse domain of narrative, theory, myth – or something else.

Another domain of discourse which co-exists with the ones I have mentioned so far (theoretical, factual and normative) is that of nominative talk – the naming, the logos, the use of words themselves. It is close to the project that the phenomenological philosophers particularly Merleau-Ponty (e.g. 1962), for example, articulated as a third possibility between Kantian theory on the one hand and positivistic scientism on the other. It is the discourse domain where we attempt to pay attention to experience, to the words we use, our descriptions of subjective worlds, to the naming of relationships before they become saturated with assumptions, theories, norms or even facts. It is the realm of 'a rose is a rose is a rose'. In ethics talk a complainant may be referred to as 'borderline' which may influence whether his or her complaint gets heard – whether or not it is valid. I have witnessed a small outbreak of righteous ethical outrage at a recent professional meeting when a trainee was explaining that his group analyst would not interpret his dreams. 'Not interpreting dreams' in some people's opinion was almost like an ethics violation and certainly judged incompetent in the judgement of some mature professionals there. There is a world of difference between a 'freedom fighter' and a 'terrorist'; an 'abortion' and a 'termination'; 'flirting with daddy' and 'incest'; 'resistant' in one case and 'giving the therapist feedback on their unconscious desire to murder the patient'; and 'having a cup of tea with a client' and 'breaking boundaries or behaving seductively as a psychotherapist'. Influenced from our theoretical positions (6) and our imbedded values (4), we as psychotherapists speak such different languages (3) (see Figure 10.1). Metaphorically some psycho-languages have as many meanings for snow as the Eskimos, some, like the Japanese, no real word for self.

For example, a client may be considering aborting the baby which she conceived of as result of a genocidally motivated rape. She may hold religious values which are morally against abortion, considering it murder. She may be emotionally revolted and fear hating the baby, while her friends and family members who have survived the atrocities are urging her to abort it. The baby can be clearly seen on the scan with his little penis. Yet she may want to kill him when he is born. There is still time for him to be aborted before her life becomes endangered. She has already chosen a name for him – the name of the revolutionary leader in whose name the war is being fought. She wishes to hang herself in her red cardigan and summer dress from a tree. She always believed the romatic stories of Prince Charming and read Barbara Cartland as soon as she could get her hand on these stories. She also loves the film *Pretty*

Woman although she believes that communism is no longer viable. She was an unwanted child conceived out of wedlock by her mother and father when they were just 16. All of these are true. All levels co-exist and mutually influence each other.

So far, I have pointed out four different domains of discourse which can usefully be separated (see Fig. 10.1) : the factual/rational/logical level (5), the theoretical/narrative/hypothetical level (6), the normative/evaluative level (4) and the nominative or phenomenological level (3). Level 2 is that of the emotional in which we are very like other mammals. In psychotherapeutic language this may refer to transference or countertransference, resonance or empathic attunement, desire or dislike, fear or fatal attraction. It is the world of feeling which co-exists in every practitioner along with the other levels – and which may or may not be in conflict or harmony with them at experiential levels. Yet we have to learn to tolerate our multivalences. Very close, of course, is the epistemenological world of the body, the discourse of sensation, physiology, our sense of smell and most primitive intuitions, the kind of experience where we are similar to most other living creatures where we respond with arousal, fight or flight or boredom, hunger, fatigue and the 'thousand other ills and pleasures that flesh is heir to'. Sometimes there is simply a visceral revulsion for a patient which makes it impossible to work with them in an ethical way, sometimes we feel in our marrow the empathy which permeates an intersubjective field with knowledge and experience and from which deep unconscious images may rise to assist the healing in ways which are not susceptible to reasoned and logical explanation, but which are felt with all the earthy force of gravity.

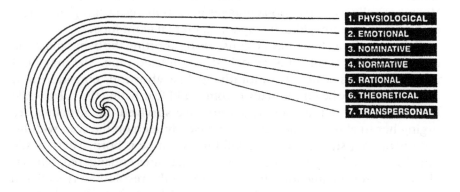

Figure 10.1 Diagrammatic representation of the seven-level model.

This brings us to the possibility of the seventh level (or domain of discourse) which is simply the category where we can rest all those things which are inexplicable at the moment. This would include such examples as dreaming the same dreams as your patient, knowing what they will say or do before they say or do it, or having your patients tell your life's stories or echo your own struggle with a particular problem. Sometimes one sees how parents' behaviour changes as adult children understand their own psyches better. And then there is Jung's famous scarab beetle tapping on the window when the patient is taking off her psychological and interpersonal armour. I include all the worlds of modern physics and complexity in this realm of epistemological discourse – because we cannot yet articulate or place them anywhere else at this moment in the history of this eurocentric culture. Perhaps we never will.

These seven levels, or 'domains' of discourse as Maturana (in a personal communication 1998) suggested I call them, co-exist in human experience and in human epistemologies with different kinds of truth values applicable for different domains, mostly holding ambiguities, conflicts and contradictions and too often bedevilled with conflation, confusion and miscommunication as we flounder linguistically, experientially and professionally in our particular Tower of Babel. The seven levels appear to have an historical evolutionary, phylogenetic and ontogenetic sequence in unfolding. It is vital to note, however, that I do not in any sense concur with the privileging of any one of these levels above another nor do I consider that the transpersonal level 7 is intrinsically better or more evolved than level 1 or level 4 for that matter. We need, and are, them all. They are descriptive categories for the human condition and supposed to be helpful in exploring the kinds of human knowledge we have and can have. They co-exist for me from the beginning, unfolding each in their own way, and always co-existing. When we apply this structure (or any other) to ethics problems or psychotherapy treatment planning or decisions about life and death there is only one criterion – is it useful?

Ethical dilemmas concerning supervision, training and organisations

- A trainee in supervision with you had been seeing a patient with manic depression for some 2 years of long-term intensive psychodynamically oriented psychotherapy. The GP who had referred her to the student then referred her to a consultant psychotherapist at the local university hospital at the patient's request, but without discussion with my the trainee. The consultant advised four ECT sessions which the patient had previously resisted but his time agreed to. The consultant then told the patient that she would like to take over her psychotherapy and adopt a cognitive-behavioural approach. The patient felt that she had no choice but to agree. This is a trainee's training patient – one of the two needed for her to qualify.

- A client who had terminated psychotherapy with you some time ago gave you written permission to publish a clinical paper using his case material. Just before the paper gets published, the client phones you to tell you that he still feels bad and wants to explore the work you had done together and how it ended. You feel that you ought to tell him that the paper would be coming out soon and that he may see it. On the other hand you don't want to worry the client unncessarily.

- You are the ethics chair of a training organisation when one member complains about publicity misrepresenting qualifications of tutors to trainees and members of the public. The management committee refuse to investigate the complaint and forbid the questioning member to come on the premises. Subsequently one of the tutors is sent to prison for misrepresenting his qualifications. What do you do?

- You are the training analyst of a trainee whom you are convinced will be dangerous to clients if they were ever left unsupervised. The training body does not require any information from you apart from the fact that the trainee is seeing you regularly. The trainee is relying on the fact that therapy with you is totally confidential. What options do you have? Would these be different if the trainee was currently dangerous to the clients they are seeing under supervision now?

- You hear from a client that colleagues from another training institute are making disparaging remarks about your orientation and your approach and encouraging your trainees and clients to transfer to practitioners from their approach.

- You hear via a trainee that a friend is yours is having sexual relationships with his patients. What do you do?

- You work for an agency where you know that files with client records are not kept confidentially or safely. You have complained to the management, but were told that there is no money or space to improve this at the moment. You are uncomfortable about this, but fear that if you say or do anything more you may lose your job.

- The receptionist at the surgery seem to be on very intimate terms with all patients coming for counselling. You overhear her discussing 'how the session went' and 'how the new counsellor is doing?'

- You are the tutor on a course and supervision reports written by students are kept safely locked in your briefcase. One day, your briefcase with all this confidential material regarding clients and trainees is stolen. It appears irretrievable. What do you do?

- A client's wealthy husband is suing your supervisee for alienation of affection, claiming that since she came into therapy the counsellor has encouraged her to break up her marriage and divorce him. There are four young children involved.

- You came to regard a particular trainee-patient as deeply damaged but cannot inform the training committee, since given the circumstances, it would involve the trainee not being allowed to qualify. It is quite contrary to your role as a therapist to play such a crucial part in your patient's affairs. Nor can you actually be sure that the trainee would really be damaging to future patients.

- As their supervisior you know that junior staff in training as therapists are being referred cases from psychiatrists that are completely beyond the competency/expertise level of those trainees. You think that it is potentially abusive to trainees and to the clients, but feel that it is important to stay on good terms with the psychiatrists in terms of safeguarding the counselling placements in his hospital.
- You are dependent on a particular professional organisation for your referrals of supervisees. You notice that this organisation is misrepresenting the qualifications of these supervisees, but none of the supervisees have noticed this. What do you do?
- You are on the training committee and give a report expressing your doubt that this person would qualify, although they are already working as a specialised counsellor. Later details of sexual misconduct of this trainee with clients emerge. The complaint of the client is dismissed and your views are disregarded. What do you do?
- A trainee, whom you know to have been disciplined for falsely claiming to be qualified when she was not, comes to you for psychotherapy. Do you tell her what you know or not? She clearly needs specialist help.
- You are a staff member of an organisation where one of the other staff is conducting a secret sexual relationship with a trainee. What do you think is the effect on the organisation and what do you do?
- A trainee brings for supervision the fact that she has been seeing a man weekly for 18 months who is now awaiting trial charged with sexual abuse of minors. His sessions are mostly concerned with exploring his sexual feelings and fantasies. The man had previously held a respected position in the education field. Your supervisee wants to know whether to break confidence since she is aware of the local scandal and her children are at school with the children of the man awaiting trial.
- You are supervising employee counsellors who are conflicted by offering 'stress-management' to employees – 'fixing them to put them back at work to be put under pressure by the company once more'. This is particularly severe since the recession.
- Patient who is attending a counselling course informs you as supervisor that he will from now on be providing therapy for students junior to him on his course so that he can pay your fees.
- A supervisee is breaking the ethical code in continuing to counsel a client with whom she is in another relationship (boundary issues). If you withdraw supervision or initiate the complaints procedure, she

will continue to counsel the client unsupervised. Should you continue to address the unethical behaviour and/or continue (in the interests of client safety) with the supervision?

- You are the psychotherapist of two students from the same psychotherapy training course. Envy arises between them and they start interfering with each other's therapy and end up complaining about you to the training body. How do you protect your own reputation and resolve the conflicts of confidentiality and professional accountability?

References

Merleau-Ponty (1962) Phenomenology of Perception (trans. C. Smith) London: Routledge.

Milgram, S. (1963) Behavioural study of obedience. Journal of Abnormal and Social Psychology 67: 371–8.

Milgram, S (1974) Obedience to Authority. New York: Harper and Row.

Further reading

Clarkson P. (1975) The Seven Level Model, Lecture delivered at Pretoria University.

Clarkson, P. (1995) The Therapeutic Relationship. London: Whurr.

Clarkson, P. (1996) The Bystander. London: Whurr.

CHAPTER 11
Whose Idea is it Anyway? (and Writing for Publication)

PETRŪSKA CLARKSON

Ethical dilemmas

> Trying to learn to use words, and every attempt
> Is a wholly new start, and a different kind of failure
> Because one has only learnt to get the better of words
> For the thing one no longer has to say, or the way in which
> One is no longer disposed to say it. And so each venture
> Is a new beginning, a raid on the inarticulate
> With shabby equipment always deteriorating
> In the general mess of imprecision of feeling,
> Undisciplined squads of emotion. And what there is to conquer
> By strength and submission, has already been discovered
> Once or twice, or several times, by men whom one cannot hope
> To emulate – but there is no competition –
> There is only the fight to recover what has been lost
> And found and lost again and again: and now, under conditions
> That seem unpropitious. But perhaps neither gain nor loss.
> For us, there is only the trying. The rest is not our business.
> Eliot (1940/1963), *East Coker*, lines 174–89)

This part of the chapter will explore some of the difficulties and dilemmas that affect counsellors and psychotherapists as more and more people begin to publish in a growing field. It may be very helpful for all of us to understand and get appropriate education on copyright law as it may affect our institutions, our private practices, and our work as teachers and supervisors.

Copyright

As the teacher, clinical or managerial employer and supervisor of several hundred counselling and psychotherapy trainers, trainees, supervisors and supervisees, I am quite accustomed to hearing words, ideas,

199

concepts, workshop and management structures, exercises, points of philosophy and standards in ethics being incorrectly attributed, where I often know the exact origin within the professional community. Sometimes intervention to correct misapprehensions seems important, sometimes not.

Also, as the sole or senior designer of most of the counselling and psychotherapy courses at Metanoia Psychotherapy Training Institute in London, and many of the workshop prototypes there, I learnt that the writing down of the course design and indications or course material to be used, selected from, improved, or have new or better components is a vital part of establishing copyright. I eventually kept all copies of such designs. Other employees or supervisees contributed in some cases and all trainers would be expected to add their own colour, individuality, references and exercises to improve such material. Such newly inserted components would ideally have the names of the later contributors on them as well as the original sources, whether personally communicated from a supervisor, trainer, or other workshop leader, or taken from a written source.

Of course ideas *per se* cannot be copyrighted. Having 'a bright idea' or participating in a mutually generative discussion is simply not the same as joining that idea with the hard work of thinking it out, writing it down, developing it for publication, or piloting it as an overall academic course design, for example. My partners and I, for example, sold my copyright to the courses (from the BAC recognised counselling course to the validated diploma course in Supervision, as well as the outline for several of the psychotherapy courses for which I initiated university validation) at Metanoia as part of the process which I publicly initiated in 1989 to put the fruit of two decades of my life's work completely into a charity.

Ideas only become subject to copyright once they have been written down – and can be bought sold or licensed in part or in whole. 'This means that person whose skill and effort produced the work – the writer of the book, not the secretary who types it out, the composer rather than the amanuensis' (Crone, 1991, p. 99).

The making of editorial comments, suggestions or improvements – whether or not these are used – cannot be construed as sharing the copyright unless explicitly and contractually so agreed beforehand **and** unless the suggestions materially change the originality of the work. The American Psychological Association's *Publication Manual* (1984) advises that someone is only entitled to joint authorship by making 'major contributions of a professional character' to the work (p. 20).

The area of intellectual property rights is one of the fastest growing specialisms in law. My legal advisers inform me that it is not necessary but advisable to put a copyright sign on every page of every document in order to secure copyright. The fact that it is a work with an original author secures copyright in law. They also say that it is advisable to use the international copyright sign with the author's name and the date of first publication coupled with the statement: 'All rights reserved. No part of this publication may be reproduced or transmitted in any form or by any means electronic, mechanical, photocopying, recording or otherwise or restored in any retrieval system of any nature, without the written permission of the copyright holder and the publisher, application for which shall be made to the publisher.' The effect of this is intended to remind others that this right has indeed been asserted (Osborne, personal communication).

Moral rights

The Copyright Act 1988 introduced:

> for the first time into English law, the European idea of an author's moral right over a work. The author of a literary dramatic, musical or artistic work has a right to be identified as the author. This also applies to the director of a film. The identification must be clear, reasonably prominent, and in a form (which may include use of a pseudonym) approved by the author or director. The identification must appear in, or on, each copy of the work, or in some other way likely to be brought to the notice of people who obtain copies of the work, or see the film.
>
> This right does not apply automatically. The author must assert *in writing* the right to be identified in this way, whenever the work is made available commercially to the public.
>
> Damages are available if the author's right to be identified is ignored. There are no guidelines about the appropriate measure of damages. They are meant to cover any financial loss suffered.
>
> The same authors and directors will have a right not to have their work subjected to 'unjustified modification'; that is, to any addition, deletion, alteration or adaptation. Modifications are justified only if 'reasonable in the circumstances, and not prejudicial to the honour or reputation' of the author or director. There are no guidelines about what will be considered reasonable by this definition. Publication of unjustifiedly modified versions of copyright works to the public infringes this right. (Crone, 1991, pp. 110-111)

As a professional in the full joy of my mature powers I have personally experienced the meaning of being legally prohibited from teaching my own material as a result of a specific copyright agreement which I made to benefit future professionals. Fortunately this was only a 3-year restriction which expired in April 1997. This was a small price to pay for the pleasure of bringing a very satisfying 20-year project to a completion as well as the opportunity to develop a new life which continues as consultant, supervisor and available trainer *complementary* to my history at Metanoia, in an independent new life at PHYSIS where I now have my practice and teach.

In the case of transferring the assets of the Metanoia partnership to the Metanoia charity, I did not assert my *moral rights* to be identified as the sole or senior author on the works whose copyright I handed over. I felt, however, that out of honourable respect and as a good example to our mutual junior colleagues, my previous employees, trainees and supervisors would be scrupulous in acknowledging my original design and conceptualisation, as well as any other aspects of my work as they continue to use it. (Unfortunately this has not always proved to be the case.)

Plagiarism

The definition of plagiarism as given in the *Shorter Oxford English Dictionary* is 'the taking and using as one's own of the thoughts, writings, or inventions of another'.

I conceived the idea of making provision in one's will for an executor of one's psychotherapeutic estate, so that someone would take responsibility for the client care expected of counsellors and psychotherapists to extend beyond their death or to continue in the event of illness or becoming incompetent to practice. I can well remember the event that precipitated the awareness of this need; it was the death of a colleague which focused me on the emotional difficulties of dealing with the grief of clients, the practicalities of disposing of confidential records, and the general unpreparedness of the individual's community. The spouse, children, loved ones or legal advisers of counsellors/therapists may have little or no preparation in dealing with such obligations. The provision of suitable counselling referrals or bereavement work for the clients of the therapist who is no longer effectively present is very important.

In many cases insufficient attention is paid in our codes of practice, our training literature or our supervision to provision for the execution of the duties of the therapist when they are unable to do so. I could find nothing in the literature that addressed this issue. By 1986 I was already communicating this idea of planning for the contingencies of death or incapacity as good professional practice to students and staff who were working for me at Metanoia, and by February 1990 I had included the concept as an item in the professional code of practice.

My colleague Barbara Traynor and I decided to prepare a paper for publication to make these ideas available for further professional discussion, and Barbara in particular outlined in considerable detail the ways in which she had made arrangements for her clients, in case of her death or incapacitation, including the appointment of a 'psychotherapeutic executor'. In February 1992 our paper entitled 'What happens if a psychotherapist dies?' appeared in *Counselling* (Traynor and Clarkson, 1992). (This paper also appears in a collection of key papers from that journal (Palmer, Dainow and Milner, 1996) and as Chapter 9 in this present book.)

A colleague subsequently brought to our attention a paper published in *Counselling* by Andrew Kitching (1995) – 'Practical approaches: our duty of care goes beyond the grave' – which seemed remarkably similar to our material. He made no reference to our paper and there was no acknowledgement in the text of where he had first learnt about this procedure. It is possible that the same ideas can arise (and they do) at different places in the world (see Koestler, *The Roots of Coincidence*, 1972). Was this what happened in this case? The publication of pretty much the same material (with no reference to the first paper) within the space of about three years, *and* in the same journal, is indeed extraordinary. I am aware that there was a change of editorship of *Counselling* and similarities between the two papers could have escaped the notice of the new editor. (It may also be instructive to note that Mr Kitching put a copyright sign on his paper, whereas Barbara Traynor and I did not.)

As part of a current research project I am asking a number of professional people to compare these two papers for the purposes of exercising our judgement as to what may or may not constitute plagiarism in professional literature. Apart from the idea, the conceptualisation, many of the action steps and idiosyncratically individual expressions, there are several examples of unreferenced direct textual quotations from our paper.

Of course, we all borrow ideas, and the more we learn the more likely it is that we will not only have our own ideas but also those of many others – some of these may have been forgotten, neglected or never properly sourced in the first place. Often ideas and expressions may feel like our own. Indeed, in our postmodern situation the notion of the self as an independent centre of initiative is in itself severely problematical. Perhaps the texts are indeed speaking to us – but they don't pay the account at the newspaper shop!

Many writers, particularly in postmodern literature, consistently and astonishingly plagiarise, pastiche or borrow from multiple other, unreferenced, sources. To some extent they may be able to rely on their readers having the background information to provide the necessary references from their own reading. Many postmodern films draw massively from others. Some respected authors in psychotherapy such as van Deurzen-Smith simply mention their sources at the beginning of a book:

> My ideas have been generated through living, studying, working with clients, teaching, supervising and training. It goes without saying that I am therefore indebted to all those people who have been there with me in that process... much else was inspired by the works of some of my favourite philosophers, including Socrates, Spinoza, Kierkegaard, Nietzsche, Heidegger and Sartre. It will be obvious that I take the contributions of many practitioners for granted although I seldom refer to them specifically. Freud, Binswanger, Boss, Laing and May are a few of the most influential ones. (van Deurzen-Smith, 1988, preface)

Others, like Wittgenstein (1922), make a clear statement that they are
ignoring them:

> How far my efforts agree with those of other philosophers I will not decide.
> Indeed what I have here written makes no claim to novelty in points of detail;
> and therefore I give no sources, because it is indifferent to me whether what I
> have thought has already been thought before me by another. (p. 27)

I have myself been criticised for referencing too much. My transactional
analysis book eventually contained some 400 references and my book
on the therapeutic relationship had close on 800. I meant this to be
helpful to teachers, practitioners and trainees alike, and some reviewers
of *The Therapeutic Relationship* (Barnett, 1995; Hauke, 1996; Rowan,
1999) perceived this to be the case.

I have also had the dubious honour of being involved in an official
academic investigation where someone was charged with plagiarising
my work. I have also been falsely accused of taking someone else's ideas,
but the accuser had got their sources wrong (for example, confusing
Boyd with Berne) and was mistaken in thinking that now common terms
within a body of knowledge, for example, ego and id in psychoanalysis,
need on every occasion to be referenced with page numbers in Freud's
works. On another occasion some vital quotation marks were omitted;
as soon as this was brought to my attention, I undertook to have it
corrected in the next edition. However, in the process of having my work
translated into around 21 languages to date, I can imagine that other
such oversights have occurred or may yet occur. So this piece is not
meant as a counsel of unreasonable perfection.

Then there are the many ways in which *teachers* of other people's
material sometimes get accredited as the originating sources of those
ideas. I have had such reason on several occasions to nudge a colleague
into correcting attributions. Unacknowledged use of lecture notes by
students in essay reports and dissertations are of the same order. Such
confusion of tongues and a multiplicity of discourses is part of the joy
and excitement of our postmodern, information-rich, multi-narratived
time, but how are we to navigate it with honour as well as respect?

Scholarship

A delightful article called 'The academy of the dead' by Simmer (1981)
makes the case for our awareness of our sources and the honouring of
our teachers in a beautiful and imaginative way. Drawing on myths and
archetypal psychology he writes that:

> Seen through the footnotes the essay is a dialogue of the dead. The thought
> appropriated as the author's own in the text above the line may be re-
> imagined from below as a collaboration of ghost-writers, each placing his
> own demand on the work. Scholarship is *daimonic* in its original meaning of
> 'divided.' (p. 103)

Reference footnotes are a criminal record. In them we confess our guilt to crimes of theft, fraud, extortion and murder. We admit the poverty and dishonesty of our own insight; little or nothing of what we say really belongs to us. In footnotes we are revealed like a criminal in the stocks, with our crimes displayed below for all to see. 'I have pillaged the grave of Plato, I have stolen from Emerson, I have maimed and slaughtered Freud, and you can see for yourself how wretchedly I have wronged them.' (p. 101)

On first glance, the reference footnote seems to give credit to the origi-nator of an idea. But ideas are not like veins of ore that wait passively to be discovered. Ideas are active, powerful, and autonomous. They, not the writers, create the work. The ideas may achieve momentary expression in the scholar's work, but they lived before and continue to live after the date of publication. To attach a name, date, and publisher to an idea seems arbitrary and presumptuous, because ideas are daimones that we serve. (p. 100)

How can we differentiate the archetypal appreciation that there is nothing original and we are all 'thieves' at the symbolic, metaphoric and theoretical universes of discourse (Level 6) from the morality of using another's ideas and conceptualisations without due acknowledgement and references at the normative (Level 4); from the nature of inaccurate, misleading or absence of referencing of sources at Level 5 about which there is consensual agreement in academic practice? (See Item 10 in this book for further discourse analysis of these levels.) Perhaps in changes to our ethical codes and by exploring these together in workshops, for our own education and that of the students for whom we may even be role models.

Codes of ethics and professional practice

There is not much in the British Association for Counselling (1992) Code of Ethics and Practice for Counsellors which is explicit or helpful in the question of plagiarism. Sections B.2.4.1 and B.2.4.2 state that:

Counsellors should not conduct themselves in their counselling-related activ-ities in ways which undermine public confidence in either their role as a counsellor or in the work of other counsellors.

If a counsellor suspects misconduct by another counsellor which cannot be resolved or remedied after discussion with the counsellor concerned, they should implement the Complaints Procedure, doing so without breaches of confidentiality other than those necessary for investigating the complaint.

So we can question whether the use of another person's ideas in writing, which is a 'counselling-related activity', can 'undermine public confi-dence'. It certainly suggests (a) the possibility of trying to pass another's ideas off as one's own in this context, or (b) that a person can attempt to make a scientific or professional contribution by publishing a paper on a particular (unusual) topic in a particular journal without at the very least reading the previous few years' output of this journal in order to check if anything had been published on this topic in this journal.

The very public nature of this lack of accidental or intentional oversight makes it difficult to resolve or remedy the matter with the counsellor concerned. Furthermore, in the light of the ambiguity (or not) from a legal position, and the absence of ethical codes specifically addressing this issue, it seems necessary to seek some advice in a confidential manner in order to begin to know what to say to authors who duplicate not only one's ideas, but also the sequence of an argument and substantial sections in which the words and phrases are identical.

How to proceed? An inquiry, an acknowledgement, an apology, an acknowledgement of synchronicity? The latter would depend on such an author not having been in contact through training, workshops, consultancy, supervision with anyone who had been studying with or in supervision with the originating author or one of their colleagues – but surely any one of my colleagues teaching this material would have acknowledged the source. Most academic institutions have specific rules against plagiarism or passing off by students, but my investigations have so far failed to reveal any such strictures applicable to staff.

I have raised a number of issues which affect me as a professional writer, academic, and supervisor of supervisors and academic researchers at masters and doctoral levels. There may be legal issues involved. However, I sincerely trust that this can be the start of an initiative on the part of the BAC, BPS and perhaps the UKCP and other bodies as well to clarify, elucidate and problem-solve in the complex arena of appropriate honour to ancestors, the celebration of individual autonomy, and the encouragement of creativity and originality (May, 1976), along with the academic and professional standards of rigorous and meticulous acknowledgement, between the excitement of the bright new ideas and the Saturnian awareness of our existential situation as the intellectual and professional inheritors of an estate that is probably very, very much older than 2500 years.

> Why do those who are pursuing knowledge not encounter tragic knowledge, or otherwise confront the penalties of knowledge, and why do they declare themselves free of sentiment and patriotism and religious conviction, and who are they writing for anyway? (Hariman, 1989, p. 211)

This section is written in order to encourage and inform novice writers in the fields of psychology, counselling and psychotherapy to share their views, experiences and in writing to the benefit of all involved. I see writing about our work (whether client records or learned papers in peer-review journals) as an important part of subjecting our learning and what we have to learn to the ongoing conversation with our professional colleagues and as an intrinsic part of conducting accountable practice. Aspiring writers on psychotherapy have many and varied concerns, ranging on the one hand from 'not having anything new to say' to 'no one will ever want to read it' and anywhere from 'I don't have any ideas' to 'I don't have any time'. On the basis of some 25 years in these fields and having been happy to facilitate numerous junior and peer colleagues into print for the first time, I have been encouraged to share some ideas myself on this topic in this form.

Clear out common mistaken assumptions

To be published, a work must be original

In my opinion (and in the opinion of Solomon of Biblical fame) there is nothing new under the sun. It is extremely unlikely that anyone will have startlingly original and totally novel ideas in any field. We almost always stand on the shoulders of those who have gone before and the seeds of most if not all ideas are found in the questions, answers and struggles of our forebears. With ambitions to be totally original, one is most likely to fail. As Ann Craddock Jones (1975) phrased it, 'Grandiosity blocks writing projects'. For myself I have learned to look upon writing as a Yoga – a spiritual exercise in learning and relearning humility. I always fail the vision. All each of us can ever reasonably hope to do is to say something for our time in our way in our corner of the field which may be of use to others. And this is rarely so small as does not need to be done.

To be published, a work must be written by someone who is qualified

Often articles and papers in serious academic journals are reviewed 'blind'. This means that the author's name and qualifications are deleted from the paper when it is submitted in manuscript form and the journal committees who decide to publish do not know who or how well known the author of the paper is. This is indeed to ensure fair reviews so that decisions to publish are made on merit, not on 'connections' or 'fame'. Indeed many famous authors have told stories of how their papers have been rejected. A recent one concerns an American Psychological Association journal rejecting a paper by Professor Alvin Mahrer – the 1997 recipient of 'America's Most Distinguished Psychologist Award' (personal communication). On the other hand, novice trainees have succeeded in having their papers published even though they were unqualified. Unfortunately, novices or unqualified individuals often hold back out of some feelings of hierarchical inferiority on their part or mystification by their seniors of the process of writing for publication.

To be published, you must have 'time to write'

Well, I think the truth is nobody has time to write, and even those who get the time – according to a friend of mine who spent a month at a special retreat for writers – don't always get much done when they do actually have the time. (She spent most of the time preparing to divorce her husband – but she won a prize for the book she published after that.) Writing is an activity for which there never seems to be time, and yet time must be made if you're having to write essays or papers or dissertations in order to get your qualifications or progress your career in a desired direction. There are many tips and tricks to do with time management and writing. One tried and tested recipe is to get up earlier in the morning – before the interruptions start. Many, many professional writers do this. The most important tip is to give up the illusion that 'one day you'll have enough time'. That day might never come. I think our problem solving energy actually needs us to give up wishing and get directed to work on to how to get the writing done – even when there is as little time as there is.

Why should we write at all?

Writing, like research, is a way of expressing your values. In fact, it is one of the very best ways of finding out what one is thinking – or what one has learned. It is a demonstration of what we value. Although reading feeds and nourishes the ground in which the seeds are to be planted, it is only by the real active work of seeding and watering and weeding and harvesting that one ever gets to enjoy the fruits of the reading which preceded it. Reading and listening, memorising and introjecting are all important parts of education, but they tend to foster a passive education often tending towards replication and imitation rather than innovation, enquiry and creativity. That is why most training courses require writing of one kind or another.

It is in our mental and emotional conversations with others in writing that our ideas become most clarified. We can only really find out if we have learned something when our ideas and our reworking of the ideas of others can be criticised, explored and improved – away from our personal influence or 'presence' we reduce the likelihood of the overly supportive feedback or overly critical feedback from friends, enemies and rivals of either kind. Writing is the fruits of genuine relationships with one's self *and* with other internalised others.

Another reason to write is to form, develop or sustain relationships with others. The notion of writing as a way of forming, developing and sustaining relationships with colleagues particularly emphasises the interrelatedness of emotional, intellectual, spiritual and academic or professional community. For hundreds of years colleagues all over the world have been having dialogic conversations into which every discovery, every significant achievement must at some point enter. In the writing we work through problems, and in the writings of others, whether in response to ours or not, the collegial conversation continues. Through writing our young ideas are tested or rejected, our questions are answered or ignored, our findings reviled or rejected.

For myself I see writing not so much as self-expression (which I keep to myself), more as a form of service to my relationships – and part of an aspirational creative ethic. And I benefit from the generosity and courage of those who care to put their thoughts where I and others may find them and be enriched or enraged or enlightened by them. These are precious relationships – this ambivalent community of peers and teachers and students where the life of the mind is conducted in the context of collegial relationships. Through writing we can make contact with many others who share our interests, argue with those others (dead or alive) whose opinions we dispute, search and sometimes find maybe even on the other side of the world special people from whom we can learn or who may even want to benefit from our teaching.

The third reason I will highlight here has been phrased as 'publish or perish'. For good or bad reasons, academic and sometimes professional survival and abundance is connected with number and quality of publications. Publications can be especially conspicuous by their absence in a CV. These can be rather negative reasons for writing, but nonetheless persuasive. Through the choice of content, process and outlet for our publications we can create a career in the academy; become popular millionaire best-sellers; or make small but frequent accessible contributions which help others in significant but less visible ways.

The process of writing for publication

Find your unanswered question

All of us are engaged in studying, in development in professional qualification as part of the great process of 'learning by enquiry' or continuing education – as such, it is likely that there is a question in your heart. Finding the question in your heart is the beginning of writing – and you'll find you've already done a lot of that. The challenge is to turn that question into a product. Nobody can help shape or relate to the ideas in your head until they're out on a piece of paper. Write down the question (or the answer) in the middle of a big blank sheet of paper in big bold coloured letters. Pin it to your wall where you can see it before you go to sleep at night. Put it in the lid of your briefcase. Use it as a screensaver on your computer. Let it grow. Let it act as a 'strange attractor'. (This is a notion from chaos theory (Briggs and Peat, 1989) which also concerns creativity.)

Trust that physis is at work. This implies an acceptance that physis – the unconscious creative primary process – will seek to complete the gestalt. Heraclitus said that 'physis loves to hide' (Kahn, 1981, p. 105). This is in the nature of creativity. Inspiration will come and go.

Perspiration is required. Please also be careful who you talk to while an idea is brewing – people can stomp on it or you can talk it away. (Many good books are talked away.) Go about your everyday business. Do the ironing, phone your mother, tidy the linen cupboard, have the fight with your wife you've been meaning to have for a long time. These so-called procrastinating tactics are all necessary preparation for the creative process.

Do what needs to be done; when your question is ripe, you will find the time. Find or make definitions of the central terms you want to use. Then write down the title – or working title – if you haven't already done so. The title should be such that anyone looking at top speed through a long table of contents in the journal or a computer listing in your area should immediately recognise that it would be valuable to them. You may revise your title many times – or the title itself may drive the work to completion.

Make some strong physical activity to stimulate the right hemisphere of your brain

Good analysis and logical sequencing is loosely associated with left hemispheric activity in most human brains. (The opposite is usually true for left-handers.) Critics – internal or external – are often good folk just trying to help. Your left hemisphere is your editor, the person or capacity who can be relied upon to find all the faults – later. Unfortunately critics constitutionally simply cannot have a good idea without criticising it to death. Have you ever seen a monument built to a critic? (This quote is not mine, but I don't know who said it first. If you know, let me know.)

Valuable as criticism can be, it appears to be incompatible with creativity at the same moment. It's like trying to breathe in and out simultaneously. It can be done for a few seconds or so, but then you're more likely to pass out. Critic and creator in each of us have to be kept separate in order to each function at their best. Some peopie give their internal critics and internal creators completely different working spaces, or dress in different clothes for the different functions. The more these two are separated in time and place, the better they can each get on with their jobs.

Creativity is usually associated with the right hemisphere of our brain. This is actually the source of liveliness, of rhythm, of excitement, of the juice which moistens and moves all good writing – and all other creative work whether captaining industry or parenting. (This is not meant to be neurologically exact.) If you want to energise your creativity in your writing, disobey the bad teachers from your schooldays. Don't listen when any internal or external voice of authority advises you to 'Just sit down and do it', or 'just sit still and concentrate'. The teachers were wrong. That's probably why so little good writing gets done. Jump, dance, sing: thc more noisy, the more nonsensical and the more disruptive, the better.

Depending on how private you are, shake all your limbs, make silly faces or disgusting noises, breathe through the other nostril. If you're angry about something, stomp and scream until you're got so much energy you just have to write out your protest on paper. Play hard rock, Philip Glass, Stockhausen. It doesn't matter if you don't like it, it may even be better so. Get thoroughly worked up in whatever way your body wants to, without leaving the room in which your pen or computer is.

The brainstorm

Then brainstorm all the ideas you associate with your question or central idea on to the big sheet. It is important to use many different colours, different kinds of writing, different places. It is necessary to avoid writing in straight lines, in sequence or from right to left or top to bottom. It should look as chaotic as you can possibly make it. The messier, the better. Don't worry about the spelling or the grammar. Some friend or colleague can always help you fix your English later. When you've finished this and your sheet is quite full of ideas, phrases, pictures, examples, memories, etc., only then let it become quiet and sort your ideas into three groupings:

- the first third, marked with a circle, for example
- the middle and largest grouping, marked perhaps with a star
- the last third, marked with exclamation points or whatnot.

In this way a preliminary shape is found among the chaos. It is a version of the technique – 'dump everything you know about the problem in one place, then stare at it until a shape emerges'.

Using case material

Although case studies for examination and re-accreditation purposes (see Item 6) and research reports must be truthful, the safest advice for using case material in publications is: don't! If a case study is indeed necessary for your story, fictionalise, amalgamate stories, change details beyond recognition – ask your supervisor to help you with this so that you don't lose the psychological integrity of the story. My best advice at the moment (from one of the senior professional organisations) recommends that if you just use some part of a story, as in a segment of verbatim transcript or dialogue without specific identifying details or with identifying details changed, it is not necessary to ask your client's permission. Finding out (by reading the journal or attending the conference) that your analyst or psychotherapist has published your life story with their commentary without your permission can be devastating – particularly if their tone is pathologising or disrespectful. If published while the client is still in therapy, it is definitely an ethical violation. On the other hand, people often identify with case studies – as we do in novels and films – and there are many coincidences, including some of the most bizarre-sounding. People are more alike than they usually think. It is best to publish more accurate or identifying case studies (still using your clinical judgement) only after the therapy or analysis has been finally terminated and then only when you have obtained the client's written permission. If you are considering exceptions to this advice (such as taking an 'ethical risk' by publishing material on the basis that the client may never come across it) get supervision or consult with colleagues.

Who are you writing for?

This is your calling card or your website, whether real or symbolic. You have one or two sentences to get someone to start a conversation with you. Who do you want it to be? Do you want to have someone who says 'Hi!', 'Hello', or a more formal 'How do you do?' (We're speaking metaphorically, of course, depending on what kind of company you want to keep.) The better your audience is defined, the better your relationship with them will be. Imagine that you're talking with them. What do they want to know? What would interest them, grab their attention? What might help them become more successful, happier, more fulfilled? Write the last sentence of your paper first – how do you want to say goodbye to them? What kind of relationship will you have made with them? This last sentence acts as the notion of an oak tree to an acorn. It calls the work to its destination. By starting with an incomplete gestalt, energised by emotion, care and soul, a whole process of completion can be set in motion at levels well beyond ordinary consciousness.

Write the first sentence of your paper

Look at your favourite books and titles and how you came to find them; perhaps you can learn how to do it too. All the best novels have strong first sentences. They are the initial conditions for the work, setting the tone and starting the conversation. The first paragraph tells people what to look for, what to pay attention to and what they should not expect. The more clearly you specify your intentions and your own criteria, the more likely that (a) you will meet them and (b) critics who want you to have written a different paper will just sound silly. The first sentence or first paragraph is always the most important part of your paper or book. Look at your favourite books and articles and study how other people have done this effectively; perhaps you can learn from them. You may need to redo this beginning part many, many times, often after you have written the whole paper. It is extremely rare for a first sentence to come out perfectly in the first place.

Only 20 rubbish statements

Then, independent of the previous sorting exercise, write down 20 statements at top speed around the theme of your central issue or question. It does not matter whether they make sense, whether they are correctly spelled out or whether they're in sequence. If they're going from most important to least important that's grand. If you really don't know if they're higgledy-piggledy, just write them down in whatever order they come. If you suddenly come across a good idea, don't wait to admire it, write down another one that's worse, just to keep the process loose. In this part of the process it is absolutely essential not to remove your pen from the paper. Keep your pen moving or keep your fingers typing. Don't stop. If it's rubbish, write rubbish down. People build houses from rubbish. If you don't know what to write, write down that you don't know what to write or that you hate the exercise or whatever. If you're not sure of what you're writing, do it anyway. You can check up later. *This is not editing time*, this is time for the playfulness of your creative self to enjoy its own expressiveness without any restraint at all. There'll be enough of that later.

After this, identify your authorities and reference them properly NOW. Ask friends, your study group, your teacher, your supervisor, their friends, the Psych. Lit. of the library, the Internet. Find these references. *Make a list of 6 initial references*. These are the first 'author-ities' you will consult. (Whether these eventually end up as 600 or a different 6 depends on how your work grows and the balance of references to the length of the work.) As quickly and accurately as possible, do them in proper Harvard form. (Take any paper from a journal to which you would like to submit your paper as an example, and copy the format for referencing – but exactly!) Then check it carefully and slowly. If you don't write down all the publication details now title, initials of author, year of publication, number of edition, place of publication, name of publisher, page number, etc., you will waste endless time later trying to find these details. These references:

> poetically name the imaginal characters who speak, listen, argue, and evaluate in the dialogue which lies behind the essay. We can read reference footnotes as a playbill and stage directions for the drama of scholarship. Enter Plato, with trumpets. (Simmer, 1981, p. 103)

Any time saved at this point by neglecting precise notes about bibliographical details will come back to haunt you when the editors send it to you for a copy-editor check which they want answered in three days – and you're just about to go off on holiday. (Well, there are always some exceptions – but will it be you?)

Read your reference books with your question in mind. These are your teachers and first consultants. They will tell you what's been done, what's over, what hasn't worked and most importantly you will see what you're working on that's different, more or slightly differently developed from them – or what needs saying again. Acknowledge them. Read the primary sources, i.e. the people who first wrote about the theme you're pursuing. Honour the ancestors; they've been talking since the beginning of time. The challenge for you, if you want to be heard, is . . .

Getting in

Find the place where relationship can begin, where there are others who want to talk about your topic, where you can get a word in edgeways. Imagine that professional writing activity is like a cocktail party; no doubt some people are talking about your topic or question somewhere in the crowded room, but how can you get to know them? It is just the same as tea time at a large international professional conference. Hang about and listen in to other people's conversations, say hello – read their abstracts and posters, go to the 'focus' and 'special interest' groups, put yourself where these collegial conversations are happening.

You're looking for an 'in', just the same as at the firm's Christmas party. And finally, when you hear someone mention wet Wednesday afternoons, you will find just the right opening to say, 'Now that you mention wet Wednesday afternoons, you might want to hear what happened to me one wet Wednesday afternoon I went to Seville to pick me some oranges', or whatever. Or listen for somebody asking the question, 'Where can we get something useful about writing for publication?' and then the moment has come for you to say, 'Well, I've been doing some work on that recently and . . .'. And if you've picked your moment right, and you've connected up with others in that conversation, they'll all quieten down for a minute and listen to you. What happens next depends on all your preparation so far. Will what you have to say fit with their questions? You've finally got your moment. (After that, it's up to them to use it, abuse it, ignore it or treasure it.) You can get the same effect looking up Psych. Lit. on your university library computer. It's a kind of detective work, boring for much of the time but, when you finally figure out whodunnit, a rush of undiluted joy.

Connecting up

You should also find up-to-date journals where these conversations in your field or about your questions are happening. (This is how to move the quality of your work from competent to excellent.) Check these journals' conditions for considering unsolicited publications. Shape your paper to their requirements, which are usually printed on the last page of the journal. Check that you know and understand the maximum word count. Since most journals want papers only between 2000 and 5000 words, there's no need to write a book length piece. You'll only have to reduce it. (I once wrote a book *twice* the size it had to be because I made a mistake with the word count. It was not fun and half a written book is still languishing somewhere on a theme with which I am finished.)

Suppose your target is 3000 words. That's 6 single-spaced pages, 12 double-spaced ones. Look over your brainstorm again. Move, jump, do push-ups. Shout your frustration at all the injustice in the world, or the teacher who shamed you in grade school. Write your paper now in sentences – only some two or three sentences per point. You'll soon fill up 6 pages. Imagine that you are a painter working with the canvas as a whole, covering it completely, then working on parts of it, then reworking it again and again. Find illustrations, diagrams to make it easier for your readers – and for you. Put the paper away for a month or so and rewrite it again. By now you'll want to. If your topic needs more life, it will keep coming up again and again in a synchronous way. You'll also have come across new references and interesting examples you may want to incorporate. Revise it again. Don't be surprised if the title, the order or the content changes completely. We never really know what shape a creative piece of work wants to be until it is finished.

If you get stuck, welcome the impasse or the block – even though you don't want to. Often it is true that the longer and more uncomfortable this blocked period, the better the quality of the eventual product. Do other things. If your paper is true, it will *ask* to be written in the end. (If it wakes you up in the middle of the night, just get up and do it then. It helps to keep the draft or the laptop by the bed.) If you want to get on with something and you're in a critical editing frame of mind, check that your references are in the style which the journal wants, then check your quotes and check the references again. As Simmer (1981) writes:

> Perhaps there is action only when there is stoppage. When the writing is not blocked nothing is really moving. There is only the caricature of movement, 'busy work'. Writing of this kind really evades writing, because the work is without the weight of dilemmas. The block causes profound movement in writing, agitating its depths like Hecate's earthquake. (p. 94)

Then follow the journal instructions on how to do it. Presenting research results, for example, almost always follows a standard form: Introduction; Aims and objectives of the study; Literature survey; Method; Qualitative and/or quantitative research; Selection of respondents; Instrumentation; Research questions; Research protocol; Data collection; Organising, analysing and synthesising data; Discussion of findings; Relationship of study findings to findings of literature review; Possible future research; Personal outcomes; Relationship of the study to professional outcomes; Relationship of study to social meanings and relevance; Future direction and goals; and References (or some such). These are also PhD research proposal headings.

Now organise. Put ideas in sequence. Now be logical and ordered. If you can't or won't, ask someone else to do it with you or for you. Then you may want to rewrite your paper again. Give your seventh (sic) draft to your friends in draft form, then to your supervisor, to your teachers. Give it to anybody who is going to be kind and generous enough to give your piece of work their time and attention. Offer them favours in return – lunch, baby-sitting, reading their manuscripts. Ask the first readers of your rough draft manuscript not to give you global appreciations or rejections or whether they 'like it' or not, but rather ask them for comments and suggestions for improvements by a certain date after which you can no longer incorporate their suggestions.

Request that they please be specific. Value and appreciate such people. Acknowledge them if they help to the extent that they do so. It is an absolute myth that writers are solitary. Nothing ever gets written by one person. (This may be a very slight exaggeration.) Read the preface to almost any book or footnotes and acknowledgements to most papers and you'll notice how many people participate – and those are only the named ones. The writer is only the funnel through which the collective awareness of a cultural nor scientific moment is expressed. The writer works for everybody.

Finally, on to the starting line

Redraft again. Check your paper for errors. Number your pages. Standardise headings and subheadings. Check it against the journal requirements. Every single journal seems to be different and they may have remarkably and sometimes frustratingly different demands on the author. What is just right for one, may come in for considerable rudeness from another. Consult an expert for the *correct placing* of your paper – which journal is likely to want it or welcome it? Consult the journal editor(s) on what the likely turnaround time is likely to be if you're factoring time in as an element in deciding where to place it. Check your paper again for word count, for headings and sub-headings, for accuracy of diagrams, tables and references and quotes, for title and subtitle, for your biographical description and where you may be contacted.

Use the spellcheck function on your word processor and have someone else proofread it again. Correct the errors (or clarify the ambiguous or misleading statements) they found *after* you thought there were no more errors to be found and everything was perfectly clear. (Better now than after they appear in print.) Send it off. You could get or ask for an acknowledgement of receipt. Then all you can do is wait. Eventually they'll reject it outright or give you suggestions for improvement. This can take anywhere from months to years. It's better to have several papers on the go at once in order to minimise the importance attached to any one rejection or acceptance. You also get more practice and can become a better writer as well. The more prestigious the journal, the longer it takes and the more corrections they may want. Very few papers in the world get accepted without changes. Choose whether you want your paper published with these changes or not. If you want it published, make the changes they want and send it back.

A long time after, they'll send it back – finally in page proof form. This is the first time you get to see what your paper will look like in its printed form as if in the actual journal. This is the way other people will see it. It's often a bit of a shock. You might tend to see many things you would still like to change. You may actually be prohibited from making any of your own changes at this point – or be charged what may feel like exorbitant sums for re-typesetting such changes – so try to imagine this moment well before it happens and iron out all possible errors and misunderstandings before the final paper goes to the printer for the first time. The purpose of the proofs is to give you an opportunity to check whether the *typesetters* have made mistakes – so your job is proofreading them, not making last-minute improvements to your own writing. (You can of course always make some private notes for the next edition or a future paper at this stage.) Then, since you are even more than usually fallible at this point, get someone else to proofread it again.

Afterwards

Do not be concerned about being misunderstood. You *will* be misunderstood. Then you may just have to write another paper or another book. This is how many keep writing. Fear of being misunderstood can mute you forever. If you don't want to risk being be misunderstood, you should never write – or speak. Then there will also never be the opportunity to be – once in a glorious while – understood, helpful, appreciated, part of the great creative process which is our world.

Do not be concerned about falling short of perfection. You *will* fall short of perfection.

> No man [or woman] ever puts down what he intended to say: the original creation, which is taking place all the time, whether one writes or doesn't write, belongs to the primal flux: it has no dimensions, no form, no time element. In this preliminary state, which is not creation and not birth, what disappears suffers no destruction; something which was already there, something imperishable like memory, or matter, or God, is summoned and in it one flings himself like a twig into a torrent. (Miller, 1964, p. 23)

A thought . . .

If this chapter helps you to publish (even if you end up proving me wrong) consider acknowledging the author.

References and further reading

APA (1984) Publication Manual of the American Psychological Association. Washington, DC: American Psychological Association.

BAC (1992) Code of Ethics and Practice for Counsellors. Rugby: British Association for Counselling.

Barnett, R. (1995) A 'gust of fresh air' – book review of P. Clarkson's The Therapeutic Relationship. Counselling News, 19.

Briggs, J. and Peat, F.D. (1989) Turbulent Mirror. New York: Harper & Row.

Clarkson, P. (1998) Dieratao – learning by inquiry – concerning the education of psychologists, psychotherapists, supervisors and organisational consultants. In P. Clarkson (ed.), Counselling Psychology: Integrating Theory, Research and Supervised Practice, pp. 242–72. London: Routledge.

Clarkson, P. (1998) Writing as research. In P. Clarkson (ed.), Counselling Psychology: Integrating Theory, Research and Supervised Practice, pp. 242–72. London: Routledge.

Craddock Jones, A. (1975) Grandiosity blocks writing projects. Transactional Analysis Journal, 5(4), 415.

Crone, T. (1991) Law and the Media. Oxford: Butterworth-Heinemann.

Deurzen-Smith, E. van (1988) Existential Counselling in Practice. London: Sage.

Dillard, A. (1990) The Writing Life. New York: HarperPerennial.

Eliot, T. S. (1963) Collected Poems 1909–1962, pp. 196–204, London: Faber and Faber.

Hariman, R. (1989) The Rhetoric of Inquiry and the Professional Scholar. In H. W. Simons (ed.) Rhetoric in the Human Sciences, pp. 211–32. London: Sage.

Hauke, C. (1996) Book review of P. Clarkson's The Therapeutic Relationship. British Journal of Psychotherapy, 12(3), 405–7.

Kahn, C.H. (1981) The Art and Thought of Heraclitus: An Edition of the Fragments with Translation and Commentary. Cambridge: Cambridge University Press.

Kitching, A. (1995) Practical approaches: our duty of care goes beyond the grave, Counselling, 6(4), 269–70.

Koestler, A. (1972) The Roots of Coincidence. London: Hutchinson.

May, R. (1976) The Courage to Create. New York: Bantam.

Miller, H. (1964) Henry Miller on Writing. New York: New Directions.

Palmer, S., Dainow, S. and Milner, P. (eds) Counselling: The BAC Counselling Reader, London: Sage.

Rowan, J. (1999) Book Review: The Therapeutic Relationship. P. Clarkson. AHP Perspective, 17th July.

Rudestam, K.E. and Newton, R.R. (1992) Surviving your Dissertation – A Comprehensive Guide to Content and Process. London: Sage.

Simmer, S. (1981) The academy of the dead – On boredom, writer's block, footnotes and deadlines. Spring – An Annual of Archetyal Psychology and Jungian Thought, 89–106.

Sternberg, R.J. (1988) The Psychologist's Companion – A Guide to Scientific Writing for Students and Researchers. Leicester: British Psychological Society.

Traynor, B. and Clarkson, P. (1992) What happens if a psychotherapist dies? Counselling, 3(1), 23–4. Reprinted (1996) in S. Palmer, S. Dainow and P. Milner (eds) Counselling: The BAC Counselling Reader, pp. 483–6. London: Sage.

Wittgenstein, L. (1922) Tractatus Logico-Philosophicus. London: Routledge & Kegan Paul.

ITEM 11
A Code of Ethics for Counselling and Psychotherapy Publications

PETRŪSKA CLARKSON

The work of counselling and psychotherapy publications is to promote education, debate and information in the fields of counselling, psychotherapy and adjacent disciplines. In their dealings therefore such publications will be guided by the law of the land and the spirit of the ethical codes of these professions.

Therefore this suggested code is not to be seen as a final set of rules, but more as a live working document to stimulate the aim towards good standards of conduct and debate about good practice as well as ongoing professional and ethical developments in the field.

Publishing or submitting material for publishing is considered acceptance of the contract clause that such acts are done by professionals currently subscribing to and in adherence with a professional code of ethics – i.e. BAC, UKCP or BPS, for example.

Certain items are of particular interest in the regard to an endeavour such as this:

- *Confidentiality*: Editors and contributors shall communicate information and opinion in ways which protects the identity of specific individuals or organisations obtained in the course of professional work. It is understood that ethical decisions sometimes involve complex or even conflicting ethical values. In this case, as in all the others, the opinions of experienced practitioners or supervisors will be sought in all situations where the welfare, safety and the reputation of others are concerned.
- *Respect*: Editors and contributors shall conduct themselves in such a way so as not to inappropriately undermine public confidence in either their role as a practitioners or in the work of other practitioners. Criticism and negative feedback will not be derogatory of individual professionals, but differences expressed will be based on

219

ideas, opinions about practice and conduct and should be balanced
with appreciation where possible.

- *Responsible involvement*: If a practitioner suspects misconduct by
another practitioner or organisation which cannot be resolved or
remedied after discussion with the individuals concerned, they
should bring it to the attention of those charged with the responsibility to investigate/implement the Complaints Procedure relevant to
this situation, doing so without breaches of confidentiality other than
those necessary for investigating the complaint.

- *Accuracy of information*: Scrupulous honesty and accuracy should
be observed and immediately corrected in all publications and
communications should false and misleading statements be identified. The contributor is responsible for checking typographical errors
and other potential sources of misinformation in material they
submit. Sensational, exaggerated or unjustifiable claims will not be
published.

- *Equal opportunities*: Contributions from all sections of the populations will be considered subject to ordinary journalistic standards. In
particular there will be no discrimination on the grounds of race,
gender, sexual orientation, ability, culture, religion or any other such
category. Contributions from disadvantaged groups will be actively
encouraged and facilitated where possible. An awareness of such
issues will be expected in written work.

- *Appropriate acknowledgement*: The editors and contributors will
refrain from claiming credit for the research and intellectual properly
of others and give due credit to the contributions of others in collaborative work. All work will be appropriately referenced and in case of
errors or omissions immediately rectified.

- *Obtaining consent*: In all cases where appropriate such as identifiable case studies, the written consent of clients should be obtained
wherever possible. Where the opinions and views of others are
published, the contributor is responsible for checking the accuracy
and obtaining consent where possible.

- *Professional honesty*: Statements or implications which are false and
misleading about qualifications, abilities, experience or by association make misleading implications about practitioners or the organisations constitute a serious offence. It is therefore expected that all
concerned will take responsibility for ensuring accuracy and appropriateness of claims, and for ensuring that their qualifications,
capabilities or views are not misrepresented by others, and to
immediately correct such misrepresentations when noticed.

- *Competency*: Editors and contributors will acknowledge the limits of
their competence in experience, or forming opinions and express
their views and findings within such limits, specifying what communications are based on fact and what based on opinion or personal

experience – rather than making generalisations on behalf of others without their consent.

- *Honourable intention*: In all understanding and practice of our work, to seek to value as well as critique our profession, its institutions, practices and ideas with demonstrated respect for persons and evidence and to endeavour to promote the highest ethical and professional standards in our work. This code item includes making suggestions for improvement to this code which will be updated on an annual basis in consultation with our Advisory Editorial Board.

(c) Drawn from BPS, UKCP and BAC codes and research by Professor Petrūska Clarkson, Physis, 1997.

CHAPTER 12
Psychotherapy Ethics in the Context of 'Schoolism'

PETRŪSKA CLARKSON

> A most painful possibility is that our ethical codes are but hollow symbols of a
> myth of professionalism. . . . As long as it appears to courts and to the public
> that psychology [or counselling or psychotherapy] is a cacophony of
> competing claims to workable procedures, the judgement of the members,
> regardless of the profession's highest minded ethical standards, will be open
> to challenge. Psychology is fragmented into many different schools each
> espousing its own theoretical orientation, a state of affairs which may
> motivate research and enliven the professional journals by which may inspire
> little confidence in society. With the field so divided it is not difficult to
> explain why codes of ethics remain vague and abstract and wide a wide
> variety of specific behaviour is tolerated. (Bersoff, 1995, p. 104)

It has been said that modern medicine began with the appearance of
rationalism in treatment exemplified in the early writings of Egyptian
and Babylonian physicians between 2000 and 3000 BCE.

The ancient 'physicians' (from the Greek 'physis' – the life force)
prescribed remedies of herbs, stone, amulets, charms, incantations.
Always the most powerful agent in activating organismic healing forces
was the relationship with the doctor, the medicine man, the powerful
priest/healer who usually shared or derived power from the ruling class
and state religions. Frank's book (1973) *Persuasion and Healing* investigated commonalities across so-called primitive approaches to healing
which maintain traces of the ancient practices. He observed that
religious conversion, primitive healing, brainwashing, altered states of
consciousness, creative furore, ESP and placebo effects all involve
similar processes of change.

A reasonably common professional view now holds that
psychotherapy and its allied disciplines have developed in response to
three essential human needs – prevention, cure and development, or:

- to prevent mental and emotional pain and distress
- to heal or cure it
- to develop or evolve human capacities for overcoming suffering and creating or improving lives which are fulfilling and satisfying.

Already in the Greek myths there are echoes of modern-day psychiatric problems and attempts to solve them.

Demeter, the earth goddess, grieved so long and so deeply for the loss of her daughter Persephone that the earth became dry, barren and lifeless. Her depression threatened to end not only her life, but the lives of all around her. Being taken seriously (by Hecate) and the family therapy mediation of Hermes restored her (and the earth) to health.

The other well-known madman in the occidental tradition is Hercules. He lost his mind (through Hera's doing) and murdered his entire family in a violent fit of mania. After completing the twelve labours he eventually emerged both heroic and healed. The ancients of all cultures have always taught that time is a great healer – and so is work. Chiron, the Centaur trained at least three nascent healers: Achilles who was both warrior and doctor, sometimes both, and Jason who also had healing powers. We are more familiar with his third student, Apollo.

In ancient Greece many of the mentally ill are reported to have gone to the temples of Asclepius (Apollo's son) where they fasted and purified themselves. Then they went to sleep on the couches or *kline* (hence our modern word clinic) waiting for Apollo, the god of healing, to appear to them in a dream. Temple priestesses or Pythia would interpret these dreams and the patients left for home to implement the directions thus received – but not without the offering of some gold or treasure. Today counselling, psychiatry, psychotherapy and so on have become multimillion pound businesses, costing state and ordinary people fortunes although still largely reliant on herbs (or their modern chemical equivalent), teaching people to forego their negative thinking – or the interpretation of dreams.

Nebuchadnezzar as reported in the Old Testament also looked to Daniel to interpret his dreams when his spirit 'was troubled'. Even in the books of the New Testament Jesus is described as driving the devils out of two possessed men: 'And the unclean spirits went out, and entered into the swine: and the herd ran violently down a steep place into the sea . . . and were choked in the sea' (Matthew 8: 32). Exorcism of one kind or another is still part of many societies that have not been infected with western European ways of looking at the world, and in some societies it co-exists. The driving out of devils still plays a part in many societies today and is practised, where deemed necessary, by clergy from most of the minor and major religious traditions in most parts of the world. (It is still not always an humane procedure. In 1994 in Britain, a young Muslim woman was beaten to death with blunt instruments over several days by her family and the local spiritual healer/teacher to drive the devil out of her – she was hearing voices.)

Centuries were to pass during which the comparatively enlightened ideas of Hippocrates, Galen and Asclepiades (who thought that personality problems were often caused by emotional disturbance) became buried in the atrocities of the European Middle Ages. During this 300 year period the fires of the inquisition and mob rule based their authority on the Dominicans' book *Malleus Maleficarum* (the hammer of witches). The people in power (and those who feared them) tortured and burnt an estimated nine million people – mostly women. The name 'faggot' for male homosexuals came from the practice of tying them to the lower end of the burning stake. (There are still psychotherapy training schools today who teach that homosexuals are mad or bad – or they will not acknowledge them as teachers or training analysts.)

The French physician Philippe Pinel (1746–1826) eventually succeeded against great popular disapproval on removing the chains from the mentally ill patients in the Bicetre Hospital for the Insane in Paris in 1793. They had been chained there to posts, walls and beds, jeered at and humiliated by regular sightseers who paid to visit the asylum as people pay today to visit zoos. Pinel was reputedly the first doctor to see the work of the 'soul healer' of the mentally sick as liberation – not punishment. He saw them as human beings capable of relationship. It took a while for his views to be accepted and taught in the great schools for physicians in our world – and only after great adversity and much criticism. Only comparatively recently (and then only in some places) have most of humankind begun to think about mental illness in other terms than possession; understanding instead of blame and mental health as the fostering of free choice and creativity in a therapeutic relationship rather than obedience to the status quo.

The word psychotherapy derives from a person attending or tending the psyche or soul. Psychotherapy grew from this mystical/religious tradition on the one hand and on the other hand from the rationalist experimental tradition which can be said to have truly begun with the Enlightenment. The first experimental psychology laboratories of Wundt was founded in 1879 and one of the first so-called psychological clinics founded by Witmer in March 1896 in Pennsylvania, USA.

The first three twentieth century 'schools'

The view of mental illness as being of psychological origin was the foundation for the work of Bernheim, Janet, Charcot and eventually *Freud*. The experimental tradition was the guiding spirit in the experimental laboratories of *Pavlov* and his associates at the beginning of this century and the self-questioning tradition of the philosophers the

ground for the work of Moreno – the iconoclastic original group therapist of Vienna's latchkey children and prostitutes who had the existen-
tialist belief that humans could change their lives by their own choice.

These three traditions, stemming from the turning of the world clock
almost 100 years ago have shaped the forms of psychotherapeutic
practice in most western countries (and many others). These three men
'fathered' all the major schools of psychoanalysis and psychotherapy,
adopted and adapted academic psychology, and in their individual
dominions held sway over the forming of the minds, hearts and imagina-
tions of novice soul-doctors for most of this century. Almost everything
known or taught today in the universities or private institutions in this
field derives directly or indirectly from the distinctive concentrating
forces first articulated by these three men in particular. This genealogy
can be debated in its details for example when and where the existentialists joined the effort, but in general it holds true.

Some 100 years after Freud, Moreno and Pavlov birthed the three
great lineages of psychotherapy, more than 450 different approaches
have been identified (Karasu, 1986). Polkinghorne's (1992) words
summarise those of many thinkers since: 'The large number of theories
claiming to have grasped the essentials of psychological functioning
provide *prima facie* evidence that no one theory is correct' (p. 158).

The contemporary situation in psychotherapy

'Pure' forms of psychotherapy seem to exist only in the minds of people
not part of current insider debates, however the orthodox party lines are
defended to outsiders (Malcolm, 1981). There is in any case substantial
evidence to indicate that most schools of psychotherapy or psychoanalysis continue to challenge and integrate within these forms
(Hinshelwood, 1990; Gee, 1995).

In the USA and several other countries 'integrative psychotherapy' is
now being hailed as the most popular descriptive term of psychotherapists (Norcross, 1997). However, this is also leading to another infinite
proliferation. In 1984, Windy Dryden estimated that there were about a
dozen different forms of integrative psychotherapy, and I would think
the figure today would be around 28. Unfortunately, many of these
integrative theories have little to recommend them and consist of a
hotchpotch of other people's theories brought together without coherence or systematisation – and by their very nature prohibiting such tests.

So in contemporary psychotherapy we could have the polarisation of
a defensive fundamentalist orthodoxy on the one hand and an infinitely
expanding relativity on the other. (By analogy, Latin died as a spoken
language and Esperanto is not gibberish but has both a structure and a
grammar.) There is a third possibility – the pluralistic or postmodern
engagement with the co-existence of many different languages
(Samuels, 1993). This will require some patience in the translation.

However, there are always structural, utilitarian and aesthetic differences between pidgin and poetry, between superstition and science – whatever one's preferences may be. Many, if not most, of the cherished beliefs of theorists and practitioners of particular methods of psychotherapy remain largely unsupported by the kinds of evidence preferred by those who control the budgets of health care systems across the globe.

However, 'head-to-head' comparisons among treatments differing in the strengths of their respective evidential support show surprisingly modest differences. For most of the disorders reviewed here, there is little evidence to take us beyond the paradoxical 'Dodo bird verdict' of equivalent outcomes from very different treatment methods. (Shapiro, 1996, p. ix)

By contemporary positivistic scientific standards, there are currently five major findings – and all of them raise ethical concerns:

• Eysenck's challenge from the 1950s has been overcome. There is substantial evidence of various kinds that psychotherapy seems to help many people (Parry and Richardson 1996; *Consumer Reports* 1995).

> Long-term treatment did considerably better than short-term treatment . . .
> No specific modality of psychotherapy did better than any other for any
> disorder . . . Patients whose length of therapy or choice of therapist was
> limited by insurance or managed care did worse. (Consumer Reports,
> 1995, p. 965)

• There is no significant evidence that theoretical approach is relevant to the successful outcome of psychotherapy – no matter how measured (Heine, 1953; Norcross and Goldfried, 1992; Barkham, 1995; Seligman, 1995; Parry and Richardson, 1996; Shapiro, 1996; Arundale 1997; Clarkson 1997b; Norcross 1997). In discussing what Barkham (1995) has described as 'the pinnacle of research efforts in researching psychotherapy', Elkin (1995) concludes that there appears to be no significant difference which can be particularly ascribed to specific differences in approach, and she is now focusing 'on the actual patient-therapist interactions in the videotaped treatment sessions' (p. 183).

• According to Roth and Fonagy (1996),

> Each model has its advantages and disadvantages though in our judgment
> there may be arguments favoring training of clinicians in more than one
> modality (i.e. in both an exploratory and a more structured
> psychotherapy). There is some evidence . . . indicating that therapists may
> have better outcomes if they are able to adapt their technique to match
> client characteristics (which may mean at times employing a different
> modality of treatment). (p. 374)

• There is substantial evidence that it is the psychotherapeutic relationship rather than diagnosis or technique which potentiates the beneficial effects of psychotherapy. (See Fiedler, 1951; Clarkson, 1990, 1995a, 1997b and Norcross, 1997 for more detail.) The special issue of the journal *Changes* (Vol. 13, No. 3), on outcome in psychotherapy, is well worth reading in this regard. In it Russell (1995) considers the work of Smith and Glass (1977), Strupp (1979), and Lipsey and Wilson (1993) and finds that they all seem to point to the conclusion that 'positive change was generally attributable to the healing effects of a benign human relationship' (p. 215).

* It has been found that different kinds of relationship are required for different kinds of patients and this factor is more important than diagnosis in predicting effectiveness of psychotherapy (Norcross, 1997). My extensive qualitative research showed five different universes of discourse or kinds of psychotherapeutic relationship spanning all approaches: working alliance, transference/counter-transference, developmentally needed or reparative, person-to-person, and transpersonal (Clarkson 1975, 1990, 1996b, 1997b).
* Evidence exists that there are experiences of psychotherapy by which people feel harmed. One of the most salient facts here is that the harmfulness seems to have to do with the extent to which a psychotherapist entrenches into a theoretical position when challenged or questioned by their client (Winter, 1997).

A puzzle: why are psychotherapists privileging theory?

Several psychotherapy organisations, most training schools and many conferences are organised around the notion of different theoretical approaches – whether integrative or not. Psychotherapy school syllabuses and curricula specify theory. Few, if any, specify demands for research capability, understanding or evidence of effectiveness. At conference after conference dozens of intelligent people passionately expound on the differences (usually 'theory') and the commonalities (usually 'high standards') between their schools. Numerical and geographical popularity arguments abound. There is the semiotically rich use of loyalist 'flag' statements as distinguishing emblems of theories. *Yet there is no significant evidence to date that theory is actually relevant to the delivery of effective psychotherapy.*

It may sometimes appear as if psychotherapy's standards are judged by democratic votes, not accountability to internal and external critique. Indeed standards ordinarily applicable to judging academically account-able theories are usually not mentioned – elegance, economy, explana-tory power, academic rigour or effort (judging by the number of quality texts), freedom (or awareness) of presumptive and logical errors, provability, freedom from undue political or financial influence, the relationship to research (whether scholarly, quantitative, qualitative, or philosophical), critical self-reflection and freedom of expression, the relationship to other theories – or even to the scientifically proven facts within the contemporary culture and sciences.

Much of psychoanalysis and academic psychology is handicapped by being harnessed to exclusively Newtonian and Cartesian models which the hard sciences such as physics actually relinquished some 70 years ago. The new paradigms of quantum physics, chaos and complexity (Clarkson, 1995a) as well as developments in computer and qualitative methodology (Denzin and Lincoln, 1994) have opened possibilities of research upon which psychotherapy can thrive. By using these with conceptual shifts such as Shotter's (1992) meta-methodology, we could make a genuine contribution to the next millennium, rather than attempting to emulate a historically passé ideal of science or religion (exclusively logical positivism or exclusively ideological beliefs) (Hauke, 1996).

Tantam, at the 1996 UKCP professional conference (as reported in the *Psychotherapist* by Smith, 1997) confirmed that:

> 1. Differences in technique are increasingly trivial and unimportant 2. theoretical knowledge has been over-emphasised and 3. we have overlooked that kind of practical knowledge that the media is interested in, the knowledge of outcomes. We each have our particular myths and rituals of healing; so long as they are valid for us and our patients, which we use does not really matter. This can also be said of theoretical knowledge. (p. 6)

This is consistent with the quantitative and qualitative psychological research evidence reviewed in this chapter and with the psychotherapy values and practice which I have elsewhere called 'beyond schoolism' (Clarkson, 1997a,b). This is a working title to refer to a situation in psychotherapy where 'schools' or 'orientations' or 'approaches' will be acknowledged as less important than the therapeutic relationship itself, and when a common value commitment to the alleviation of human suffering and the development of human potential will have replaced factionalism, rivalry and one-up-one-down politics. The attendant destructiveness to creativity and innovation of the latter tendencies hardly needs pointing out.

Schoolism in psychotherapy is the result of passionately held convictions of being right that fly in the face of the facts. Schoolism outlaws questioning and expels dissidents. In 1950 Bowlby compared the Kleinian group of analysts to a religious sect (Rycroft called it the Ebenezer Church) 'in which, once one had espoused the doctrine, one was welcomed to the fold. If one deviated, if one did not subscribe totally to the doctrine, one faced the terrible threat of excommunication' (Grosskurth, 1989, p.428). (Not all Kleinians are of such mind; nor is this syndrome confined to Kleinians or Gestaltists.)

Schoolism fails to see that if passionately held beliefs, weight of numbers, influence with the authorities and volume of academically rigorous effort are to be the deciding criteria, orthodox psychoanalysis and cognitive-behavioural clinical psychology are demonstrably superior. It is only by stepping outside of this inherited frame that psychotherapy can offer something equivalent or better. It is, of course, usually in the interstices and liminal spaces where the creative discoveries of any art or science are made (Koestler, 1989; Gleick, 1992).

> The major problem with the notion of 'school' is its relative inflexibility in response to new ideas in psychotherapy. Schools have responded to varying degrees of psychotherapy innovation, but the value of schools has been to preserve good ideas. At this point in psychotherapy's history, these good ideas within schools have been preserved well enough. (Beitman, 1994, p. 210)

Reasons/rationalisations for schoolism

An Italian dictionary defines science as: 'il resultato da pensiero'. *Science is the result of thinking*. Thinking is hard work. It is easier to adapt, introject, claim or modify other people's ideas – with or without appropriate academic acknowledgement – as your own model.

Information in psychotherapy and psychology is being produced at the rate of hundreds of books and thousands of papers and research reports per year – that's a lot of reading. If you are unable or unwilling to read, you have a problem. Research of any kind is notoriously difficult. It's far more comfortable to avoid its multiple risks by adherence to ideological statements claiming the status of 'philosophy'. Philosophy is an ancient academic discipline; it is not a gratuitous statement of unquestioned preferences. It is indeed very difficult to make research relevant to practitioners (Morrow-Bradley and Elliott, 1986). *But, this bridge between the academy and the clinic is precisely what psychotherapy organisations who take research into account are uniquely equipped to sponsor* (Clarkson, 1995b; Lepper, 1996).

Schoolism is comfortable because it can relieve the existential burden of thinking and free choice (see the Grand Inquisitor's speech in Dostoevsky's *The Brothers Karamazov*). It makes it possible for a professional psychotherapist to say (as was found in recent research, Lindsay and Clarkson, in Chapter 2): 'in my 30 years of clinical practice I have never had the misfortune to encounter an ethical dilemma'. As the histories of our world and our professions prove, it is infinitely more comfortable to be a *bystander* to malpractice and injustice than to risk the responsible engagement with such demanding issues (Clarkson, 1996a).

It is patently uncomfortable to live up to the House of Lords statement that 'professionals, whether in practice or in employment, must be independent in thought and outlook, willing to speak their minds without fear or favour, and not be in the control or dominance of any person or organisation'. Can one speak of psychotherapy as a profession in this sense? (See Chapter 13.)

As the Oxford philosopher of psychology Farrell pointed out in 1979, participants, 'trainees' or clients are usually considered to be 'cured' or 'trained' or 'analysed' or 'qualified' by one single criterion – they have adopted the WOT or the 'way of talking' of the leaders, governing bodies, examination boards and others of perceived status or power. An empirical study by Silverman (1997) also found repeatedly that 'rather than being a deviant case, such adoption by clients of the professionals' rhetoric is common... each centre [of counselling] offers an incitement to speak structured according to its own practical theories' (p.209).

The statement that 'we must give the trainees a secure base' has enormous face validity. It is perhaps even true at a certain level. However, the epistemological nature of this vaunted security deserves profound investigation, not an unquestioning culture-blind acceptance (Ani, 1994). Every western European psychotherapeutic narrative minimises the 'radical differences between egocentric western culture and socio-centric non-western cultures and disclose *that culture exerts a powerful effect on care*' [italics added] (Kleinman quoted in Helman, 1994, p. 279). Helman continues: 'Whether this narrative is short (as in spirit exorcisms) or lengthy (as in psychoanalysis) it summarizes *post hoc* what had happened to them, and why, and how the healer was able to restore them to happiness or health' (p. 280). (See also Gergen, 1994.)

All these perspectives are in line with the seminal work of Foucault (1980, 1988) who laid bare the power of social processes to constitute certain kinds of realities and distinctive kinds of human subjects in situations where professional knowledge is used, such as clinics and prisons. Unless psychotherapy training and supervision are done with these considerations in mind, they are likely to suffer from the very defects and destructive consequences entailed by short-sighted ignorance of these issues or adoption of unquestioning compliance with potentially fundamentalist ideologies. Indeed, what research there is of acceptable standard about psychotherapy supervision suggests, for example, that developmental models of supervision are not empirically supportable, but it has been found again that it is the 'quality of the supervisory relationship [which] is paramount to successful supervision' (Watkins, 1997, p. 495).

Or in the lyrical words of Lyotard (1993):

> . . . is this correct? is it authorized? Is this statement acceptable? These become the 'right' questions. . .What does the theoretical text offer its fascinated client? An *impregnable* body, like a thief, a liar, an impostor who can never be caught. Everything stated in this text is in principle capable of being derived from its set of axioms. A text which is utterly consistent within its own terms and can be derived from itself by explicit procedures, a wide-open organic

body, which the client is supposed to be able to go through without the *solution of continuity*, repeating it or replying to it without error, a body which tolerates no erring, which defines the apparatuses of exclusion and channels of implication. Every statement form within it has *right* on its side: the client may in principle derive it from the others. Nice tautological body of the theoretical test, without any external reference, without a risky interior region where roads and tracks may be lost, a model sealed up in its blank identity, exposing itself to repetition.' (pp. 246, 247)

In my view it is perhaps even more important to subject all our theoretical and philosophical assumptions to continuing critical analysis and to ongoing research enquiry – not separately in the academy, but as the very heart of the ethical activity which characterises as well as nourishes the consulting room. Practitioners have often criticised psychotherapy research mostly by ignoring and frequently refusing to be involved with it, saying that it has little or no relevance to their work. Morrow-Bradley and Elliot (1986) found that practitioners feel that research incorporating the complexities of psychotherapy is rarely done, that important variables are ignored and that traditional research methodologies . . . derived from the physical sciences, are not usually appropriate for the investigation of psychotherapy. Most significantly for me it was felt that: 'Often researchers focus on specific techniques while ignoring the importance of the relationship between therapist and client' (p. 17). Such considerations over the years have led me to collaborate with, study and encourage practice clinically and professionally relevant research as shown in several chapters in this book and elsewhere. In particular I have pleaded for the seamless integration of theory, supervision, practice and research (Clarkson, 1995b). This is now beginning to become more widespread. I also hope that I have shown in this book and particularly in *Counselling Psychology – Integrating theory, research and supervised practice* (1998) some of the ways in which to integrate research into our practice.

The time may be ready for a transcultural, transtheoretical, trans-disciplinary perspective which is genuinely based on learning by enquiry (dierotao) – research in the widest, most philosophical, objective and most subjective sense of the term, because there is:

- little if any evidence that theory has an appreciable effect on the effectiveness of psychotherapy
- an increasing valuing of exploratory research
- an increasingly felt need for professionals to associate, collaborate, interact and research across disciplines, across orientations and across cultural divides
- although not necessarily wanting to give up specialisations and loyalties to specific 'psycholanguages', there is an increasing number of people who want instead, or also, to be *independent* of such

languages, concentrating on transtheoretical and epistemological aspects as well as fundamental empirical questions and methods (see Clarkson, 1997b)

This moment might even mean recognising and celebrating our essential and inescapable *interdependence* on each other (Hahn, 1997). As Stewart (1996) pleaded:

> We must get away from the simplex [or even complex] emphasis on the differences between areas of human culture, and begin to construct a multi-plex vision founded on their similarities. (p. 80)

We will have to come to terms, as we stagger into the postmodern era, with the hard-to-avoid evidence that there are many different realities, and different ways of experiencing them, and that people seem to want to keep exploring them, and that there is only a limited amount any society [or psychotherapy organisation] can do to ensure that its official reality is installed in the minds of most of its citizens [members] most of the time (Anderson, 1990, p. 152).

Conclusion

The narratives of theory are located in a different universe of discourse from that of facts or even research. However beautiful, theory cannot properly substitute for these or be conflated with them. Theories are the stories we tell about the facts, about how we constitute the phenomena, about how the observer perceives and co-creates the field of the research. Even in law. Clare Dalton (1988), a member of the Criticial Legal Studies group at Harvard Law School, wrote: 'Law like every other cultural institution, is a place where we tell one another stories about our relationships with ourselves, one another, and authority.'

Every theory carries it assumptions about culture, language, gender, ability, race and class – our relationships with ourselves, one another and authority. It surely behoves psychotherapy to avoid the simplistic category errors which Gilbert Ryle (1960) pointed out decades ago in his philosophy classes at Oxford. To honour the value of theory appropri- ately, it should not be abused in the service of work it is ill-equipped and perhaps even dangerous to do. When we use our theories, we need to do so ethically – with a wholehearted commitment to questioning the imbedded values and ideologies which our theories carry in their very constructions – no matter how much we want to believe that our prefer- ences represent some kind of truth.

These ideas are emphatically not intended as a call to the abandon- ment of theory. *It is an invocation to take philosophical and empirical research seriously* – not as a luxurious special interest, but as a depth charge challenge to our foundational assumptions, our moral values and organisational structures – our ethics. Each well-developed theory, like each well-developed question, has its own language, grammar, rhetoric and poetry. At the very least they can be beautiful and useful as tools are to the artist and the craftsman. They can live, die or be improved. When we shirk this work of questioning, we are in danger of being unethical in the most profound sense of the term.

The Greek word *theoreo* (the root of theory) indicates a show, a spectacle or the sacred procession around the temple – a story told or performed for the audience. The concept is closely linked to the ancient idea of theatre. A *theoros* was an ambassador sent by the state to consult the oracle. *Theoria* was the office of such an ambassador. But we all know how oracles can instruct *or* deceive. Indeed, contemporary psychotherapy theories could be equated to what we would now understand as their socially constructed narratives or stories (Harré and Gillett, 1994). As the map is not the territory, so the story is never what actually happened. Furthermore there are also the silent narratives: 'Whereof one cannot speak, thereof one must be silent' (Wittgenstein, 1922, p. 189).

When we bridge the academy/clinic divide through research, we find that it is about relationship again – the questioner and the question, the researched itself with the researcher (Einstein – see Schlipp, 1949). As Jung (1928) wrote: 'Learn your theories as well as you can, but put them aside when you touch the miracle of the living soul' (p. 361).

There is a mystery here whether we call it God, physis (the healing force), *élan vital*, Heisenberg's uncertainty principle (1959), the emergent order in positivistically, scientifically measured chaos and complexity, or Schrodinger's cat (Clarkson, 1993; Black, 1996; Marshall, Zohar and Peat, 1997). *And it is very scientific to acknowledge that we don't know, when in truth, we do not know. It's also ethical.* Separating our philosophical universes of discourse for their proper differential uses of theoretical language, forms of rational research and experientially based beliefs, the mystery remains intact (Marcel, 1950; Tillich, 1973).

References

Anderson, W.T. (1990) Reality Is Not What It Used To Be. San Francisco, CA: Harper & Row.

Ani, M. (1994) Yurugu – an African-centred Critique of European Cultural Thought and Behavior. Trenton, NJ: Africa World Press.

Arundale, J. (1997) Editorial. British Journal of Psychotherapy 13(3), 305–6.

Barkham, M. (1995) Editorial: Why psychotherapy outcomes are important now. Changes 13(3), 161–3.

Beitman, B.D. (1994) Stop exploring! Start defining the principles of a psychotherapy integration: Call for a consensus conference. Journal of Psychotherapy Integration, 4(3), 203–28.

Bersoff, D.N. (1995) Professional ethics and legal responsibilities: on the horns of a dilemma. In D.N. Bersoff (ed.) Ethical Conflicts in Psychology, pp. 104–6. Washington, DC: American Psychological Association.

Black, D.M. (1996) Abiding values and the creative present: psychoanalysis in the spectrum of the sciences. British Journal of Psychotherapy 12(3), 314–21.

Clarkson, P. (1975) Seven-Level Model. Paper delivered at University of Pretoria, November.

Clarkson, P. (1990) A multiplicity of psychotherapeutic relationships. British Journal of Psychotherapy, 7(2), 148–63.

Clarkson, P. (1993) New perspectives in counselling and psychotherapy (or adrift in a sea of change). In On Psychotherapy, pp. 209–32. London: Whurr.

Clarkson, P. (1995a) The Therapeutic Relationship. London, Whurr.

Clarkson, P. (1995b) Counselling psychology in Britain – the next decade. Counselling Psychology Quarterly, 8(3), 197–204.

Clarkson, P. (1996a) The Bystander (An End to Innocence in Human Relationships?). London: Whurr.

Clarkson, P. (1996b) Researching the 'therapeutic relationship' in psychoanalysis, counselling psychology and psychotherapy, Counselling Psychology Quarterly, 9(2), 143–62.

Clarkson, P. (1997a) Integrative psychotherapy, integrating psychotherapies, or psychotherapy after Schoolism?. In C. Feltham (ed.), Which Psychotherapy?, pp. 33–50. London: Sage.

Clarkson, P. (1997b) The therapeutic relationship beyond Schoolism. In Psychotherapy in Perspective, post-conference seminar at the 7th Annual Congress of the European Association for Psychotherapy, Rome, 29 June.

Consumer Reports (1995) Mental health: does therapy help? Consumer Reports, November, pp. 734–9.

Dalton, C. (1988) An essay on the deconstruction of contract doctrine. In S. Levinson and S. Maillous, (eds.), Interpreting Law and Literature. Evanston, IL: Northwestern University Press.

Denzin, N.K. and Lincoln, Y.S. (eds) (1994) Handbook of Qualitative Research. Thousand Oaks, CA: Sage.

Dryden, W. (ed.) (1984) Individual Therapy in Britain. Milton Keynes: Open University Press.

Elkin, I. (1995) The NIMH treatment of depression collaborative research program: major results and clinical implications. Changes 13(3), 178–85.

Farrell, B.A. (1979) Work in small groups: some philosophical considerations. In B. Babington Smith and B.A. Farrell (eds.),Training in Small Groups: A Study of Five Groups, pp. 103–15. Oxford: Pergamon.

Fiedler, F.E. (1951) A comparison of therapeutic relationships in psychoanalytic, nondirective and Adlerian therapy. Journal of Consulting Psychology, 14, 436–45.

Foucault, M. (1980) Power/Knowledge: Selected Interviews and Other Writings 1972–1977. New York: Pantheon.

Foucault, M. (1988) Politics, Philosophy, Culture: Interviews and Other Writings 1977–1984 (ed. D.L. Kritzman), London: Routledge.

Frank, J.D. (1973) Persuasion and Healing, 2nd edn. Baltimore, MD: Johns Hopkins University Press.

Gee, H. (1995) Supervision: relating and defining (the essence of supervision). Talk delivered at Spring Conference and Special General Meeting of Group for the Advancement of Therapy Supervision (now the British Association for Psychoanalytic and Psychodynamic Supervision), London, 20 May.

Gergen, M. (1994) Free will and psychotherapy: complaints of the draughtsmen's daughters. Journal of Theoretical and Philosophical Psychology, 14(1), 13–24.

Gleick, J. (1988) Chaos: Making a New Science. London: Heinemann.

Gleick, J. (1992) Genius: Richard Feynman and Modern Physics. London: Abacus.

Grosskurth, P. (1986) Melanie Klein: Her World and her Work. New York: Alfred A. Knopf.

Hahn, H. (1997) Meeting of Choreo Committee, 21 June 1997.

Harré, R. and Gillett, G. (1994) The Discursive Mind. Thousand Oaks, CA: Sage.

Hauke, C. (1996) Book review of The Therapeutic Relationship by Petruska Clarkson. British Journal of Psychotherapy, 12(3), 405–7.

Heine, R.W. (1953) A comparison of patients' reports on psychotherapeutic experience with psychoanalytic, nondirective and Adlerian therapists. American Journal of Psychotherapy, 7, 16–23.

Heisenberg, W. (1959) Physics and Philosophy. New York: Harper & Row.

Helman, C.G. (1994) Culture, Health and Illness: An Introduction for Health Professionals, 3rd edn. Oxford: Butterworth-Heinemann.

Hinshelwood, R.D. (1990) Editorial. British Journal of Psychotherapy, 7(2), 119–20.

Jung, C.G. (1928) Analytical psychology and education. In Contributions to Analytical Psychology (trans. H.G. Baynes and F.C. Baynes, pp. 313–82. London: Trench Trubner.

Karasu, T.B. (1986) The psychotherapies: benefits and limitations. American Journal of Psychotherapy, 40(3), 324–43.

Koestler, A. (1989) The Act of Creation. London: Arkana. (First published 1964.)

Lepper, G. (1996) Between science and hermeneutics: Towards a contemporary empirical approach to the study of interpretation in analytical psychotherapy. British Journal of Psychotherapy, 13(2), 219–31.

Lipsey, M.W. and Wilson, D.B. (1993) The efficacy of psychological, educational and behavioral treatment. American Psychologist, 48(4), 1181–209.

Lyotard, J-F. (1993) Libidinal Economy (trans. I.H. Grant). London: Athlone Press.

Malcolm, J. (1981) Psychoanalysis: The Impossible Profession. New York: Knopf.

Marcel, G. (1950) The Mystery of Being (trans.G.S. Fraser and R. Hague). Chicago, IL: Regnery.

Marshall, I., Zohar, D. and Peat, D. (1997) Who's Afraid of Schrödinger's Cat? New York: William Morrow.

Morrow-Bradley, C. and Elliott, R. (1986) The utilization of psychotherapy research by psychotherapists. American Psychologist, 41(2), 188–97.

Norcross, J.C. (1997) Emerging breakthroughs in psychotherapy integration: Three predictions and one fantasy. Psychotherapy, 34, 1: 86–90.

Norcross, J.C. and Goldfried, M.R. (1992) Handbook of Psychotherapy Integration. New York: Basic Books.

Parry, G. and Richardson, A. (1996) NHS psychotherapeutic services in England. London: Department of Health.

Polkinghorne, D.E. (1992) Postmodern epistemology of practice. In S. Kvale (ed.), Psychology and Postmodernism, pp. 146–65. London: Sage.

Rilke, R.M. (1993) Letters to a Young Poet (trans. M.D. Herter) (revised edn.) New York: W.W. Norton.

Roth, A. and Fonagy, P. (1996) What Works for Whom? A Critical Review of Psychotherapy Research. New York: Guilford Press.

Russell, R. (1995) What works in psychotherapy when it does work? Changes 13(3): 213–18.

Ryle, G. (1960) Dilemmas: The Tarner Lecture. Cambridge: Cambridge University Press.

Samuels, A. (1993) What is a good training? British Journal of Psychotherapy, 9(3), 317–23.

Schlipp, P.A. (ed.) (1949) Albert Einstein, Philosopher-Scientist. Evanston, IL: Northwestern University Press.

Seligman, M.E.P. (1995) The effectiveness of psychotherapy. American Psychologist 50(12), 965–74.

Shapiro, D.A. (1996) Foreword to What Works for Whom? A Critical Review of Psychotherapy Research (A. Roth and P. Fonagy), pp. viii–x. New York: Guilford Press.

Shotter, J. (1992) Getting in touch: the meta-methodology of a postmodern science of mental life. In S. Kvale, Psychology and Postmodernism, pp. 58–73. London: Sage.

Silverman, D. (1997) Discourses of Counselling – HIV Counselling and Social Interaction. London: Sage.

Smith, E. (1997) Knowing what we're doing. The Therapist, 8, 6.

Smith, M.L. and Glass, G.V. (1977) Meta-analysis of psychotherapy outcome studies. American Psychologist, 32, 752–60.

Stewart, I. (1996) Signing off. Tate Magazine, Winter, 80.

Strupp, H.H. (1979) Specific versus non-specific factors in psychotherapy. Archives of General Psychiatry, 36, 1125–36.

Tillich, P. (1973) The Boundaries of Our Being. London: Collins.

Watkins, C.E. (ed.) (1997) Handbook of Psychotherapy Supervision. New York: Wiley.

Winter, D.A. (1997) Everybody has still won but what about the booby prizes? Inaugural address as Chair of the Psychotherapy Section, British Psychological Society, University of Westminster, London.

Wittgenstein, L. (1922) Tractatus Logico-Philosophicus (trans. C. K. Ogden). London: Routledge and Kegan Paul.

ITEM 12
Physis – or 'a Pleasing Illusion'

PETRŪSKA CLARKSON

Freud ([1920]1973a) expressed his doubt about the existence of a general creative force of evolution (such as physis), terming it as 'a pleasing illusion'. Freud was none too sure at one time, however, that something like physis did not assist Ananke (necessity) as the motive force in evolution. 'This appreciation of the necessities of life need not, incidentally, weigh against the importance of 'internal developmental trends' if such can be shown to be present' (Freud, [1916–17]1973b, p. 400). Freud seemed to have much more conviction about the death instinct, and later he gave equal weight to Eros and Thanatos – metaphoric personifications of the sexual and death instincts (Rycroft, 1968, pp. 45–6 and 165).

In this psychoanalytic process of emphasising the human drives toward sexuality and death, a person's unconscious drive towards health, wholeness and creative evolution was ignored, denied or neglected. Berne, along with Jung and several of the humanistic psychotherapists, had a larger vision which took account of the healing and creative instincts which can transform both the sex and death drive. Berne (1968) thought that physis, as the evolutionary healing growth force of nature was 'only one aspect of inwardly directed libido, *but it may be a more basic force than libido itself* (p. 370) [italics added]. In this respect I agree with him and conceptualise physis as onto- and phylogenetically prior to the other drives.

Berne (1968) therefore added physis to the other two great, unconscious forces (energies) – Eros and Thanatos – in human life, and he saw all three as the background of psychological life. Physis is not a derivative of libido or mortido energies, although aspects of each can be used to understand it. Physis is larger and more impersonal, infusing eros and thanatos (and their more individual needs) in its creative, healing and evolutionary quest. Physis is at least an equal and probably a much more

237

fundamental and basic force than the other two in individual and collective evolution (see Table 12.1).

Table 12.1: Characteristics of Physis, Thanatos and Eros (from Lapworth in Clarkson, 1992b, p. 205)

Physis	Thanatos	Eros
Life	Death	Survival
Life instinct	Death instinct	Life or sexual instinct
Creation/creativity	Destruction	Procreation
Self-transformation	Self-destruction	Self-preservation
Libido (inwardly directed) Mortido (outwardly directed)	Mortido (inwardly directed)	Libido (outwardly directed)
Seeks fulfilment/realisation	Seeks freedom from striving gratification	Seeks pleasure
Evolving	Ending	Beginning
Aspiration	Expiration	Inspiration

Ethics is concerned with the physian aspects of relationship. The heart of relationship is *physis*, a physian ethic involved in ongoing constant involvement and evolvement with ethics – the good *and* the better.

> The Greeks called it phusis, a word which has been too narrowly translated by 'Nature' but which seems to mean more exactly 'growth', or 'the process of growth'. It is Physis which gradually shapes or tries to shape every living thing into a more perfect form what Bergson calls la vie or 'elan vital' at the back of *l'Evolution Creatrice* (1965), though to the Greeks it seemed still more personal and vivid, a force which is present in all the live world, and is always making things grow toward the fulfilment of their utmost capacity – and that includes their utmost ethical capacity. (Murray, 1915, pp. 33–4)

Berne referred to *physis* (sometimes spelled as *phusis* [Berne, 1968, p. 91]) in his first major work, *A Layman's Guide to Psychiatry and Psychoanalysis* as follows:

> The growth force, or Physis, which we see evidence of in the individual and society, if properly nourished in infancy, works along with the Superego, so that the individual has an urge to grow and to behave 'better'—that is, in accordance with the principles of the adult stage of sexual development which takes the happiness of others into consideration. Both Superego and Physis, if normal, oppose crude or brutal expressions of Id wishes. They start the individual off in not soiling his diapers, and end up in the ideals of the United Nations. (Berne, 1968, p. 129)

Thus *physis* as the life force – life itself – refers to the forces of growth and evolution— individuals' independent aspirations as well as the sense in which *physis* in concerned with the collective evolution of our ethics.

A good bootmaker is one who makes good boots, a good shepherd is one who keeps his sheep well, and even though good boots are in the Day-of-Judgement sense entirely worthless, and fat sheep no whit better than starved sheep, yet the good bootmaker or good shepherd must do his work well or he will cease to be good. To be good he must perform his function; and, in performing that function, there are certain things that he must 'prefer' to others, even though they are not really 'good'. He must prefer a healthy sheep or a well-made boot to their opposites. It is this that Nature or Physis, herself works when she shapes the seed into a tree or the blind puppy into a good hound. The perfection of the tree or the blind puppy is in itself indifferent, a thing of no ultimate value. Yet the goodness of Nature lies in working for that perfection. (p. 43) . . . It is your play that matters, not the score you happen to make. . . What interests God is not success or failure, it is the action of your free and conscious will.

For the essence of goodness is to do something, to labour, to achieve some end; and if goodness is to exist, the world process must begin again . . . Physis must be moving upward, or else it is not Physis. (Murray, 1915, p. 43)

We see now what goodness is, it is living or acting according to Physis, working with Physis in her eternal effort towards perfection . . . it means living according to the spirit which makes the world grow and progress . . . it is at work everywhere. it is like a soul, or a life-force, running through all matter as the 'soul' of a man runs through all his limbs. It is the soul of the world . . . this Physis, the life of the world, is from another point of view, the law of nature; a natural law . . . a law which is itself alive, which is itself life. (Murray, 1915, p. 34)

The *physis* of the Pre-Socratics of course, is wonderfully echoed in some of the most recent work to come out of *complexity theory*; for example, Brian Goodwin (1994, p. xiv) writes: 'And we are biologically grounded in our relationships which operate at all the different levels of our beings at the basis of our nature as agents of creative evolutionary emergence, a property we share with all other species.'

The directive stimulus of joy and the *aspiration* [italics added] of our moral nature are not contradictory of any science, even the most abstract or the most exact. Intellect and intuition are not opposed, except when the one refuses to adopt precision through contact with facts that have been scientifically questioned and arraigned, or the other, instead of keeping within the limits set to it by science, makes for itself, more or less unawares, a metaphysic falsely pretending to be based on science. (Bergson, 1914, p. 241)

All the world is working together. It is all one living whole, with one soul though it and, as a matter of fact, no single part from modern quantum Physics (for example, entanglement theory; Isham, 1995) teaches us that it is impossible not to be in a relationship. If at any one time our lives have touched any other, it is likely not only that we will be influenced by that person because of what happened in the past, but also that there will continue to be a mutually reciprocal relationship for the rest of time. We remain involved with each other, even when we are 'not speaking' to or when we exclude people; we still continue to be in relationship with them. As we evolve and improve ourselves, we evolve and improve others our profession and the world.

Goodwin writes that:

> These not romantic yearnings and utopian ideals; the arise from a re-thinking of our biological natures that is emerging from the sciences of complexity and is leading towards a science of qualities which may help in our efforts to reach a more creative relationship with the other members of our planetary society. (p. xiv)

As students of history, human nature and statistics we are well aware of the apparently overwhelming presence of determinism as it affects the individual and the group. Based on similar observations we have also participated in and witnessed individuals, groups and societies making profound and lasting changes in directions which few, if any, observers would have predicted (Clarkson, 1990b). So, although we value insight, analysis and understanding, we see these as in service of the processes of *individual transformation and collective evolution*. In considering large scale changes in countries such as the former Soviet Union, South Africa and Germany, we can also see physis at work. Despite the inevitable disappointments, their regressions and failures, there is also always present:

> . . . the removal of limitation and the burgeoning of horizons and the resurrection of the questing, insurgent, indomitable force for hope and health and human aspiration which Berne referred to as Physis. (Clarkson, 1990b, p. 8)

Thus we can hope and work for an evolution in our individual, professional and collective ethics.

> The man who does not see that the good of every living creature is his good, the hurt of every living creature is his hurt, is one who wilfully makes himself a kind of outlaw or exile: he is blind, or a fool. (Murray, 1915, p. 37)

Physis is our inextricable connection with all of life – outside, but also inside ourselves.

In Heraclitus (Guerriere, 1980, p. 96) physis equals Zeus, equals God. It can be seen to assist the struggle for a definition of God as a constantly evolving process. The transpersonal relationship is potentially present in all healing encounters in individual psychotherapy. It is characterised by its timelessness and a sense of numinousness. In Jungian thought (Guggenbühl-Craig, 1971) this aspect of psychotherapy is conceived of as the relationship between the unconscious of the analyst and the unconscious of the patient.

> My whole tendency, and I believe the tendency of all men who ever tried to write or talk ethics or religion, was to run against the boundaries of language.

This running against the walls of our cage is perfectly, absolutely hopeless. Ethics so far as it springs from the desire to say something about the ultimate meaning of life, the absolute good, the absolutely valuable, can be no science. What it says does not add to our knowledge in any sense. But it is a document of a tendency in the human mind which I personally cannot help respecting deeply and I would not for my life ridicule it. (Wittgenstein, 1994, pp. 14–7)

References and further reading

Aristotle, (1933) Metaphysics: Books I–IX, XVII (trans. H. Tredennick, ed. G.P. Goold). Cambridge, MA: Harvard University Press.

Bergson, H. (1914) An Account of his Life and Philosophy. London: Macmillan.

Bergson, H. (1965) Creative Evolution. London: Collier-Macmillan.

Berne, E. (1968) A Layman's Guide to Psychiatry and Psychoanalysis, 3rd edn. New York: Simon and Schuster. (first published 1947, revised 1957).

Clarkson, P. (1990a) A multiplicy of psychotherapeutic relationships, British Journal of Psychotherapy, 7, 148–63.

Clarkson, P. (1990b) What was your contribution to bringing down the Berlin Wall? ITA News, 26, 6–8.

Clarkson, P. (1992) Transactional Analysis Psychotherapy: An Integrated Approach. London: Routledge.

Corballis, M.C. (1991) The Lopsided Ape. New York: Oxford University Press.

Edwards, P. (ed.) (1967) Encyclopedia of Philosophy. New York: Macmillan.

Freud, S. (1973) Beyond the pleasure principle. In A. Richards, (ed.), J. Strachey (trans.), On Metapsychology: The Theory of Psychoanalysis. (Pelican Freud Library, Vol. 11, pp. 275–338). Harmondsworth, Middlesex: Penguin. (Original work published 1920)

Freud, S. (1973) Some thoughts on development and regression—aetiology. In A. Richards (ed.), J. Strachey (Trans.), Introductory Lectures on Psychoanalysis. (Pelican Freud library, Vol. 1, pp. 383–403). Harmondsworth, Middlesex: Penguin. (Original work published 1916–1917)

Goodwin, B. (1994) How the Leopard Changed its Spots. London: Weidenfeld & Nicholson.

Guerrière, D. (1980) Physis, Sophia, Psyche. In J. Sallis and K. Maly (eds.), Heraclitean Fragments: A Companion Volume to the Heidegger/Fink Seminar on Heraclitus. Tuscaloosa, AL: University of Alabama Press.

Guggenbühl-Craig, C.A. (1971) Power in the Helping Professions. Dallas, TX: Spring.

Isham, C. J. (1995) Lectures on Quantum Theory, London: Imperial College Press.

Maslow, A.H. (1963) Toward a Psychology of Being. Princeton, NJ: Van Nostrand.

Murray, G. (1915) The Stoic Philosophy. London: Watts.

Murray, G. (1955) Five Stages of Greek Religion. Garden City, NY: Doubleday Anchor.

Rogers, C.R. (1980) A Way of Being. Boston, MA: Houghton Mifflin.

Runes, D.D. (ed.). (1962) Dictionary of Philosophy. Totowa, NJ: Littlefields, Adams.

Rycroft, C. (1968) A Critical Dictionary of Psychoanalysis. London: Thomas Nelson.

Weiss, E. (1950) Principles of Psychodynamics. New York: Grune and Stratton.

Wittgenstein, L. (1994) A lecture on ethics. In P. Singer (ed.), Ethics, pp. 140–7.

Winter, D.A. (1997) Everybody has still won but what about the booby prizes? Inaugural address as Chair of the Psychotherapy Section, British Psychological Society, University of Westminster, London.

Wittgenstein, L. (1922) Tractatus Logico-Philosophicus (trans. C.K. Ogden). London: Routledge & Kegan Paul.

CHAPTER 13
Judicial Review of Psychotherapy Self-regulation

PETRŪSKA CLARKSON AND VINCENT KETER

> Clarity of structure and of the constitution make it possible to assess whether
> or not the system of authorisation is functioning, and what steps would need
> to be taken to withdraw authorisation, should that be decided. This is, of
> course, not possible in authoritarian regimes, where the constitution either
> does not exist or else is subverted, and rule or management is on the basis of
> power rather than of law. Furthermore, there needs to be a match between
> authority and power, and responsibility. Responsibility for outcomes involves
> being answerable or accountable to someone, either in the organisation or
> else in one's own mind as part of an inner world value system. A sense of
> responsibility without having adequate authority and power to achieve
> outcomes often leads to work related stress and eventually burn-out. In
> assessing the nature and function of an organisation, whether as a member or
> as an outside consultant, the time used in clarifying the nature, source and
> routing of authority, the power available, and the names describing various
> organisational functions is time well spent. (Obholzer, 1994, p. 43)

> Professionals whether in practice or in employment, must be independent in
> thought and outlook, willing to speak their minds without fear or favour, and
> not be in the control or dominance of any person or organisation. (Lord
> Benson, Hansard 618, LD92/93 July 6–11, 1207)

Self-regulation

In Britain the professions of psychotherapy, counselling and psychology
are self-regulated. Self-regulation means that the systems of regulation
are set up and run by the profession itself and not yet externally
imposed by legislation. Whether or not this state of affairs benefits the
profession more than the public is often a matter of heated debate.
Doubtless there are benefits and drawbacks. A definite advantage of self-
regulation is that the development of the profession in terms of the
variety and nuance of practice is often preserved to a greater extent in
unregulated or self-regulated professions. Legislative intervention often

tends to inhibit this development and so the services on offer tend toward the more sterile and safe and are slow to take on advances or innovation.

The willingness of the profession to honour its published promises as regards the fairness of complaints procedures and the outcomes produced by those procedures is often a key factor in retaining the trust of the public in the profession and its ability to address misconduct or malpractice. If this fails then government may be pressured into intervening in ways that can only reduce the variety and choice of services. Demand for the services may also be affected if the promised protection against bad services or professional abuse appears to be cosmetic. Public awareness of instances of professional abuse by psychotherapists or counsellors has been growing steadily in recent years. The kinds of abuse that can take place are now widely understood and accepted. Organisations such as the Prevention of Professional Abuse Network (POPAN) have become established to help individuals make complaints or negotiate resolutions when they have negative experiences of a professional's services or conduct.

The regulatory structures are also an important way in which standards are upheld and fairness maintained between the members of the profession. Professionals have the right to ensure the integrity of their qualifications is not eroded by misleading, false or inflated claims by other professionals. They also have the right to have their reputation safeguarded by the profession and there are invariably items in ethical codes which address derogatory treatment or marring statements about colleagues. These are subject to the important exception of statements made in the course of laying a confidential formal complaint. These are likely by their very nature to be negative.

The largest important body for the regulation of psychotherapists in Britain is the United Kingdom Council for Psychotherapy (UKCP). The UKCP comprises a membership of organisations with varying rights, affiliation and status within UKCP. The actual handling of complaints takes place within the systems and procedures of each respective member organisation. There are UKCP guidelines and common understandings in respect of how such procedures should be run. Appeal lies to UKCP on the basis that a member organisation's procedures were not properly followed or were unfair or unjust. In February 1999, the President of the British Psychological Society, Ingrid Lunt referred to a psychologist who admitted to sexual abuse of a number of his patients when she wrote:

> Following a number of widely publicised cases, including that of Peter Slade, there are plans to consider how far existing arrangements of professional bodies can ensure protection of the public, rather than protection of the profession. The question will be asked how far the bargain struck a century ago between professionals and society, in which they exchange competence, integrity and self-regulation for trust and relative freedom from external

control and interference, is appropriate for the current professional and consumer context. The question, posed by the poet Juvenal in the first century, *'quis custodiet ipsos custodes?'* (who will guard the guardians themselves?) is again apt.

The Cabinet Office's Better Regulation Task Force, chaired by Lord Haskins, is about to announce a review of the effectiveness of self-regulation. This task force has developed five clear principles for evaluating direct government regulation and intends to use these test systems of self-regulation in five sections. These five principles are transparency, proportionality, targeting, consistency and accountability.

Government

The position of the government with regard to the regulation of psychotherapy is founded on the Foster Report (1971). The basic position set out in this official government report is that regulation is necessary because the practice of psychotherapy is capable of causing harm if done badly or abusively. This position has remained unchanged and has now become assumed whenever the subject comes up in the views put forward by Ministers or government officials. The method by which the profession should be regulated is less clear. The inherent difficulties involved in drafting legislation and then getting Parliament to pass it, militate against direct statutory control. The current position appears to be that the best method of regulation available is to allow the profession to regulate itself. The existence of UKCP and other such bodies could remove the need for externally imposed legislation if they can be seen to be operating effectively and under clearly articulated public aims.

Judicial review

Judicial review is the procedure which allows judges of the Queen's Bench Division of the High Court to review the decisions of inferior courts or public bodies to ensure that they are legal, rational and fair, and to intervene, if necessary, to put matters right. The need for such jurisdiction arises primarily from the imbalance of power between the individual and the organs of the state. The process of judicial review is thus there to ensure that those who wield the powers of the state in the public interest do so fairly and properly. The principles of law that operate in judicial review are of quite a different texture to the principles of ordinary civil law. The principles are often called 'public law' as opposed to 'private law'. The reasoning is much less legalistic and far more open to tactile considerations as to whether the decision being challenged was fair.

The process of judicial review evolved out of a set of legal remedies known as the 'prerogative writs'. Originally these remedies emanated from the sovereign's powers as a sovereign and came to be exercised by the King or Queen's own judges. These remedies could be characterised as the sovereign interceding on behalf of an individual in order to bring about a just and fair outcome where it appeared that to leave matters unchanged would be to tolerate an injustice for which there was no other remedy. Accordingly, these remedies were always remedies of last resort where no other recourse was available. The individual seeking these remedies had no power to issue them, but only to inform the court of the circumstances and the need. This could be done *ex parte* (i.e. without the other side having the right to be heard). The name of an action for judicial review reflects this process. The action is entitled:

[The Queen] versus [the respondent public body] *ex parte* [the applicant].

The procedure in judicial review is divided into two stages: the leave stage (which is *ex parte*) and the full hearing. The leave stage is a request for the permission of the High Court to ask for judicial review of a particular decision. Judicial review can only be applied for if leave is granted by the Court. The leave stage can be submitted on paper or by oral hearing. Documents, an affidavit and a statement of the grounds for seeking judicial review are put before a High Court judge who decides whether or not to grant leave. The respondent usually backs down if leave is granted and reconsiders their decision. A full hearing usually only takes place if the matter is very complex or there are a number of interested parties who would be directly affected by the decision (Jones, 1989). There are three main grounds for challenging a decision of a public body by way of judicial review: illegality, irrationality and procedural impropriety.

- *Illegality* means that the decision was contrary to law as set out in the relevant statute or rules. It may mean that the body taking the decision had no real power to do so or acted outside their discretion.
- *Irrationality* means that the decision is so unreasonable that no reasonable body could have come to the same decision. Such decisions are often referred to as 'perverse' or 'lacking in ostensible logic or comprehensible justification'.
- *Procedural impropriety* refers to decisions which are tainted by bias or the appearance of bias, or some other defect or unfairness in the manner in which the decision was reached.

In the pamphlet 'Judge over your shoulder' (Collis, 1995) these notions are well explained. Anyone involved in making a decision who is biased against one party or in favour of another will result in the decision being set aside by the Court. Such cases of 'real' bias are rare, however, and most cases that reach the Court are concerned with the *appearance* of bias: the question to ask yourself is not 'am I biased?' but 'would any of the parties have reasonable cause to think I favoured one party or disfavoured another?' The example quoted refers to a coroner who expressed the view that a mother bereaved in the *Marchioness* tragedy was 'not acting rationally' and described some of the relatives and survivors as being 'mentally unwell'. He was also alleged to have referred to the mother as 'unhinged'. The Court of Appeal held that there was a real possibility, judging by the remarks attributed to the coroner, that he had unconsciously allowed himself to be influenced against the applicants by a feeling of hostility towards them and had therefore undervalued the strength of their case to resume the inquest. The coroner's decision was quashed (R v. Inner West London Coroner ex parte Dallaglio, 1994, 4 All ER 139, pp. 18 and 19).

Another type of bias is direct 'pecuniary interest', however slight. Receiving referrals, donations or other benefits – such as payments for conference attendances, for example – would all fall under this type of bias. Furthermore, the recent ruling in the case of Lord Hoffman showed that even undeclared connection with a charity is considered to be enough bias to invalidate decisions on the grounds of bias in which such a person(s) was involved.

Club or profession?

Writing in *The Psychotherapist*, the house magazine of the UKCP, the UKCP Ethics Officer reporting on a conference with the legal firm Walker Martineau published a claim that 'some would be heartened to hear that the UKCP is not subject to judicial review' (Palmer Barnes, 1998, p. 4). This seems to claim that the UKCP governing body is above the law or is merely a 'club'. It was unclear why some member organisations of UKCP would be 'heartened' by such a statement, since judicial review exists in order to ensure that bodies with public responsibilities are legally accountable for how they carry these out – particularly if complaints processes are based on claims that these exist for the protection of the public. The UKCP (1998) claims that:

> the purpose of a Code of Ethics is to define general principles and to estab-
> lish standards of professional conduct for psychotherapists in their work and
> to inform and protect those members of the public who seek their services.
> Each organisation will include and elaborate upon the following principles in
> its Code of Ethics. (p. 2)

A club represents itself to the public as a private club; it is not amenable by judicial review and is for the benefit of the members only. It is governed solely by laws of contract or tort and there is no significant element concerning the public in its decisions. There is no particular interaction with the state other than being subject to general laws.

Membership is entirely within the discretion of existing members or the governing committee and membership is terminable under club rules subject to discretion of existing club members. No codes of ethics apply other than simply the internal rules of the club to which outsiders are not privy and a club may therefore exhibit arbitrary and even unprincipled decisions and actions simply because it suits them. A profession, on the other hand, represents itself to the public as a professional body whose decisions can be judicially reviewed since it claims protection or assistance to the public as a stated aim or published objective and thus there is a 'public element' in its decisions.

> The professional's possession of knowledge and expertise can be warranted by diplomas, certificates and degrees, but only up to a point. Thereafter, trust becomes extremely important and trust will be accorded to those whose outward appearance and manner fits in with the socially accepted standards of repute and respectability. (Macdonald, 1995, pp. 30–1)

A profession usually has a history or seeks a relationship with the state or specifically acknowledged in statute, e.g. the Courts and Legal Services Act. Membership is based on professional standards and fixed criteria and such membership is terminable only pursuant to breach of ethical codes. Codes of ethics and procedures exist which can be invoked by a member of the public or other member of the profession and it is expected that such a profession would display principled decision making and actions.

In an attempt to clarify the distinction between club and profession further, a table of key characteristics has been drawn up (Table 13.1).

Judicial review of the UKCP

Judicial review is the legal process whereby the judiciary exercise some control over the powers of decision-makers which arise in a public context in that their source, function or consequences disclose a public law duty to act judicially. The principal reason for this is to ensure that public powers and functions are performed justly. Accordingly, the principles of natural justice are the governing standards upon which judicial review is based.

Certain complaints regarding professional, academic and professional concerns of Professor Clarkson (and others) had not been satisfactorily dealt with by two UKCP member organisations. Only a brief outline of the of the circumstances can be given here.

It has only recently been established that the organisations that make up the self-regulatory framework for psychotherapy are subject to challenge by way of judicial review. The UKCP's published position (Palmer Barnes, 1998) was that its decisions could definitely not be taken to judicial review in the High Court.

Table 13.1:

Profession	Club
Represents itself to the public as a professional body	Represents itself to the public as a private club
Decisions can be judicially reviewed	Not amenable to judicial review
Protection or assistance to public a stated aim or objective	For benefit of members only
Subject to principles of natural justice	Governed by contract or tort only
'Public element' in decisions	No significant public element in decisions
History/relationship with the state (Foster and Sieghart Reports) or specifically acknowledged in statute, e.g. Courts and Legal Services Act	No particular interaction with state other than being subject to general law
Membership based on professional standards and fixed criteria	Membership entirely within discretion to existing members/ governing committee
Membership terminable only pursuant to breach of ethical codes	Membership terminable under club rules subject to discretion of existing members
Codes of ethics and procedures which can be invoked by a member of the public or other member of the profession	No codes of ethics other than simply internal rules of the club to which outsiders are not privy
Principled decision-making and action	May exhibit arbitrary and unprincipled decisions and actions

However, the second author of this chapter (Vincent Keter) made an application for judicial review in respect of a decision of the Governing Board of UKCP and was granted permission by Mr Justice Collins in October 1998. At the final hearing of the application on 18 February 1999 the UKCP were still arguing that they were not a body that could be taken to judicial review. However, it became clear from the Judge's comments that this argument could not be sustained and UKCP agreed to reverse its decision to drop complaints that had been laid against two member organisations.

The Application was 'consolidated' with an application for committal for contempt of court against the professional development officer of UKCP, Geoff Mothersole, for 'acts intended to prejudice the due course of justice'. The Judge said that Mr Mothersole's actions were *prima facie* contempt of court and that Mr Mothersole had had an opportunity of contemplating his committal to prison. Mr Keter accepted an apology expressing profound sorrow from Mr Mothersole and agreed not to press for committal.

The significance of this particular judicial review action has been to establish an accountability of the Governing Board of UKCP (and potentially other similar organisations) to the High Court, both in terms of placing undue pressure on complainants and also in terms of hearing complaints. As far as the possibility of statutory registration for psychotherapists goes, the success of the application raises the public importance of maintaining proper controls over the self-regulatory framework, but probably also takes some pressure off government creating legislation, since the High Court is clearly willing to intervene where decisions are biased, improper, illegal or perverse.

Conclusion

The significance of this application is that this is the first time that judicial review has been applied for in respect of any professional body representing counsellors, psychologists or psychotherapists. The implications for such bodies are manifold and are mainly positive. This outcome should be in the best interests of such bodies since it will lend weight to their status in terms of providing clear force to their public accountability. Because they can be seen to be under the supervisory jurisdiction of the High Court, trust in their functions of protection of the public can only be enhanced, notwithstanding the questioning of the current UKCP Governing Board's actions. Careful consideration will need to be given to all complaints procedures and processes to ensure that decisions taken within them can stand the scrutiny of the High Court on judicial review and meet the standards of accountability of public law.

As the president of the British Psychological Society recently wrote,

> In seeking legislation, we need to find ways not only to prevent psychologists such as Peter Slade from practising, but also to monitor competence, minimum standards of practice, and continuing professional development. We might otherwise be vulnerable to the accusations sometimes levelled at professional bodies that Chartered status and legislation are for the protection more of their members than of the public. (Lunt, 1999)

References

Collis, W. (1995) Judge over your shoulder – Judicial Review: Balancing the scales, revised May 1995. The Treasury Solicitor's Department in conjunction with the Cabinet Office (OPSS) Development Division.

Foster Report (1971) London: HMSO.

Jones, B.L. (1989) Garner's Administrative Law, 7th edn. London: Butterworths.

Lunt, I. (1999) Disciplining psychologists. Psychologist 12, 2:5.

Macdonald, K. (1995) The Sociology of the Professions. London: Sage.

Palmer Barnes, F. (1998) Club or profession? Psychotherapist, 3, p. 4.

UKCP (1998) United Kingdom Council for Psychotherapy Register of Psychotherapists. London: Routledge.

ITEM 13
Thought Experiments and Imaginary Dilemmas for People Involved in Complaints Procedures

1. You are appointed as a member of an investigatory panel into a complaint from a trainee against a trainer. You have yourself successfully pleaded not guilty to a similar charge – on the basis that a code for trainers did not exist at the time of the offences. Your colleague is disciplined by your professional association for 'canvassing students', with most severe consequences for health and livelihood. Later, a different colleague, who is also the financial backer and chair of the organisation, is not challenged when exhibiting identical behaviour. What do you do?

2. You (as ethics chair of one organisation) are approached by the ethics chair of another organisation to confirm in writing to the validating body that a mutual colleague was unethical in making a formal confidential complaint against the other organisation. No hearing has yet taken place.

3. Your organisation has received substantial financial input from a donor who is also a member and office holder on the Board of an organisation. How would it be possible to process a complaint against this person/charity according to the principles of natural justice?

4. You are the chair of an organisation's council who expels a senior colleague on the basis of anonymous letters from colleagues who are 'too frightened' to meet and discuss concerns with the colleague who is being expelled. The teachers and supervisors of the 'school' stress personal responsibility for one's actions.

5. A colleague who is also a friend refers a client with whom they have had a sexual relationship to you. You are also on the organisation's ethics committee. This colleague is your most regular source of referrals and would expect you to 'contain' this situation for them.

6. You are aware that a particular organisation has draconian methods of intimidation and retaliation against potential complainants. This organisation refers people discouraged from supervisory or

therapeutic relationships with a colleague who has made complaints to you and your friends. Yet you are aware of other ethics violations in this organisation which no one else is prepared to challenge.

7. You belong to an organisation of organisations. Many of these organisations are dependent on maintaining their financial position in order to remain belonging to the umbrella body. This thus resembles a trade association (e.g. all chemist shops) rather than a profession (all doctors). Is a complaints process possible at all in this situation which would meet the criteria of a judicial review?

8. The umbrella body is dependent on the membership fees of the organisations – the larger the organisation, the more money is provides to the umbrella body. You notice that smaller organisations are expelled for the same kind of issues (trainer–trainee sexual misconduct and not following their own ethics procedures) whereas larger organisations (who provide more fees to the umbrella organisation) are protected in a variety of ways (e.g. interminable delays, then changing the regulations, prejudging the complaint by the ruling council, openly attempting to influence colleagues against anyone who should raise challenges to the large organisation, etc.).

9. You are on the ethics committee of an organisation where the Chair appoints a known political opponent to the complainant as the investigator. You are informed by the complainant that this person had secretly in the past campaigned against the complainant, asking the complainant's students to vote against their teacher and/or psychotherapist.

10. The organisation publishes a commitment to protect the psychological safety of complainants. Yet you know that complainants are prohibited from attending community meetings, have their names removed from referral lists for patients and supervisees and suffer from innuendo and rumours that they are in fact the person complained against. If you question this treatment of the complainant you may be scapegoated in a similar manner.

11. Trainees who complain about misrepresentation of staff qualifications have their essays marked down and are eventually prevented from graduating. The organisation then refuses to provide them with a certificate of attendance. What would you advise?

12. As a member of a panel you discover that individuals have been disciplined and expelled for misrepresentation of qualifications, but the organisation claims that similar rules do not apply if such misrepresentation is in fact done by the management committee. The ethics code of the organisation is written in such a way as to support this interpretation.

13. An organisation claims that, because there was a change of management, ethics offences committed before that date do not fall within their purview. However, they also claim to the umbrella organisation

that there has been no substantial change and their organisational membership should therefore continue uninterrupted. This is condoned.

14. As a member of a Governing Board you are informed 'on the grapevine' about details of a certain colleague's complaint. You know that such details are claimed to be protected, but it would cause a fuss if you pointed this out to the people concerned. Furthermore you might miss out on further interesting gossip in future.

15. You are in a pub at a conference where colleagues are discussing another colleague in a derogatory way, suggesting that she or he is has been late for several appointments with clients and should be prevented from practising on health grounds. The agitator claims that the colleague under discussion 'won't listen' and therefore concerted group action where everyone supports each other against this colleague is required.

16. At a meeting a senior teaching analyst boasts to junior colleagues about their ability to get things done 'by the back door' in the organisation.

17. You discover that students can be disciplined and penalised for plagiarism at universities, but that no such rules apply to staff who therefore freely avail themselves of such liberties.

18. You know that many trainees of a certain organisation are in fear of making complaints about the fact that the academic external examiner for the validating body is actually a close friend of their teacher and the psychotherapist of participants on the course as well as members of staff. New universities do not have any body which scrutinises their validation or management of complaints processes against 'partner-organisations'.

19. As chair of an ethics board you receive a letter from a prominent member of the profession claiming to have taken money from a certain individual and at the same time testifying to his/her innocence of exerting influence because of this – stating categorically that the donor is sure to be found innocent in the investigation.

20. You are selected to sit on an ethics panel and subsequently discover that colleagues of yours (in your professional organisation) have been in receipt of work, referrals or donations from the person complained against. When the complainant objected to your participation, the ethics chair had overruled their objection. What do you do?

CHAPTER 14
Integrative Relational Research: An Approach to Ethics

One of the key assumptions of phenomenological psychology is that human consciousness is structured by an *intentional* relationship. Human consciousness is openness to a world, in the same sense that subjectivity is necessarily intersubjectivity and that personhood necessarily implies interpersonality. . . . This way of understanding consciousness in particular, and human reality as whole, is not a recent philosophical or psychological discovery, but represents a view that is probably as old as mankind itself. There is an ancient Greek proverb that says very simply and directly *Aner oudeis aner*; meaning, literally, 'none without another' or, more fully, 'One single human being, considered in the absence of a relationship to another, is in fact no human being at all.' Being human means standing in a relationship to others, to things, and to the world . . . (Jager, 1998, pp. 87–8)

Denying that relationship does not make it disappear; it *cements* it.

It is worth noting here that, despite the intoxicating attraction of scientific positivism as the best or finest sort of knowledge, most of what we know is not, and never was, of this sort. Most of what we know, most of the knowing we do, is concerned with trying to make sense of what it is to be human and to be situated as we are. The constant 'topics' of human life are, for example love and loneliness, pride and pain, and pre-eminently birth and death. We can know these things in two significantly different ways. We can 'know about' them in the sense that we can comprehend the facts of the case, or theories about the facts of the case. In this sense such knowledge is not different from 'knowing about' insects, plants, rocks or telephone numbers. We can also know them in quite a different way which is more difficult to characterize. We can know them *as human persons*. In this sense such knowledge must begin with at least some facts of the case but cannot end there. To such knowledge we add moral significance; indeed such knowledge is transformed by it. (Steedman, 1991, p. 58)

North American practitioner–researchers have for several decades been engaged in researching ethical dilemmas and practices (Bersoff, 1995). Yet despite the benefits of such efforts, in an authoritative review of ethical principles, O'Donohue and Mangold (1996) conclude about the American Psychological Association's ethics that:

> the ethical theory or premises upon which the code is based is not explicit and is poorly understood; that since no evidence or arguments for the claims within the code are provided it is epistemologically undefended; and it is inconsistent with influential scientific accounts of human behavior. This is a most unfortunate state of affairs for the public as well as for psychologists. (p. 378)

As a white child growing up in apartheid South Africa I had hoped that the other countries to which I looked for moral guidance and ethical education would have done better. I started my voluntary exile to Britain in 1976 when the schoolchildren were massacred in Soweto for refusing to speak the Afrikaans language. As a child my father had been persecuted by the English for speaking Afrikaans in the playground of his school. My ancestors were refugees from the counter-Reformation massacres in Europe. It seems as if I and mine have always been grappling unceasingly with the question of how apparently good people can do evil – and whether anything at all can be known or done about it (Arendt, 1964). Unknowing of the terminology at the time, I had grown up into a heuristic researcher.

> Heuristic inquiry is a process that begins with a question or problem which the researcher seeks to illuminate or answer. The question is one that has been a personal challenge and puzzlement in the search to understand one's self and the world in which one lives. The heuristic process is autobiographic, yet with virtually every question that matters there is also a social – and perhaps universal – significance. (Moustakas, 1990, p. 15)

I had established my credibility as a scientific quantitative researcher wearing a white laboratory coat in the early 1970s, doing obligatory rats and maze work, even counting their pellets (a measure of stress), followed by a large scale quantitative investigation into the interplay of personality, neurophysiology and environmental variables. I used state-of-the-art electronic and computer equipment to count (EEGs, ECGs, electrogalvanic skin response rate measures, and so on and so forth). I aimed for neutral objectivity, but I wanted 'the truth'. I did not find either. I did, however, learn how to do objective empirical quantitative research to doctoral standard and was awarded distinctions twice, also by my viva examiners (who included two members of the Royal Society of Medicine).

But I have moved on. And so has the field of research itself. Not that the old forms are discarded, but the new forms are gaining their own unique place as I have shown particularly in the volume *Counselling Psychology: Integrating Theory, Research and Supervised Practice* (Clarkson, 1998a). There I both plead for and demonstrate examples of integration between these indivisible aspects of our work. And my interest here is still in what possible *relationship* we can establish between knowledge and practice, between reading and thinking, between doubting and believing, between standardisation and invention, between safety and risk, between self and other, individual and profession, consumer and provider and of course – always – between body and soul (as if there ever was such artificially constructed dichotomies). And if we fail again, the search itself will bear the hallmarks of honest endeavour and soulful encounter and the possibility of hope, again.

> Heuristics is a way of engaging in scientific search through methods and processes aimed at discovery; a way of self-inquiry and dialogue with others aimed at finding the underlying meanings of important human experiences. The deepest currents of meaning and knowledge take place within the individual through one's senses, perceptions, beliefs, and judgements. This requires a passionate, disciplined commitment to remain with a question intensely and continuously until it is illuminated or answered. (Moustakas, 1990, p. 15)

Until recently, UK research on ethics in counselling, psychotherapy, psychology, supervision, training and professional organisations and complaints procedures was virtually non-existent. With the exceptions of Lindsay (1995), Lindsay and Colley (1995) and Marzillier (1999), most of what we know is based on conjecture, 'received wisdom', or the rather inadequate teaching of and adaptation to published rules and codes distinguished by their lack of coherence and evidential basis.

At a recent UK conference on ethical dilemmas in counselling and psychotherapy, Tim Bond (1999) wondered whether there is so little research in ethics because people are 'afraid to stick their heads above the parapet' or being made into 'targets' for attack themselves. Lindsay and Colley (1995), in referring to the impact of organisational settings on ethical practice, also found evidence of 'professional gagging'. As I have been actively engaged in a variety of projects throughout my adult life with ethical and moral questions, writing, practice and research, I can empirically ('from experience') testify to the risks of enquiry into ethics.

At several points in this lifelong, ongoing research (of which this book is only a preliminary report), I have been challenged by individual colleagues.

- Case one concerned a colleague who loudly proclaimed in a public meeting that I was being 'unethical' in asking practitioners to write down some short account of ethical dilemmas they had faced, even though I had asked them to do it anonymously and to take care to protect all identifying details about the case. At the time I was so shocked I interrupted the project until I found that both the President of the British Psychological Society (BPS) and several internationally known experts on ethics had already conducted research in exactly those terms. (If we were all 'unethical', at least I would be in good company.)

- Case two concerned an individual who responded to a research questionnaire giving no other reply than virulent and rather personal criticism of the project on the grounds that I was not, in her opinion, giving sufficient information about the project. She threatened to report me to an ethics board. (The cover letter and questionnaire were still largely identical to the USA prototype.)

- Case three concerned the CEO of an organisation who took such extreme exception to me sending to other colleagues – in an organisation to which I belong – similar questions about ethical dilemmas involving training or training organisations that he committed an ethics violation himself by defaming me. (Survey replies were of course anonymous and anyone wanting to be contribute a personal qualitative interviewed was also assured of confidentiality!)

Every week I personally receive research questionnaires from colleagues and students (who get my name from various published registers which are thus in the public domain) on a wide variety of topics. I often put them at the bottom of my pile unless the theme interests me, in which case I respond immediately. Why such extreme reactions when the research questions concern ethics? It certainly encourages neither veteran nor novice professionals in this field to attempt to get information about the thinking and practice of ethics in these professions.

Disappointed in my search for an infallible truth, I had already grown used to the fact that there are always multiple perspectives all seen by their proponents as 'true' even though obviously incompatible and contradictory.

> Another way of putting this is to say that pursuing this dichotomy is not the most fruitful way to think about moral knowledge. . . . We live in a pluralistic world, a world of many knowledges and many moral voices. There is no master narrative that can command the allegiance of all the moral voices that assail us. To try, falsely, to impose such a narrative can result only in rigidity and in silencing those moral voices that fail to conform to the norm. (Hekman, 1995, pp. 46 and 112).

Certainly it has been my experience from my earliest experimental training that the work of writing itself is another process of discovery, both about myself, my discipline and the work of thinking and writing itself (Richardson, 1994). It is only with an increasing grasp of the postmodernist, poststructuralist *zeitgeist* that I have begun to appreciate the possibilities – not necessarily of a wholesome final product called 'integration', but a continuing endeavour of validating all the forms of my search and my knowing – even as I subject these very processes to intuition, dialogue and objective as well as subjective enquiry.

> This is an exciting time for psychology. A number of methodologies consonant with a shift to a post-positivist, non-experimental paradigm are now emerging and they are beginning to be used in a wide range of empirical studies. As these studies proliferate and are published, there will be a real chance of fundamentally changing the discipline of psychology, of dramatically redrawing its boundaries to include a whole set of new questions, asked and answered in new ways. (Smith et al., 1995, p. 1)

In fact I have come to believe, with Havel (1990), that:

> the intellectual should bear witness to the misery of the world, should be provocative by being independent, should rebel against all hidden and open pressures and manipulations, should be the chief doubter of systems, of power and its incantations . . . always at odds with hard and fast categories. (p. 167)

However, like the multiple 'suicides' which were reported as being 'voluntarily' committed from South African police stations, the facts speak for themselves. The Prevention of Professional Abuse Network (POPAN) document indicates that it is almost impossible for clients to make complaints which are heard fairly, quickly, without imposing severe further psychological distress and which make appropriate responses to the concerns raised by the complainant. They describe, for example, the UKCP complaints procedures as 'appalling'. POPAN also reports that trainee complaints are mounting and that there exists little or no redress for trainee complainants to safely prosecute their concerns without opening themselves to severe retaliation in terms of their qualifications, their reputation and their future livelihood from their training or professional organisations. There is apparently no way to challenge the ethics and complaints procedures of the new universities who claim to 'validate' many newer training courses and recent degree awards through private or charitable institutions (M. Laugharne, personal communication, 1998).

Brown (1997) reports on the criticisms from the supposed beneficiaries of these ethics codes, our students and clients, who ask who truly benefits from organised psychologists' formal ethical guidelines.

> The critics – most frequently from feminist psychology, mental patient liberation groups, and groups of psychologists of color . . . have inquired repeatedly into whether the dominant culture's code existed simply to uphold a certain oppressive status quo within psychology and to protect psychologists from those over whom they hold power, rather than the reverse. (Brown, 1997, p. 53)

In Brown's appraisal, Lerman and Porter (1990) claim that the dominant ethics codes 'encourage passivity, existential bad faith, and the failure to be courageous when it becomes necessary to take a stand to ensure ethical outcomes' (Brown, 1997, p. 58), while for Koocher (1994) 'standards and guidelines that mandate the doing of good are potentially anti-entrepreneurial' (Brown, 1997, p. 59). As a colleague wrote to me when challenged about the integrity of his actions: 'It's normal business practice'. (Personally I think he was insulting to most of the business practitioners I know.)

In 1992 Pilgrim wrote:

> I am not satisfied that the discussion of abuse within the confines of a culture of therapists constitutes a genuine public airing. Equally, medical practitioners have researched and debated iatrogenic problems for decades but it has not stopped them plying their trade of prescribed dangerous drugs and surgical procedures. The lesson from this is that professionals, including psychotherapists, cannot be trusted to police themselves. (p. 251)

As a participant in the world of psychotherapy who also observes this my world, I have noticed that some colleagues have been sanctioned for similar ethics violations for which others have been excused. I have seen struggling individual colleagues shamed and disciplined for matters for which large and financially well-off organisations have been pardoned. I have seen small organisations expelled while larger organisations have donated money or other services to the professional bodies who did not expel them (although their actions were similar or worse than those of the small organisation who could not distribute benefits, nor threaten expensive legal action). I have seen some individuals punished and die either spiritually or physically subsequent to such persecution while others have flourished having committed similar offences apparently with immunity from the consequences of their actions. I have interviewed numbers of these people confidentially in terms of how they have experienced our ethics and complaints processes (these interviews are still to be subjected to discourse analysis). All have been relieved to be heard confidentially and non-judgementally since all respondents reported pain and distress as result of having been a participant in an ethics investigation.

In this I was following a naturalistic and field study approach where

> observations are made of a process as it occurs under natural conditions. The researcher may play the role of an outside observer (not part of the process being studied) or may be a participant observer whose identity as a researcher is either known or unknown to other participants. (Anderson and Braud, pp. 275–6)

This way of doing *lived research*, more usual in social activists, was prefigured for me in the work of Dryden and of Barber. Windy Dryden's

Reflections on Counselling (1993) is an exemplary document of researching into personal adversity and as result transforming it into creative activity with social benefit. Loss of a full-time job was followed by redundancy and then the dole. Instead of descending into despair or hopelessness, he applied for job after job, logging how long it took for letters to be answered, whether he was interviewed or not, and how. Of course, he did not tell every potential employer that he was actually conducting research on their conduct towards him. Some *fifty-five* rejections later, Windy turned these experiences into personal and professional learning by publishing a paper of his findings. And his professional success has since spoken for itself.

Barber (1994) did something similar when he found himself in hospital by researching the length of time nurses would take to attend to him after he had rung the bell. As a nurse researcher, he had found this way of *living research*, bridging what has been called the academy–clinic divide and transforming a difficult personal experience into professionally valuable learning for many. Mahrer (1996) analyses tapes of other psychotherapists after the event and retrospective studies of documents such as meetings, correspondence, therapy or court transcripts, recollections of significant events (like growing up with an alcoholic parent) and other recorded material often only become interesting in retrospect when these can be subjected for example to discourse analytic procedures.

Kiesler (1966) furthermore noted that therapy researchers are coming to believe 'that we need to return to an essential first step that we bypassed in our rush to nomoetheic respectability – to wit, careful naturalistic observation guided by clinical judgement' (p. 528).

Gee (1998) researched his own psychoanalytic supervision sessions by tape-recording his supervisees, and Sarason (1988) professes that his life as a psychologist and his life at large are intertwined. As Clandinin and Connelly (1994) comment,

> it is not that he fails to make a distinction between his job as a psychologist and the rest of his life. Rather, it is impossible to separate them in practice: he is a human being as a psychologist and a psychologist as a human being. (p. 415)

Ulichny (1997) describes her engagement in the process of critical theorising with reluctant or opposed participants. Ulichny sees this as 'my attempts at what Fine (1994) calls "working the hyphens" in qualitative research between Researcher–Researched and Self–Other, and I would add, between Researcher–Activists, in an attempt *"to pry open a conversation in need of public shaping"'* [emphasis added] (Ulichny, 1997, p. 164).

These are not the kinds of research opportunities for which one plans meticulously, does a literature search, draws up a research design and waits for an university ethics committee to pass, blinding oneself to all data until that day. Of course it helps to have done research training and have those investigative muscles at peak fitness when these opportunities come one's way. These papers and others like them are examples of lives examined in the here-and-now of existence by professional people to serve others as well as to help themselves.

My engagement with the ethical and professional ambiguities and inequalities of psychotherapy's ethical dilemmas and complaints procedures can also be described as a form of critical ethnography. Thus:

> it is disruptive, it is often about giving voice to the unheard. It is also about the play of power–knowledge relations in local and specific settings. . . . It enables the analyst [researcher] to focus upon and explore 'events', spaces which divide those in struggle. It is very much about local memories and marginalized perspectives. (Ball, 1994, p. 4)

Should one therefore simply avoid researching professional ethics? It certainly is safer and less likely to attract criticism to focus on unproblematic areas of one's discipline. There is also always the danger of being misinterpreted and for data to be misused. Researchers should be aware of the ethical and moral implications of using such dangers as excuses for suppressing material. Such solutions have their drawbacks, however. Defensive research sticks to the tried and true and refuses to consider the ethical implications of failure to conduct important but sensitive studies. 'It is impossible to know the costs of experiments not done or research not undertaken. Who speaks for the sick, those in pain and for the future?' (Kaplan, 1988, pp. 839–40). This is the valid charge of *bystanding* – not getting involved when someone else is in trouble (Clarkson, 1996a). By all accounts there are numbers of 'others in trouble' as result of our professional ethics and it requires the most concerted effort to keep turning away from this problem – which is in my opinion at the very heart of our business.

For example, both the UKCP and the BPS have been judicially reviewed in the English High Court during 1999 – thus leading to the (kindest) conclusion that these bodies leave much to be desired in their handling of complaints and ethics processes. This is as a direct consequence of my conscious participation in the process of exploring and investigating our codes and our practice because my research concerns are:

> to work for a view which recognises the diversity an complexity of real life, which pays attention to socio-political factors and the cultural constitution of experience, which takes seriously the terms in which people make sense of their lives. (Salmon 1992, quoted in Marshall and Woollett, 1997, p. 43)

Notwithstanding the UKCP's published claims (Palmer Barnes, 1998) to the contrary, it is now properly established that the UKCP is not in fact 'above the law'. There *is* in fact 'a Judge over your Shoulder' – as the leaflet on judicial review is entitled (Collis, 1995). Officers of regulatory bodies such as the UKCP cannot threaten complainants while legal actions are pending (or retaliate later) without facing the consequences of being in criminal contempt of court.

Action research has in this way led to such 'objective facts' now being established in the public domain. Professional outcry and private pain reach us through newsletters of organisations (such as Marianne Fry's resignation letter at the beginning of this book) and publicity in the national press (such as about damage done and professionals shielded by the professional bodies rather than protecting the public, as we claim to do). I have acted in accordance with the belief that 'the social responsibility in research transcends the academic discipline or profession to which the researcher belongs' (McLeod, 1994, p. 174).

Following on my review of the evidence (Clarkson, 1998b), *if*:

- 'schools' or theoretical orientations do not make much difference to the effectiveness of psychotherapy – no matter how measured (e.g. Fiedler, 1950; Orlinsky and Howard, 1980; Luborsky et al., 1986)
- there is serious doubt about whether training (e.g. Strupp and Hadley 1979; Hattie et al., 1984); or personal therapy (e.g. Greenberg and Staller, 1981) makes much difference; and
- our professed professional organisations are so blatantly failing to uphold reasonable criteria of 'self-regulation' (as explained in Chapter 13)

then, for me, the only remaining bastion of integrity lies in our individual attempts to question ourselves and others, and our organisations ethically *all the time*.

So, *not* to research these areas would then mean turning away from these kinds of ethical and professional problems and concentrating perhaps on investigating the 'efficacy' of one's preferred brand of psychotherapy – ignoring all those reports which also validate the efficacy of other approaches. As Frank and Frank (1993) so trenchantly observed: 'No training institute has yet disbanded because it concluded that its theory was inferior to that of another school' (p. 162).

Then there is the fact that emotional and mental healing has been with us since the beginning of recorded times (e.g. the madness of Hercules and Nebuchadnezzar) as well as the fact that emotional and mental healing is currently taking place in many cultures (and sub-cultures) through so-called traditional medicine means (such as throwing the bones, psychic surgery, voodoo and other shamanic practices). We can simply outlaw such non-Eurocentric experience or we can allow the implications of such facts to permeate our consciousness and raise questions about our work.

Furthermore, according to Frank and Frank (1993), to be effective, the therapeutic myth (or theory) must be compatible with the cultural world view shared by the patient and the therapist. The infrequent use of counselling and psychotherapy services provided by Eurocentric psychology practitioners for people from minority cultural or racial backgrounds substantiates this finding. Indeed recent studies are beginning to acknowledge traditional healing methods alongside or instead of Eurocentric practices such as the work of Ince (1999) and Moodley (1998): 'inclusion of traditional healing methods would also dispel many of the notions regarding Western health care as knowing what is best for black clients' (p. 54).

Frank (1973; also Frank and Frank 1993) found that psychotherapists and other healing artists such as magicians and scientists had in common that:

- There is 'an emotionally charged confiding relationship with a helping person (often with the participation of a group)' (Frank and Frank, 1993, p. 40).
- The setting is designated as a place of healing.
- Therapy is based on 'a rationale, conceptual scheme, or myth that provides a plausible explanation for the patient's symptoms and prescribes a ritual or procedure for resolving them' (Frank and Frank, 1993, p. 42).
- 'A ritual or procedure that requires the active participation of both patient and therapist and that is believed by both to be the means of restoring the patient's health. The procedure serves as the vehicle for maintaining the therapeutic alliance and transmitting the therapist's influence' – a form of persuasion (Frank and Frank, 1993, p. 43).

The field may or may not be transformed as results of the efforts of my colleagues and me, but I certainly am.

> Having made a discovery, I shall never see the world again as before. My eyes have become different: I have made myself into a person seeing and thinking differently. I have crossed a gap, the heuristic gap, which lies between problem and discovery. (Polyani, 1962, p. 143)

Method

The method used is the interweaving of researcher and researched, folding in on the self and out into the practice. 'It is through this spiral movement, through experiencing lived space with others, that the researcher would learn, illuminate, and generate data' (Shelef, 1994, p. 3). Also of course, test the data. In this sense it reflects a contemporary post-modernist attempt to give validity to all the 'different stories about stories' (Anderson, 1990, p. 267) which currently constitute the body of knowledge and practice we call psychotherapy. It also allows for future development.

The exploration of the moral situatedness of the researcher/clinician/supervisor in psychotherapy is thus crucial to the research project. According to Rudestam and Newton (1992),

> Because the researcher is regarded as a person who comes to the scene with his or her own operative reality, rather than as a totally detached scientific observer, it becomes vital to understand, acknowledge and share one's own underlying values, assumptions and expectations. (p. 38)

This exploration is all part of *triangulation*. Triangulation is a method of improving the quality of research – not merely to improve its 'accuracy' and trustworthiness, but also to illuminate the work from different angles – much as facet cutting shows the qualities of a diamond. In this way the work acquires 'the advantages of allowing a multiplicity of voices to speak to the research issues of concern' (Gergen and Gergen, 1991, p. 79).

> Triangulation [therefore] has as much to do with the choice of methodology as it has to do with validity. The essential rationale is that, if you use a number of different methods or sources of information to tackle a question, the resulting answer is more likely to be accurate (or useful). For example, a study of bullying in schools might involve carrying out separate interviews with teachers, the head teacher and the children, and then go on to obtain personal accounts in the form of essays or diaries from the participants as well. Finally the researchers might attempt to gain access as participant observers and include their own reports on the activities within the school as a source of data. (Smith, 1996, pp. 193–4)

Denzin (1978) identified four basic types of triangulation:

> (a) the triangulation of data which involves the use of a variety of data sources; (b) investigator triangulation which refers to the use of several different researchers or evaluators (c) theory triangulation involves the use of multiple perspectives to interpret a single set of data and (d) methodological triangulation: the use of multiple methods to study a single problem. Qualitative researchers seek alternative methods for evaluating their work, including verisimilitude, emotionality, personal responsibility, and ethic of caring, political praxis, multivoiced texts and dialogues with subjects . . . see the everyday social world in action and embed their findings in it. . . . Qualitative researchers use ethnographic prose, historical narratives, first-person accounts, life histories, fictionalised facts and biographical and autobiographical materials among others. (pp. 5–6)

On the advice of Denzin and Lincoln (1994), it was my hope to 'seek out groups, settings and individuals where (and for whom) the processes being studied are most likely to occur' (p. 200). Thus it is a discovery-oriented kind of research where opportunistic sampling becomes similar to what Barfield (1957) called 'systematic investigation of phenomena by way of participation' (p. 138). This is analogous to ethnographic research where a researcher observes and interacts at the same time as participating in the life of the community. As member of several of the metaphorical tribes of psychotherapy (thus being multilingual in this tower of Babel) and also experiencing some measure of independence,

> The naturalist is likely to eschew random or representative sampling in favour of purposive or theoretical sampling because he or she thereby increases the scope of range of data exposed (random or representative sampling is likely to suppress more deviant cases) as well as the likelihood that the full array of multiple realities will be uncovered. (Lincoln and Guba, 1985, p. 4)

Five kinds of relationship in research

Bor and Watts (1993) wrote that researchers in counselling psychology should conduct their research using a methodology which is congruent with their theoretical framework and approach to counselling and psychotherapy.

Since my psychological psychotherapy approach is based on the vast volume of research findings privileging *different kinds of relationship* as the primary common factor across healing practices, I will therefore here briefly highlight aspects of using the five kinds of relationships which I identified (Clarkson, 1990, 1995) as a framework for theory and practice, supervision and training as well as in organisational and cultural life. It should not be necessary to have to point out that each of these relationships includes the sociocultural, ethical and philosophical implications specific to themselves and that such aspects cannot be logically or ethically separated out from their embeddedness in human discourse (Clarkson, 1996b).

We know that the work of therapy is *not* primarily technical. It occurs neither *in* the client, nor *in* the therapist, but in the between of their encounter. It is not mechanical, but a live and human process (Mair, 1989). Research such as reported in this book, to be congruent with my approach, is also a live and human process. This squares well with Clandinin and Connelly (1994) who have also commented on the way in which research itself is about relationship, conducted in relationship and through relationship.

> Personal experience methods inevitably are relationship methods. As researchers, we cannot work with participants without sensing the fundamental human connection among us; nor can we create research texts without imagining a relationship to you, our audience. Voice and signature make it possible for there to be conversations through the texts among participants, researchers, and audiences. It is in the research relationships among

participants and researchers and among researchers an audiences, through
research texts that we see the possibility for individual and social change. . . .
We see personal experience methods as a way to permit researchers to enter
into and participate with the social world in ways that allow the possibility of
transformations and growth. (p. 425)

Relationship is *fractally* understood here, i.e. intrapsychically at
microscopic scales and interpersonally, organisationally or culturally at
macroscopic scales. *All* these at different levels are implied whenever the
notion of relationship is used. The five kinds of relationship were discovered on the basis of another 20 year research project described in
Clarkson (1996c). This kind of discourse analysis in terms of the five
relationships can also be applied in any psychotherapy approach which
seeks to take account of perspectives more inclusive than single secular,
ideologically provincial concerns. Hinshelwood (1990), the then editor
of the *British Journal of Psychotherapy*, described my work as:

a careful analysis of the various levels of the psychotherapeutic relationship in
an *attempt to find a perspective from which an overview might become
possible*. She [Clarkson] offers a way of circumventing the inherent contradictions and incompatibilities that exist *between* different psychotherapies;
instead of incompatibilities we have different priorities and emphasis. (p. 119)

However, this perspective also applies to any one approach because the
five kinds of therapeutic relationship can be found (as is to be expected)
in any well developed theory and practice of psychotherapy from
Kleinian analysis to hypnotherapy. It also serves well for supervision,
consultation, family and couples' work. Therefore what follows is an
acknowledgement of a multiplicity of relationships in ethics research –
not a simplistic dichotomy which can be culturally disconnected – but a
pluralistic matrix which cannot absolve us from ongoing moral ethical
and legal responsibilities.

The therapeutic relationship takes on the capacity to create new ways of
being. . . . The opportunity for creating new inter-subjectivities, which
depend on various interpersonal relationships, allows for old versions of the
autonomous individual to be retired, along with its components – agency,
self-determination, and free will. This move to relationship selves does not
eradicate the necessity of pondering issues of moral choice and action.
Rather, these alternative conceptions suggest the need for revisioning what
constitutes moral action. (Gergen, 1994, p. 21)

This section is not designed to be a comprehensive overview of
ethical considerations in research practice, but to indicate ways in which
the five kinds of relationship framework can be used to illuminate and
mine this important area. It presents an integrative research methodology hoping to combine aspects of all important dimensions of the

research relationship. On the other hand, the research and approach that I have used in this book can be said to merely reflect specifically on the five different kinds of relationships and their ethical implications as an example of the kind of thinking and questioning which I hope readers will themselves take much further and deeper.

This is in the spirit of Kvale's (1992) suggestion: 'by discarding a modern legitimation mania, justification of knowledge is replaced by application, with a pragmatic concept of validity' (p. 39). Of course he does not mean indiscriminate pragmatism. The criterion of validity is ethically particularly applicable in this case where usefulness of the framework is its *raison d'être* – not its 'truth' *per se*. 'Anyone over the age of twelve knows there is no such thing as certainty, right?' (Jim Hartle in Hawking, 1992, p. 177).

However, there are errors of confusion, conflation, abuse and neglect which can affect the responsible and effective use of all research relationships – particularly when they are not differentiated and distinguished from each other. We have noticed how emphasis on each draws in specific universes of discourse, encompassing different worlds of values, perspectives on human nature, assumptions about free will and determinism, individuality and commonality, prejudices, blind spots and particular gifts of caution and vision. I hope I have pointed out at least a significant number of these throughout the therapeutic relationship book (Clarkson, 1995) to inspire and alert readers to their own most favourite and their own most avoided concerns.

To recap, the five kinds of therapeutic relationship are:

- the *working alliance* (the contractual consensual agreement)
- the *transference/countertransference* relationship (the possible distortions of the working alliance)
- the *developmentally needed or reparative* relationship (the intentional provision of deficits or growth opportunities)
- the *person-to-person* (the existential dialogic) relationship
- the *transpersonal* relationship – (the dimension that allows for the unknowable, the auto-poetic and the transcendent in our relationships) (Clarkson 1975, 1990, 1996a, 1997). According to Maturana and Varela (1987) *autopoiesis* literally means the self-generating poetry of living systems (*auto* means 'self' and *poiesis* means 'poetry' or 'making'). It is another name for *physis*, the life force.

Different theoretical and ideological approaches to research privilege some of these (e.g. the quantitative aspects of the working alliance in quantitative research) and ignore or deny or attempt to control the others (e.g. transpersonal or chance elements). Other approaches concentrate on the developmentally needed aspects such as action research in the form advocated by Reason and Rowan (1981). Probably these five dimensions (under whatever names) exist potentially in every piece of research – and explicitly in all lived research.

> Experience, in this view, is the stories people live. People live stories, and in the telling of them re-affirm them, modify them, and create new ones.. . . . Stories such as these, lived and told, educate the self and others, including the young and those, such as researchers, who are [always] new to their communities. (Clandinin and Connelly, 1994, p. 415)

The objective aspects of the research relationship

• Ethical issues around the working alliance: the researcher as objective technician

The working alliance aspect of research is often considered as *the primary if not the only* relationship operative or acknowledged in quantitative methods. The researcher is conceptualised as a technician who is doing the experiment impartially and 'objectively'. It is that dimension of the researcher–researched relationship which is concerned with boundaries, contracts, legitimate expectations, the explicit or implicit cultural context in which the research is conducted – the university laboratory or the clinical couch. In order to show that their personal influence is either absent or properly controlled, 'quantitative researchers use mathematical models, statistical tables and graphs and often write about their research in impersonal third person prose' (Denzin, 1978, pp. 5–6). Unfortunately in psychotherapy it has been said that the better the research in terms of meeting positivistic criteria, the less useful the results. It is essential to remember that such research is valuable and important and can have its own unique place in integrative research. However, vast volumes have been written about such scientific research methods, so I will here concentrate on other aspects closer to our theme.

Of course there is a sense in which all research is ethics research because no research – notwithstanding all claims – can be ethically neutral. McLeod (1994) is clear: 'It is impossible to design ethically neutral research. All research necessitates making value decisions which may be in conflict with the beliefs and values of some other people' (p. 166).

Furthermore, what may be ethical is not always legal and it may or may not be moral. Objective scientific research was conducted in South Africa by white psychologists during the apartheid era to 're-channel the aggression of young black men' (personal knowledge). It was both legal and ethical. Was it moral? If a researcher secretly videotapes parents abusing their children in a hospital ward – without the parents' consent – to get evidence of such abuse it would be unethical – but is it legal or moral?

If evidence of bias emerges during subsequent studies of the transcripts of ethics hearings transcripts, should these ever be made public? If information about warden brutality and widespread drug abuse emerges during a study of a prison population, is it legal or ethical to keep their confidence as the researcher had promised?

Some research (for example into psychotropic drug treatments) gets done because it can attract funding – other areas remain undone (for example, prejudice and racism inherent in our Eurocentric psychology curricula and assessment systems) because it might 'rock the boat?' (See for example Teun van Dijk's (1987) studies of ethnic prejudice in thought and talk.) How can any researcher claim to be objective?

From physics we learned than we 'cannot measure or observe physical events, except in ways that must interfere with the events themselves. Any experiment becomes an interaction with the physical world, so that the physical world is not just observed, but changed. We cannot know exactly what form the physical events would have taken if we had made no attempt to interfere with them by observation' (Eiser, 1994, p. 94).

The continuum which ranges from defensiveness to coercion is a prevalent consideration in considering the ethical implications of the working alliance. When can it be said that a person has given informed consent? When cataloguing the experiences of children growing up with parents who were mentally ill – do the parents have to give their consent?

When videotaping infants or psychoanalysing children – have they really given their consent?

> The usual reponse of traditional liberal humanist (male elite) philosophers . . . is to assert that it makes no difference how truth gets produced. and what its consequences are – truth is independent of the truth-teller. Congealed in this view are beliefs concerning the objectivity of truth of many western philosophers, including Kant, Descartes and Locke. (Gergen, 1994, p. 17)

The problems with claims of objectivity in research has been only too well demonstrated by the consequences of the scientific objectivity of those who made the atom bomb, as in the case of Robert Oppenheimer (Gleick, 1992). Scientists who still claim to be objective are in the minority – and often associated with exactly the kind of research which is questionable in terms of social responsibility (e.g. cloning and genetically modified food). According to Smith et al. (1995), 'research is one form of social interaction . . . not divorced from everyday social practices' (p. 6). Also:

> Or as Woody Allen put it: 'Can we really "know" the universe? My God, it's hard enough finding your way around Chinatown'. The point, however is: Is there anything out there? And why? And must they be so noisy? Finally, there

can be do doubt that the one characteristic of 'reality' is that it lacks essence. That is not to say it has no essence, but merely lacks it. (The reality I speak of here is the same one Hobbes described, but a little smaller). [Source unknown]

The projective aspect of the research relationship

• Ethical issues around the transference/countertransference relationship: the researcher as projective screen or interference (noise)

The *transference/countertransference relationship* (one could also call this the anticipated relationship or 'schema' from a cognitive perspective or 'bias' from an existential perspective) is concerned with the experience of the researched transferring (carrying over) or projecting (pushing out) wishes, experiences and fears from their past on to the researcher or research project. Depending on the relevant 'way of talking' (WOT) (Farrell, 1979), it can also be described as essentially concerned with distortion of or interference with the experimental measurements due to uncontrolled variables or unaccounted for influences on the research findings. As we know from eye-witness account studies (e.g. Loftus and Palmer, 1974; Kassin et al., 1989) humans often see what they want to see rather than what is actually happening.

Child observation studies in psychotherapy trainings invariably support the theoretical bias of the observers – Kleinians see Kleinian babies, Jungian analysts see Jungian ones, and self-psychologists observe baby behaviour that seems to fit self-psychological explanations. (See Gergen et al., 1990 on the cultural construction of the developing child.) Since the babies can't really tell us what is going on we are free to project on to them mother's mouth, father's chin or Freud's ideas. (It is probably just another case of unexamined WOTs.)

The research of Gelso et al. (1995) on the influence of theory on distorting countertransference reactions in psychotherapy bears this out.

The surprising finding was that high use of theory combined with low awareness of countertransference feelings resulted in the greatest amount of countertransference behaviour. In reflecting on these findings, the researchers theorised that when counsellors are unaware of countertransference feelings, their use of counselling theory may serve a defensive function. They may intellectualise about the client and the relationship, but there is a lack of emotional understanding. The use of counselling theory in the absence of emotional self-understanding is ineffective in deterring counsellors from enacting countertransference behaviour with clients [or research respondents]. . . . We should not forget the role of personal or clinical experience in guiding the theoretician and researcher. Our experiences in the world, and with clients if we are in practice field (and/or as clients ourselves, if we are theorising about and studying therapeutic interventions), guide us in a profound way in our selection of theories to generate hypotheses and explain findings. Although these experiences must be guided by reason and managed (not unlike countertransference management) if they are to most effectively lead us, they are an inevitable part of the process. (Gelso, 1996, p. 367)

Generally double-blind studies are designed to *exclude* this distorting effect. However, analysis of many hundreds of scientifically controlled studies show that 25–35% of patients recover from severe depressive illness due to the placebo effect. Response to the anti-depressant medication itself is only some 45% for fluoxidine (M Lader, personal communication, 1999). Although it may apply reasonably in some other research situations, psychotherapy research is even less amenable to this form of reducing distortion in the working alliance. Furthermore, it is even questionable if many such procedures are effective for this purpose – for example, the finding that experimenters expectation of rats' intelligence seem to affect even the rate at which the rats learnt mazes! (See Feather, 1982.)

Transference effects from respondents or 'experimental subjects' can impact findings dramatically skewing them. On the other hand, by paying attention to precisely the distorting effects, as in psychoanalysis, enormous value can emerge. One thinks, for example, of the Milgram (1974) experiments (authority transferences 'absolved' people from responsibility for their destructive actions) and the Hawthorne studies (Roethlisberger and Dixon 1939) where workers' productivity kept improving not as a result of experimental changes to the lighting in the factory, but because they felt valued.

Countertransference is one of many words which can loosely be used to refer to the feelings, attitudes and behaviours of the researcher towards the researched or the research project. As in clinical work, there are usually at least two kinds of countertransferences:

- *pro-active*: those introduced by the researcher's own past experiences (for example, humiliating schoolteachers or rote reproduction of learnt formulas)
- *reactive*: those experienced in response to the material raised in the research project (for example, the acute distress experienced when interviewing parents about their child's brain damage with a highly structured questionnaire).

Both kinds of countertransferences can create distortions and both kinds can provide most valuable insight into the research itself. It is always necessary to explore these possibilities and to involve other researchers who bring different eyes and different perspectives to such questions. Because of this the presences of my supervisors, colleagues, journal reviewers, critical and appreciative colleagues and my analyst accompanies and permeates every aspect of my work.

In a recent small opportunistic study (Clarkson, 1999) conducted with psychologist researchers using the five-relationship model, every participant found, upon invitation to explore, significant personal investment in their supposedly objective studies. Each one was in some way attempting to resolve painful, conflicting or confusing experiences from their own lives through doing their particular research project. This is another way of talking about countertransference. The value of the exercise was that up to that moment, they had not known or acknowledged the potential of such distorting subjective influences. Whether such personal investments (e.g. having suffered from abuse oneself) culminate in better or worse results is largely up to the honesty and willingness of the researchers to becoming aware of their own internal processes which may skew their findings. Often a counter-phobic reason emerges upon questioning, e.g.: 'My own experience of being depressed and a failed suicide bid was very terrifying and maybe I will feel I can understand the experiences of people going through something similar more fully and therefore be of greater help.' Such considerations may also highlight the importance of psychotherapeutic exploration of themselves for all researchers – even objective quantitative researchers.

Rather than denying or attempting to avoid such distorting effects, I believe it is much more effective and enriching the research findings themselves when these influences are acknowledged, welcomed and explored *as part of the research*. This is why I have advocated that all researchers should have clinical training and all clinicians constantly be engaged in research (Clarkson, 1998b). Naturally, the worst case is when any researcher imagines that they are free of these or that they have fully accounted for them. The question of integrity is not 'if', but 'how' are my own issues and my noise helping or hindering this account? The qualitative researcher is 'historically positioned and locally situated [as] an all-too-human [observer] of the human condition' and meaning is 'radically plural, always open, and . . . there are politics in every account' (Bruner, 1993, p. 1).

The reparative aspect of the research relationship

• Ethical issues around the developmentally needed or reparative psychotherapeutic relationship: the researcher as offering social remedy

The *reparative or developmentally needed relationship* therapeutic dimension is relevant when the researcher or researching team intentionally provides a corrective, reparative, or replenishing experiences (for themselves *and* others) in doing the research. The express intention is to hopefully improve the functioning of the organisation or the understanding of ethical and moral dilemmas through the doing of the research. It concerns the intentional provision of deficit-replenishment where the researcher also functions as therapist or developer. It is concerned with educational or reparative effects for the researcher and/or the researched and with the ethical principle of beneficence.

As result of such research, not only may other individuals change, but smaller and larger groups, organisations, institutions, societies and culture – even the planet as a whole – may change as well.

> This is the social action component – the political component of the process. . . . Aspects of this transformation of others are suggested by the Greek term *diakonia*. Diakonia involves service or ministering to others, or attending to a duty. Here, the service resides in presenting and making available what is helpful or needed for the change and transformation of others and of society at large. (Anderson and Braud, 1998, p. 245)

> There is a social responsibility in research that transcends the academic discipline or profession to which the researcher belongs. The ultimate moral justification for research is that it makes a contribution to a greater public good, by easing suffering or promoting truth. This wide horizon introduces further challenges and demands on researchers. . . . Many feminist and qualitative researchers argue that one of the aims of research should be to empower those who participate in it. (McLeod, 1994, p. 174)

> Action, feminist, clinical, constructivist, ethnic, critical, and cultural studies researchers are all united on this point. They all share the belief that a politics of liberation must always begin with the perspectives, desires and dreams of those individuals and groups who have been oppressed by the larger ideological, economic and political forces of a society, or a historical moment. (Lincoln and Denzin, 1994, p. 575)

An absolutist stance argues that social scientists should not withhold information or mislead participants

> if the participants are typically likely to object or show unease once debriefed. Where this is in any doubt, appropriate consultation must precede the investigation. Consultation is best carried out with individuals who share the social and cultural background of the participants in the research, but the advice of ethics committees or experienced and disinterested colleagues may be sufficient. (BPS, 1993, section 4.2)

> The researcher should always first consider whether there are alternative procedures available which do not require deception. If so such alternatives are available, and if it is judged that the intended deception is an ethically permissible procedure then the subjects should be debriefed at the earliest opportunity. (Barrett, 1995, p. 31)

Social scientists have a responsibility to contribute to a society's self-understanding, and it could be argued that any method that contributes to this understanding is thereby justified – as long as it does not cause harm. However, sometimes deceptive techniques may be justified 'because frequently people in power, like those out of power, will attempt to hide the truth from the researcher' (Denzin and Lincoln, 1994 p. 21). This is in agreeement with Becker's (1967) call to 'take sides' (cease bystanding); and Douglas' (1979) persuasive argument that it may sometimes be ethical to deceive the 'establishment' in order to expose it. An example may be researchers who had themselves admitted to mental hospitals – without the administration's consent – in order to expose malpractice and abuse (Goffman, 1961). Another is a real patient who keeps detailed notes and tape-recordings of all staff conversations with her – to publish after discharge in a publication for mental health users.

Sometimes it seems as if there is a pretence at or denial of a real presence and natural undulations of life, love and existence and their impact on the course and the conduct of a psychotherapy or psychoanalysis, their ethics and their research. Elsewhere (Clarkson, 1995, 1996a), there have been reviews and explorations of the ethical and moral consequences of this 'scientific' attitude in the clinician – as well as its impossibility. It has been argued that a value-free practice is as impossible as a value-free science and that all of us are involved in the structuring and construction of our world, complicit with its ideological assumptions and never free from the moral and epistemological consequences of our acts of commission *and* omission. Mary Gergen (1988) puts it quite bluntly: 'The claim that science is value-free is a self-deception or an attempt to deceive others' (p. 91).

The subjective aspect of the research relationship

- Ethical issues around the person-to-person or real relationship: the researcher as involved person

This dimension of the research relationship focuses on engagement and dialogue of the kind which qualitative research valorises. It can also be described as the real or core relationship most concerned with our intersubjectivity. It shows the humanity of the researcher and deals with the genuine presence of the researcher as person equally human with the people with whom the research is encountered. The *subjective* (as contrasted with the *objective* of the working alliance) becomes the focus. According to Wolman (1965) empirical scientists must study all data – including introspective private data. The researcher's self becomes the instrument in this kind of research. Partisanship or engagement is an essential tool of such research. 'Heuristics is a passionate and discerning personal involvement in problem solving, an effort to know the essence of some aspect of life through the internal pathways of the self' (Douglass and Moustakas, 1985, p. 39).

> Qualitative researchers . . . seek to examine the major public and private issues and personal troubles that define a particular historical moment. [They] self-consciously draw upon their own experiences as a resource in their inquiries. They always think reflectively, historically, and biographically.

They seek strategies of empirical inquiry that will allow them to make connections among lived experience, larger social and cultural structures, and the here and now. (Denzin and Lincoln, 1994, p. 199)

The qualitative researcher is not an objective, authoritative, politically neutral observer standing outside and above the text (Bruner, 1993, p. 1).

[The] false division between the personal and the ethnographic self rests on the assumption that it is possible to write a text that does not bear the traces of its author. Of course, this is not possible. All texts are personal statements. (Lincoln and Denzin, 1994, p. 578)

As I have shown before (Clarkson 1996a), values permeate everything and every action or non-action of the contemporary psychotherapist researcher. This also includes texts (or research reports) which claim to be 'impartial', objective and positivistic. The 'personal statements' cloaked by such 'scientific' adjectives, may merely have somewhat more aspects hidden, less conscious, or less acknowledged. Informal research, for example, asking quantitative researchers easily disclose personal agendas, subjective concerns, even childhood influences. (Try it yourself.) Perhaps a formal study of the biographies of scientists would corroborate these preliminary findings?

Most researchers, except where it is merely for the money/status or actually being forced (as in the mid-century Russian asylums), choose to some extent what they will study, whether they are researching IQ differences between white and black people, or doing an ethnographic study of lap dancers, or the amount of neurological damage caused by psychotropic drugs on prisoners, quality of life in the elderly housebound and so forth. In particular, metaphorically every PhD title speaks a biography. In a sense it has to – because often only those themes which *move* us (such as spina bifida in a daughter) can interest most of us long enough to sustain the kind of long-term committed interest required in the frequently arduous and sometimes boring work of bringing a major research project to conclusion. Whatever I choose to know and how (epistemology) has moral (ethical) implications.

Hekman (1995) contrasts feminist ways of research – which cannot exclude the subjective knower – from patriachal ideologies which suppose that 'morality' can be disembodied, neither in relationship, nor localised:

It is my contention that particular moral theories are inextricably linked to particular epistemologies. More specifically, I am arguing that the epistemology that informs modernist moral theory necessarily assumes a disembodied knower that constitutes abstract universal truth. The individual who occupies Kohlberg's stage 6 is such a knower. The moral truth that this knower constitutes is singular, universal, and absolute; it is a truth that is disembodied, removed from the relationships and connectedness of everyday life that, on this view, distort moral judgements. [p. 30] Morality is constitutive of subjectivity: my moral beliefs make me who I am. (pp. 30 and 157)

Many kinds of qualitative researchers, including those who call themselves phenomenological or heuristic researchers, would agree with her. Empirical means by experience, experience is only possible through the body, through relationship, through intersubjectivity. In the process of phenomenological research we also engage in a relationship with each other, which cannot but be conceptually separated from who we are, and when and why and who else is listening or turning away.

> Qualitative researchers . . . understand the social, political, cultural, economic, ethnic and gender history and structure that serve as the surround for their inquiries. . . . [They] self-consciously draw upon their own experiences as a resource in their inquiries. They always think reflectively, historically and biographically. They seek strategies of empirical inquiry that will allow them to make connections among lived experience, larger social and cultural structures, and the here and now. (Denzin and Lincoln (1994, p. 199)

The ethics reseacher of whatever is defined by and in history and time – 'a contintual dynamic process of moral discourse and discovery. . . . The morals of today are not the morals of yesterday, and they will not be the morals of tomorrow' (Anderson, 1990, p. 259). What was acceptable ethically decades ago, will now be abjured; what we condemn today may be valued in twenty or ten years' time – who knows? And every researcher in every era has to deal with issues of being, knowing and method. According to Denzin (1978),

> The gendered, multiculturally situated researchers approaches the world with a set of ideas, a framework (theory, ontology) that specifies a set of questions (epistemology) that are then examined (methodology, analysis) in specific ways. That is, empirical materials bearing on the question are collected and then analysed and written about . . . [from] the personal biography of the gendered researchers, who speaks from a particular class, racial cultural and ethnic community perspective. (p. 11)

> According to the primarily theoretical framework adopted in order to comprehend the attempt to transform unruly inimically into docile obedience (Foucault, 1979), the secretly vicious 'disciplinary order is a cultural–historical process into which we are born. Psychology's methods of dealing with persons are structurally no different from those in the areas of medicine, criminal justice, education and industry . . . and yet I do argue that we as individual persons and as psychologists are responsible for our participation in this order and are free to abandon the project of domination and control, to practice a psychology that recognises, embraces, liberates and empowers the Other through a practice of open dialogue. This entails not an eradication but a respectful acknowledgement of the presence of inimicality in others and in ourselves. (Wertz, 1995, p. 451)

Instead of attempting the arguably impossible, qualitative researchers take pride in mining their own experiences and taking as data their own feelings, fantasies, hopes, subjectivities and dreams. Scholars are now 'writing about *how*, not if, our subjectivities sculpt the stories that we tell and the ones that we don't' (Kidder and Fine, 1997, p. 44).

Qualitative researchers study friendship, beauty in their own families, loneliness, moral dilemmas and other important aspects of human existence. One of the most valuable and honest accounts of homosexual experiences is Joseph Styles' (1979) discussion of his 'insider' role in researching gay baths. He contrasts the earlier phases of his study where he used an *outsider* strategy – 'observation without sexual participation, and a correspondingly heavier reliance upon informants as original sources of ideas as well as a means of testing these notions' – with an *insider* strategy – 'observation and sexual participation in the baths, the heavy use of these as a source of original typologies and images, and the employment of informants as a way of testing, revising and evaluating these typologies and images' See also Coyle, 1996, 1998; Wright and Coyle, 1996; Gergen, 1997. Lofland and Lofland (1985) have observed that 'much of the best work in sociology and other social sciences . . . is probably grounded in the remote and/or current biographies of its creators' (p. 8). This accords with the statement of Moustakas (1994) that the research questions of phenomenological research methods 'reflect the interest, involvement and personal commitment of the researcher . . . viewing experience and behaviour as an integrated and inseparable relationship of subject and object and of parts and whole' (p. 21).

Foucault (1987) called ethics 'practice of self' (p. 129). This requires the most arduous and severest form of subjectivity – to seek to know oneself by ceaseless questioning. And as we know from teachers of meditation, the hardest question of all is: who am I? And even then we may encounter again only a region of relationship which transcends itself as a kind of research at the end of it where individuality or a separate voice no longer exists. Or as the phenomenologist Merleau-Ponty (1962) put it:

> In the experience of dialogue, there is constituted between the other person and myself a common ground; my thought and his are interwoven into a single fabric, my words and those of my interlocutor are called forth by the stage of the discussion, and they are inserted into a shared operation of which neither of us is the creator. We have here a dual being, where the other is for me no longer a mere bit of behaviour in my transcendental field, not I in his; we are collaborators for each other in consummate reciprocity. (p. 354)

The transformative aspect of the research relationship

- Ethical issues around the transpersonal relationship: the researcher as conduit and custodian of the ultimately mysterious

Transformative research

> says that we are essentially spiritual beings in a spiritual universe, that humans ultimately seek meaning in their lives, and that creativity is necessary

for both psychological and spiritual growth. It represents a transpersonal approach to research, insisting on its location in a much wider context of time and place. This involves transformative changes in the fundamental nature of the research effort: it is about giving research a new kind of vision and mission. (Rowan, 1998, p. 172)

The transpersonal relationship in research attends to the unexplained areas of human interaction and experience. It is the 'kind of Knowing that is a love. Not a scholarly knowing [which says] there are certain plusses and minuses which we must carefully consider' (Rumi, 1990, p. 25). It arises within an inner locus of evaluation and experience that appears to connect with the universal and as such it is distinct from the outer locus of evaluation, which is group norm related.

The transpersonal relationship is the timeless or indescribable aspect of the research relationship. It refers to the scientific or spiritual dimensions of the relationship which we don't understand yet. Everyone puts in here what they want to from the aesthetics of the sublime (Longinus, 1899); from synchronicity or one unconscious to another (Jung, 1972); from God to entanglement theory (Isham, 1995); or there is the beginning of speaking in poetry about the region beyond dualism, beyond contradiction, beyond yes and no.

> Before going ahead, I ought to say that I am not trying to settle these matters once and for all. I am on a poetic plane where the yes and no of things are equally true. Were you to ask me, 'Is a moonlit night of one hundred years ago identical to a moonlit night of ten years ago?' I could demonstrate (as could any other poet who is master of his craft) that it was. But with the same ring of indisputable truth, I could also prove that it was not. I am trying to avoid the sort of ugly erudite data that tire out audiences; it is emotional data I shall try to emphasise. You are surely more interested in knowing whether a melody can give birth to a finely sifted, soporific breeze, or whether a song can place a simple landscape before the child's newly jelled eyes, than in knowing whether the melody is of the seventeenth century or whether it is written in 3/4 time, information the poet ought to know but not to repeat and which is, after all, within reach of anyone who dedicates himself to these matters. (Garcia Lorca, 1980, p. 8)

> As a field of research, scholarship, and application, transpersonal psychology seeks to honour human experience in its fullest and most transformative expressions. The word transpersonal has its etymological roots in two Latin words: trans, meaning beyond or through, and persona, meaning, mask or facade – in other words, beyond or through the personally identified aspects of self. Whenever possible, transpersonal psychology seeks to delve deeply into the most profound aspects of human experience, such mystical and unitive experiences, personal transformation, meditative awareness, experiences of wonder and ecstasy, and alternative and expansive states of consciousness. In these experiences, we appear to go beyond our usual identification with our limited biological and psychological selves. (Braud and Anderson, 1998, p. xxi)

This domain thus refers to the epistemological area or universe of discourse concerned with people as 'spiritual beings', or for those who want to use another nomination – with the soul. It is beyond rationality, facts and theories and concerns the paradoxical, the unpredictable and the inexplicable. It is a region of unknowability, a horizon that has to be left open for the development of future areas of discourse and reference for these currently unknown conditions. In this domain, we could present complexity as those aspects of autopoiesis (e.g. Mingers, 1995) which are still mysterious, '*physis*' or the life-force (see Sallis and Maly, 1980) which makes systems and organisms emerge and self-develop out of unpredictable circumstances – autopoetic emergence itself. As the biologist Goodwin (1994) explains it:

> We are biologically grounded in our relationships which operate at all the different levels of our being as the basis of our nature as agents of creative *evolutionary emergence* [emphasis added], a property we share with all other species. These are not romantic yearnings and utopian ideals; they arise from a re-thinking of our biological natures that is emerging from the sciences of complexity and is leading towards a science of qualities which may help in our efforts to reach a more balanced relationship with the other members of our planetary society. (p. xiv)

It is characteristic of experience in this domain that people are convinced by 'direct experience' which feels impossible to articulate or effectively communicate to others who have not shared similar direct experience – or who come to do so. It is the knowledge of the mystic, the 'peak experiences' which Maslow (1968) studied or the quantum physicist who marvels at the mysterious awesome beauty of our universe and concludes that 'God does not play dice'.

> Knowledge [of whatever kind] is not a series of self-consistent theories that converges toward an ideal view; it is rather an ever increasing ocean of mutually incompatible (and perhaps even incommensurable) alternatives, each single theory, each fairy tale, each myth that is part of the collection forcing the others into greater articulation and all of them contributing, via this process of competition, to the development of our consciousness. (Feyerabend, 1975, p. 30)

There are many ways we use discourses about such concepts, although one does not have to accept any of these given terms for talking about the 'unexplained' or the currently inexplicable. Frank and Frank (1993) open the question of *telepathy* as being a significant if under-acknowledged part of effective psychotherapy. Most human beings have experienced awe or wonder or synchronistic encounters, or sudden flashes of intuition or creativity which are not circumscribed in the other realms discussed so far.

In fact many important scientific and artistic discoveries are characterised by such sudden discontinuous shifts, portentous dreams, and fortuitous accidents which often appear as by-products of what the researcher intended to 'research' (Koestler, 1972). For example, Freud first considered the emergence of the cornerstone of psychoanalysis – transference – as 'an untoward event' (Jones, 1953, p. 246). Richard Feynman had his best ideas while in the bathroom or drumming (Gleick, 1992). This is the realm for these kinds of untoward phenomena – until we can sensibly speak about them in other ways. In fact it is characteristic of matters to do with the transpersonal relationship that it is silent or wordless and that we lack vocabulary which can truly represent what we know (or sense) at this level. In the oriental tradition it is said that the Tao which can be described is not the Tao; in the occidental tradition (which started with the Heraclitean *physis*) Wittgenstein (1922) advises: 'Whereof one cannot speak, thereof one should be silent' (p. 189).

The five relationship facets of research are summarised in Table 14.1.

Table 14.1: The five relationship facets of research in summary

Type of relationship and focus	Researcher's role	Examples of research methods	Examples of good counsel for researchers
Working alliance (objective) Surveys on ethical dilemmas, spontaneous data collection at conferences, developing new questions based on findings applied, e.g. to supervision, organisations.	Detached technician controlling variables, clustering factors, interrater reliabilities, testing hypotheses and doing statistics. Researchers should always choose research topics amenable to their methods of investigation.	Literature reviews and most quantitative methods as in studies of Shapiro et al. (1991). *Measures of validity, reliability and generalisability relate to quality of quantitative research (Woolgar, 1996).*	Learn and use quantitative methods and quantitative research results to understand how they work, what they mean and what they conceal.
Transference/ counter-transference (projective) Fear of asking uncomfortable questions managed through therapy, peer review, professional support and regular clinical and research supervision.	Projective screen to keep data clean of distortion/to control for the influence of 'noise' – or to learn about the distortion from individual and collective cultural explorations.	Most quantitative methods require that we identify, control or avoid these distorting effects – sometimes, however, they *become* the research result as in the famous Hawthorne studies.	Seek to understand yourself and your perceptual patterns, question your assumptions, your authorities, your world – seek therapy and supervision in order to know and allow for the advantages and disadvantages of such distortions.

Table 14.1: (contd)

Type of relationship and focus	Researcher's role	Examples of research methods	Examples of good counsel for researchers
Developmental (reparative) Feedback to and from writing, teaching, supervising and speaking at conferences on ethical dilemmas. Chairing and sitting on ethics boards.	Educator, social activist creating benefits for people – also for those who are classically oppressed.	Q-methodology and action research of the kind advocated by Stainton Rogers (1995) Reason and Rowan (1981), Denzin and Lincoln (1994), Critten et al. (1998).	Serve as a minister (*diakon*) to the world which you are researching *and* find people, situations and places which will nourish and repair you.
Person-to-person (subjective) Personally being engaged as complainant in ethics matters and interviewing other complainants about their experiences.	Subjective dialogic partner in the business of living your values explicitly in the uncertainty of the moral maze. *Accounts of credibility, dependability and transferability relate to quality of qualitative research (Bannister et al. 1994).*	Discovery-oriented – qualitative methods and existential phenomenological research methods, for example that of Giorgi (1975), Moustakas (1994), von Eckartsberg (1998).	Be present to the exigencies of the human dialogic encounter – be authentically and actively engaged in the work, do a reflexive analysis. Know that we can never be morally certain and yet, like Arjuna in the Mahabharata, we have to act . . .
Transpersonal (transformative) Perhaps part of autopoetic evolution of sensitised ethical awareness in our profession – and in our relationships to each other and our world.	Conduit and conductor for life's unfolding creativity, open to serendipity and the accidents of creativity and grace. (Penicillin, the Post-it note and the law of gravity were all discovered as unexpected side-effects of other research.)	Integral inquiry, intuitive inquiry, organic research, transpersonal-phenomenological inquiry and inquiry informed by exceptional human experiences. (See Braud and Anderson, 1998.)	Allow the inexplicable, the unknowable *and* the paradoxical space in your work and in your play; be attentive to the accidents of creativity; the coincidences of your life and the promptings of your intuition. Know that the end is not due to yourself, but to the grace of God – or whatever you conceive physis/life energy to be.

Conclusion

As indicated in Table 14.1, integrative research uses all five of the relationship categories in order to illuminate a problem from multiple different angles. In this chapter, I have tried to show how an integrative model of research (utilising the five kinds of therapeutic relationship which emerges from contemporary psychotherapy research) can be used to combine and reconceptualise a multifaceted research method-ology which accounts for objective quantitative as well as qualitative, educative, subjective and transformative aspects of human inquiry. Different methods and assumptions are *systemically* interrelated in that they focus on different dimensions of the same question allowing for the creative process and life's vicissitudes to shape and refine the work. This encourages a multiple triangulation (a pentagulation) from at least five relational perspectives on the problem. Integrative research therefore combines methods, epistemologies and approaches from different perspectives systemically and iteratively in order to study a phenomena in the round – as a whole.

We come now to the end of what has been here and will continue to be for the rest of my life a significant and inescapable destiny to question, to explore, to bring into the light. In an important way I do not feel that I would have chosen to engage in this work. I feel myself through the experiences which have been vouchsafed me, responsible for communicating what has transpired and what might help. I trust that the imperfect example of a scientist–practitioner–social activist I have set encourages others to attempt the journey; I hope everyone will have seen some glimpse of a new perspective at moments along the way and I wish that somehow I will have contributed to the re-evaluation and refinement of standards in ethics, in researching ethics and in the ethical practice of psychotherapy whether in organisations, in our professions or in the imaginative regions of our dreams.

> To create such standards, we must challenge the problematic assumptions at the heart of psychological ethics today and not allow them to overtake the creation of new models. . . . It asks psychologists as individuals and psychology as a discipline to move beyond self-imposed restrictions on the meaning of ethical practice to become visionary and aspirational. Psychology would no longer we construed as an abstract and empirical science apart from the political fray. Instead, it would be acknowledged a highly political endeavour whose participation in the status quo is an actual and potential source of harm to vulnerable populations and to the soul of the profession. ethical codes must become meaningful, clearly voiced documents in which lines are drawn free of the careful legalisms that protect psychologists and corporate psychological organisations. The raison d'être of an ethics code itself requires transformation. . . . The revisioned ethics code would become a map into the difficult terrain of self-knowledge, self-criticism, self-care, and

commitment to the use of psychology as a toll for making a just and free world. . . . Ultimately, psychologists and consumers of psychology must refuse to allow the discipline to rest comfortably within our current parameters. We must simply begin to insist that nothing less than an integration of personal and professional, and nothing narrower than a focus on the entire domain of psychology, will fit our definitions of the words 'ethics in psychology'. (Brown, 1997, pp. 61–7)

Acknowledgements

Thanks to Elaine Clifton and all practitioner-researchers (doctoral students or otherwise) who have helped in developing the inspiration for finishing this chapter.

References

Anderson, R. and Braud, W. (1998) Appendix C: Synopses of 17 conventional methods of disciplined inquiry. In W. Braud and R. Anderson (eds), Transpersonal Research Methods for the Social Sciences, pp. 270–83. Thousand Oaks, CA: Sage.

Arendt, H. (1964) Eichmann in Jerusalem: A Report on the Banality of Evil. New York: Viking Press.

Ball, S.J. (1994) Education Reform: A Critical and Post-Structural Approach. Buckingham: Open University Press.

Bannister, P., Burman, E., Parker I., Taylor, M. and Tindall, C. (1994) Qualitative Methods in Psychology: A Research Guide. Buckingham: Open University Press.

Barber, P. (1998) Caring: a Therapeutic Relationship. In A. Jolley and M. Perry (eds) Nursing: a Knowledge Base for Practice (2nd edn). London: Edward Arnold.

Barfield, O. (1957) Saving the Appearances: A Study in Idolatry. London: Faber and Faber.

Barrett, M. (1995) Practical and Ethical Issues in Planning Research. In G.M. Breakwell, S. Hammond and C. Fife-Schaw (eds), Research Methods in Psychology, pp. 16–35. London: Sage.

Becker, H.S. (1967) Whose side are we on? Social Problems, 14, 239–47.

Bersoff, D.N. (1995) Ethical Conflicts in Psychology. Washington, DC: American Psychological Association.

Bond, T. (1999) Keynote speech: 'Ethical Issues in Counselling', Conference at Whitelands College, Roehampton Institute, London, April.

Bor, R. and Watts, M. (1993) Training counselling psychologists to conduct research. Counselling Psychology Review, 8(4), 20–1.

Braud, W. and Anderson, R. (1998) (eds) Transpersonal Research Methods for the Social Sciences, pp. 270–83. Thousand Oaks, CA: Sage.

Brown, L.S. (1997) Ethics in psychology: cui bono? In D. Fox and I. Prilleltensky (eds) Critical Psychology: An Introduction, pp. 49–67. London: Sage.

Bruner, E.M. (1993) Introduction: the ethnographical self and the personal self. In P. Benson (ed.) Anthropology and Literature, pp. 1–26. Urbana, IL: University of Illinois Press.

Clandinin, D.J. and Connelly, F.M. (1994) Personal experience methods. In N.K. Denzin and Y.S. Lincoln, (eds) Handbook of Qualitative Research, pp. 413–27. Thousand Oaks, CA: Sage.

Thousand Oaks, CA: Sage.

Clarkson, P. (1975) Seven-Level Model. Paper delivered at University of Pretoria, November.

Clarkson, P. (1990) A multiplicity of psychotherapeutic relationships. British Journal of Psychotherapy, 7(2), 148–63.

Clarkson, P. (1995) The Therapeutic Relationship. London: Whurr.

Clarkson, P. (1996a) The Bystander (An End to Innocence in Human Relationships?). London: Whurr.

Clarkson. P. (1996b) A Socio-cultural Context for Psychotherapy. In The Bystander, pp. 157–62. London: Whurr.

Clarkson, P. (1996c) Researching the 'therapeutic relationship' in psychoanalysis, counselling psychology and psychotherapy – a qualitative inquiry, Counselling Psychology Quarterly, 9(2), 143–62.

Clarkson, P. (1998b) Beyond schoolism. Changes ,16(1), 1–11.

Clarkson, P. (1999) The five relationships framework in research. Unpublished manuscript available from Physis.

Clarkson, P. (ed.) (1997) The Sublime. London: Whurr.

Clarkson, P. (ed.) (1998a) Counselling Psychology: Integrating Theory, Research and Supervised Practice. London: Routledge.

Collis, W. (1995) Judge over your shoulder – Judicial Review: Balancing the scales, revised May 1995. The Treasury Solicitor's Department in conjunction with the Cabinet Office (OPSS) Development Division.

Coyle, A. (1996) Representing gay men with HIV/AIDS. In S. Wilkinson and C. Kitzinger (eds) Representing the Other London: Sage.

Coyle, A. (1998) Qualitative research in counselling psychology: using the counselling interview as a research instrument. In P. Clarkson (ed.) Counselling Psychology: Integrating Theory, Research and Supervised Practice, pp. 56–73. London: Routledge.

Critten, P., Portsmouth, F. Murray, T. and Blackwood, F. (1998) The change agent as shaman. In C. Combes, D. Grant, T. Keenoy, and C. Oswick (eds) Organisational Discourse: Pretexts, Subtexts and Contexts, pp. 82–3. London: KMCP.

Denzin, N.K. (1978) The Research Act, 2nd edn. New York: McGraw-Hill.

Denzin, N.K. and Lincoln, Y.S. (eds) (1994) Handbook of Qualitative Research. Thousand Oaks, CA: Sage.

Douglas, J.D. (1979) Living morality versus bureaucratic fiat. In C.B. Kockars and F.W. O'Connor (eds) Deviance and Decency: The Ethics of Research with Human Subjects, pp. 13–33. Beverly Hills, CA: Sage.

Douglass, B.G. and Moustakas, C. (1985) Heuristic inquiry: the internal search to know. Journal of Humanistic Psychology, 25(3), 39–55.

Dryden, W.D. (1993) Reflections on Counselling. London: Whurr.

Eckartsberg, R. von (1998) Existential-phenomenological research. In Valle, R. (ed.) Phenomenological Inquiry in Psychology: Existential and Transpersonal Dimensions, pp. 21–61. New York: Plenum Press.

Eiser, J. R. (1994) Attitudes, Chaos and the Connectionist Mind. Oxford: Blackwell.

Farrell, B.A. (1979) Work in small groups: some philosophical considerations. In B. Babington Smith and B.A. Farrell (eds), Training In Small Groups: A Study of Five Groups, pp. 103–15. Oxford: Pergamon.

Feather, N.T. (ed.) (1982) Expectations and Actions: Expectancy-Value Models in Psychology. Hillsdale, NJ: Lawrence Erlbaum.

Feyerabend, P. (1975) Against Method. London: Verso.

non-directive and Adlerian therapy. Journal of Consulting Psychology, 14, 436–45.

Fine, M. (1994) Working the hyphens: reinventing self and other in qualitative research. In N.K. Denzin and Y.S. Lincoln (eds) Handbook of Qualitative Research, pp. 70–82. Thousand Oaks, CA: Sage.

Foucault, M. (1979) Discipline and Punish: The Birth of the Prison (trans. Alan Sheridan). New York: Vintage.

Foucault, M. (1987) The ethic of the care of the self as a practice of freedom. Philosophy and Social Criticism, 12, 112–31.

Frank, J.D. (1973) Persuasion and Healing: A Comparative Study of Psychotherapy (rev. edn.). Baltimore, MD: Johns Hopkins University Press.

Frank, J.D. and Frank, J.B. (1993) Persuasion and Healing: A Comparative Study of Psychotherapy (3rd edn), Baltimore, MD: Johns Hopkins University Press.

Garcia Lorca, F. (1980) Deep Song and Other Prose (trans.C. Maurer). London: Marion Boyars.

Gee, H. (1998) Developing insight through supervision: relating, then defining. In P. Clarkson (ed.) Supervision: Psychoanalytic and Jungian Perspectives, pp. 9–33. London: Whurr.

Gelso, C.J. (1996) Applying theories in research: the interplay of theory and research in science. In F.T.L. Leong and J.T. Austin (eds) The Psychology Research Handbook: A Guide for Graduate Students and Research Assistants, pp. 359–68. Thousand Oaks, CA: Sage.

Gelso, C.J., Fassinger, R.E., Gomez, M.J. and Latts, M.G. (1995) Countertransference reactions to lesbian clients: the role of homophobia, counsellor gender and countertransference management. Journal of Counselling Psychology, 42, 356–64.

Gergen, K.J. (1997) Who speaks and who replies in human science scholarship? History of the Human Sciences, 10, 3: 151–73.

Gergen, K.J. and Gergen, M.M. (1991) Toward reflexive methodologies. In F. Steier (ed.) Research and Reflexivity, pp. 76–95. London: Sage.

Gergen, K.J., Gloger-Tippelt, G. and Berkowitz, P. (1990) The cultural construction of the developing child. In G.R. Semin and K.J. Gergen (eds) Everyday Understanding – Social and Scientific Implications, pp. 108–29. London: Sage.

Gergen, M. (1988) Toward a feminist metatheory and methodology in the social sciences. In M. Gergen (ed.) Feminist Thought and the Structure of Knowledge, pp. 87–104), New York: New York University Press.

Gergen, M. (1994) Free will and psychotherapy: complaints of the draughtmen's daughters. Journal of Theoretical and Philosophical Psychology, 14, 1:13–24.

Giorgi, A. (1975). An application of phenomenological method in psychology. In A. Giorgi, C. Fischer, and E. Murray (eds), Duquesne Studies in Phenomenological Psychology: Vol II, pp. 82–103. Pittsburgh, PA: Duquesne University Press.

Gleick, J. (1992) Genius: Richard Feynman and Modern Physics. New York: Abacus.

Goffman, E. (1961) Asylums. Garden City, NY: Anchor.

Goodwin, B. (1994) How the Leopard Changed his Spots.

Greenberg, L.S. and Staller, J. (1981) Personal therapy for therapists. American Journal of Psychiatry, 138, 1467–71.

Hattie, J.A., Sharpley, C.F. and Rogers, H.J. (1984) Comparative effectiveness of professional and paraprofessional helpers. Psychological Bulletin, 95, 534–41.

Havel, V. (1990) Disturbing the Peace. New York: Vintage.

Hawking, S. (ed.) (1992) A Brief History of Time – A Reader's Companion. London: Bantam Press.

Hekman, S.J. (1995) Moral Voices, Moral Selves: Carol Gilligan and Feminist Moral

Hekman, S.J. (1995) Moral Voices, Moral Selves: Carol Gilligan and Feminist Moral Theory. Cambridge: Polity Press.

Hinshelwood, R. (1990) Editorial. British Journal of Psychotherapy, 7(2), 119–20.

Ince, D. (1999) Healing and psychotherapy: African/Caribbean healers' therapeutic intervention in the United Kingdom. PhD proposal, unpublished.

Isham, C. (1995) Lectures on Quantum Theory – Mathematical and Structural Foundations. London: Imperial College Press.

Jager, B. (1998) Human subjectivity and the law of the threshold: phenomenological and humanistic perspectives. In R. Valle (ed.) Phenomenological Inquiry in Psychology: Existential and Transpersonal Dimensions, pp. 87–108. New York: Plenum Press.

Jones, E. (1953) Sigmund Freud: Life and Work, Vol. 1. London: Hogarth Press.

Jung, C.G. (1972) Synchronicity: An Acausal Connecting Principle (trans. R.F.C. Hull). London: Routledge and Kegan Paul. (Original work published 1952)

Kaplan, J. (1988) The use of animals in research. Science, 242, 839–840.

Kassin, S.M., Ellsworth, P.C. and Smith, U.L. (1989) The 'general acceptance' of psychological research on eyewitness testimony. American Psychologist, 44, 1089–98.

Kider, L.H. and Fine, M. (1997) Qualitative inquiry in psychology: a radical tradition. In D. Fox and I. Prilleltensky (eds) Critical Psychology: An Introduction, pp. 34–50. London: Sage.

Kiesler, D.J. (1966) Some myths of psychotherapy research and the search for a paradigm. Psychological Bulletin, 65, 110–36.

Koestler, A. (1972) The Roots of Coincidence. London: Hutchinson.

Koocher, G.P. (1994) The commerce of professional psychology and the new ethics code. Professional Psychology: Research and Practice, 25, 355–61.

Kvale, S. (1992) Postmodern psychology: a contradiction in terms? In S. Kvale (ed.), Psychology and Postmodernism, pp. 31–57. London: Sage.

Lerman, H. and Porter, N. (1990) The contribution of feminism to ethics in psychotherapy. In H. Lerman and N. Porter (eds), Feminist Ethics in Psychotherapy, pp. 5–13. New York: Springer.

Lincoln, Y.S. and Denzin, N.K. (1994) The fifth moment. In N.K. Denzin and Y.S. Lincoln (eds), Handbook of Qualitative Research, pp. 575–86. Thousand Oaks, CA: Sage.

Lincoln, Y.S. and Guba, E.G. (1985) Naturalistic Inquiry. Beverly Hills, CA: Sage.

Lindsay, G. (1995) Values, ethics and psychology. Psychologist, 4, 493–8.

Lindsay, G. and Colley A. (1995) Ethical dilemmas of members of the British Psychological Society. Psychologist, 8, 448–53.

Lofland, J. and Lofland, L. (1985) Analysing Social Settings: A Guide to Qualitative Observation and Analysis. Belmont: Wadsworth.

Loftus, E.F. and Palmer, J.C. (1974) Reconstruction of automobile destruction: an example of the interaction between language and memory. Journal of Verbal Learning and Verbal Behaviour, 13, 585–9.

Longinus (1899) Longinus on the Sublime (trans and ed. W. Rhys Roberts). Cambridge: Cambridge University Press.

Luborsky, L., Crits-Christoph, P. and McClellan, A.T. (1986) Do therapists vary much in their success? Findings from four outcome studies. American Journal of Orthopsychiatry, 56, 501–11.

Mahrer, A. (1996) Discovery-oriented research – or how to do psychotherapy. In W. Dryden (ed.), Research in Counselling and Psychotherapy, pp. 233–58. London: Sage.

Mair, M. (1989) Between Psychology and Psychotherapy. London: Routledge.

Marshall, H., and Woollett A. (1997) Researching Asian women's accounts of parenting and childcare: some conceptual methodological and political concerns. Changes, 15(1), 42–6.

Marzillier, J. (1999) Training of clinical psychologists in ethical issues. Clinical Psychology Forum, 123, 43–7.

Maslow, A.H. (1968) Toward a Psychology of Being, 2nd edn. New York: Van Nostrand.

Maturana, H.R. and Varela, F.J. (1987) The Tree of Knowledge: The Biological Roots of Human Understanding. Boston, MA: Shambala.

McLeod, J. (1994) Doing Counselling Research. London: Sage.

Merleau-Ponty, M. (1962). Phenomenology of Perception (trans. C. Smith), London: Routledge and Kegan Paul.

Milgram, S. (1963) Behavioural study of obedience. Journal of Abnormal and Social Psychology, 67: 371–8.

Milgram, S. (1974) Obedience to Authority. New York: Harper and Row.

Mingers, J. (1995) Self-Producing Systems-Implications and Applications of Autopoeiesis. New York: Plenum Press.

Moodley, R. (1998) Cultural return to the subject: traditional healing in counselling and therapy. Changes, 16(1), 45–56.

Moustakas, C. (1990) Heuristic Research: Design, Methodology, and Applications. Newbury Park, CA: Sage.

Moustakas, C. (1994) Phenomenological Research Methods. London Sage.

O'Donohue, W. and Mangold, R. (1996) A critical examination of the ethical principles of psychologists and code of conduct. In W. O'Donohue and R.F. Kitchener (eds) The Philosophy of Psychology, pp. 371–80. London: Sage.

Orlinsky, D.E. and Howard, K.I. (1980) Gender and psychotherapeutic outcome. In A. Brodsky and R.T. Hare–Mustin (eds). Women and Psychotherapy, pp. 3–34. New York: Guilford Press.

Palmer Barnes, F. (1998) Club or profession? The Psychotherapist, 3, p. 4.

Pilgrim, D. (1992) Psychotherapy and political evasions. In W. Dryden and C. Feltham (eds) Psychotherapy and its Discontents, pp. 225–53. Buckingham: Open University Press.

Polyani, M. (1962) Personal Knowledge. Chicago, IL: University of Chicago Press.

Reason, P. and Rowan, J. (eds) (1981) Human Inquiry: A Sourcebook of New Paradigm Research. Chichester: Wiley.

Richardson, L. (1994) Writing: a method of inquiry. In N.K. Denzin and Y.S. Lincoln (eds), Handbook of Qualitative Research, pp. 516–29. Thousand Oaks, CA: Sage.

Roethlisberger, F.J. and Dickson, W.J. (1939) Management and the Worker. Harvard: Harvard University Press.

Rowan, J. (1998) Transformational research. In P. Clarkson (ed.) Counselling Psychology: Integrating Theory, Research and Supervised Practice, pp. 157–75. London: Routledge.

Rudestam, K.E. and Newton, R.R. (1992) Surviving your Dissertation: A Comprehensive Guide to Content and Process. Newbury Park, CA: Sage.

Rumi, J. (1990) Delicious Laughter: Rambunctious Teaching Stories from the Mathnawi. (ed. C. Barks) Athens: Maypop Books.

Sallis, J. and Maly, K. (eds) (1980) Heraclitean Fragments: A Companion Volume to the Heidegger/Fink Seminar on Heraclitus. Tuscaloosa, AL: University of Alabama Press.

Sarason, S.B. (1988) The Making of an American Psychologist. San Francisco, CA: Jossey Bass.

Shapiro, D.A., Barkham, M., Hardy, G.E., Morrison, L.A., Reynolds, S., Strait, M. and Harper, H. (1991) University of Sheffield Psychotherapy Research Program: Medical Research Council/Economic and Social Research Council Social and Applied Psychology Unit. In L.E. Beutler and M. Crago (eds) Psychotherapy Research: An International Review of Programmatic Studies. Washington, DC: American Psychological Association.

Shelef, L.O. (1994) A simple qualitative paradigm: the asking and telling. The Qualitative Report, 2(1), 1–6.

Smith, J.A. (1996) Evolving issues for qualitative psychology. In J.T.E. Richardson (ed.) Handbook of Qualitative Research Methods for Psychology and the Social Sciences, pp. 189–201. Leicester: BPS Books.

Smith, J.A., Harré, R. and Van Langenhove, L. (1995) Rethinking Methods in Psychology. London: Sage.

Stainton Rogers, R. (1995) Q Methodology. In J.A. Smith, R. Harré and L. Van Langenhove (eds), Rethinking Methods in Psychology, pp. 178–92. London: Sage.

Steedman, P.H. (1991) On the relations between seeing, interpreting and knowing. In F. Steier (ed.), Research and Reflexivity, pp. 53–62. London: Sage.

Strupp, H.H. and Hadley, S.W. (1979) Specific versus nonspecific factors in psychotherapy: A controlled study of outcome. Archives of General Psychiatry, 36, 1125–36.

Styles, J. (1979) Outsider/insider: researching gay baths. Urban Life, 8, 135–52.

Ulichny, P. (1997) When critical ethnography and action collide. Qualitative Inquiry, 3(2), 139–68.

van Dijk, T.A. (1987) Communicating Racism – Ethnic Prejudice in Thought and Talk. London: Sage.

Wertz, F.J. (1995) Yerkes' rabbit and career: from trivial to more significant matters. Theory and Psychology, 5(3), 451–4.

Wittgenstein, L. (1922) Tractatus Logico–Philosophicus (trans. C. K. Ogden). London: Routledge and Kegan Paul.

Wolman, B.B. (1965) Handbook of Clinical Psychology. New York: McGraw-Hill.

Woolgar, S. (1996) Psychology, qualitative methods and the ideas of science. In J.T.E. Richardson (ed.), Handbook of Qualitative Research Methods for Psychology and the Social Sciences, pp. 11–24. Leicester: BPS Books.

Wright, C. and Coyle, A. (1996) Experience of AIDS-related bereavement among gay men: Implications for care. Mortality 1: 267–82.

ITEM 14
Extract from
Letters to A Young Poet
by Rainer Maria Rilke

Be patient toward all that is unsolved in your heart and try to love the *questions themselves* like locked rooms and like books that are written in a very foreign tongue. Do not now seek the answers, which cannot be given because you would not be able to live them. And the point is, to live everything. *Live* the questions now. Perhaps you will then, gradually, without noticing it, live along some distant day into the answer.

Appendix 1
A Traveller's Guide to Psychotherapy: A Companion for Clients and Patients

Petrūska Clarkson

Dedicated to all the people, but especially those who, in the period 1–12 March 1995, have asked me these questions. Happy landings!

Contents

- This guide is for those people who are thinking of, are, or have been in counselling, psychoanalysis and psychotherapy.
- Potential or actual consumers of psychotherapy want information and knowledge.
- Every week people contemplating the adventure of therapy ask me, 'How do I find out what's right for me?'
- I believe consumers can use information and knowledge well.
- All knowledge, like cars and alcohol, can be used or abused.
- I believe this knowledge and information should be available to all.
- If people can get the information in a straight way, they will take responsibility for their choices.
- This guide is a beginning of providing such knowledge and information.
- It is written by an independent chartered counselling and clinical psychologist, psychotherapist, counsellor and supervisor who has trained in many different approaches in several countries.
- The back-up information to this booklet is contained in my book *The Therapeutic Relationship* (1995) which contains references to some 9000 books and papers in this field.
- I have shaped courses, and trained and supervised thousands of people in these professions in many different countries.
- I have originated and chaired and taught for and consulted to many organisations – everything seems to make a kind of sense in its context.
- I also have long-term – almost 30 years – of in-depth personal experience as consumer of these disciplines – both as patient and as trainee.

289

- Some experiences have been bad and some have been good.
- It has cost me thousands of pounds, dollars and rands and nearly 30 years of my life.
- I would like to make your journey cheaper, easier, less destructive and more productive.
- It's up to you how you use it.

Key to symbols

! This sign means caution – be careful, be aware.

* This sign means take notice, there are exceptions.

? This sign means think further about it, wonder why, speculate further.

1. What is? (psychotherapy, psychoanalysis, counselling psychology, etc.)

- Psychoanalysis, psychotherapy, counselling, therapeutic counselling, counselling and clinical psychology are similar terms. These professions are all related.
- Usually they mean that one person is providing their professional services to another person on the basis that 'talking' can help or 'cure' the person who is buying or receiving the service.
- These professions have only been in existence for the last 100 years or so.
- They are all different from psychiatry.
- A psychiatrist is a medical doctor who has also trained in the medical treatment of mental and emotional disorders – particularly those which may end up in a mental hospital.
- So, a psychiatrist is trained to be able to prescribe drugs such as valium, lithium, antidepressants or largactyl. These are the major types of drug treatments available through psychiatrists for mental disorder.
- Psychiatrists may or may not have training in psychoanalysis, psychotherapy, psychoanalysis, counselling or clinical psychology. This would be important to find out.
- A psychiatrist will have to be involved for any admission to a mental hospital. Such an admission can be because the person requested it themselves, or because someone in their family, their family doctor and/or the social services organise it.
- Try to avoid this. Mental hospital staff usually do their best in their current conditions. But they should be seen as a last resort.
- Many people think secretly that they are mad and may end up in a mental hospital. This is very rarely the case. There are many other less drastic ways of getting help.
- Psychotherapy, psychoanalysis, counselling, and psychological treatment are the additions (to hospital admission) or alternatives to this available to everyone.

- You may have to exercise some nous and imagination to get at the right thing for you, your friend, employee or relative.

! Long-term use of any or all of the major psychiatric drugs has serious side-effects and sometimes permanent destructive after-effects. Always ask your doctor and read more about it yourself before you take any medicine.

* A psychiatric record may count against people applying for jobs or medical insurance. This should not be the case. But, take this into account when you make decisions or give/seek advice.

? Why have psychotherapy and its cousins only arisen as professions in this century? May it have something to do with the decline in religious faith or the disappearance of the extended family?

2. What for? (Claims, goals, objectives, change, cure and growth)

- People think about coming into therapy (including psychoanalysis, psychodynamic psychotherapy, counselling of many kinds, psychotherapy or psychological treatment) for many reasons.
- Some people are in despair, even wanting to commit suicide. Some people feel crazy. Some people are so burned up with jealousy or hate that they can't function any more.
- Some people want out of an addiction of some kind – for example, to a bad love or a hard drug.
- Some people want to be better lovers, better parents, better at their jobs or get through a block to their creativity in writing, dancing, painting, making money.
- Some people are lonely and never learned how to make (or be) friends, talk comfortably to new people, stand up for themselves in arguments and negotiations.
- Some people have terrible memories, flashbacks or hurts from their childhood abuse, experiences in a war or a hospital, school traumas of being humiliated for being the wrong colour, wrong kind of kid, wrong kind of brain or gender.
- Some people just want to understand themselves and other people better.
- Some people want to be better managers, better consultants, better leaders in their field to the benefit of the people and/or the benefit of the stockholders.
- Sometimes they may even want to be the best – golfer, actor, themselves.
- Some people hate themselves, their bodies, their appetites.
- Some people hate others, or they feel both and never relax.
- Human motivation is mixed. People always have good and bad feelings.

- When these mixtures become overwhelming, people should seek help. It's easier and better before there's a crisis.
- In summary, people come into therapy for reasons of cure, change or growth.
- Make sure you try to get the help that's best for you. If you have doubts, get a second opinion. Often. It may not always work, but it's better than waking up several years from now, thousands of pounds and hundreds of hours of time later, regretting the investment.

! Watch out for any person or organisation's claim to the 'magic cure' guaranteed success. No such remedy exists yet. If it did, mental or emotional problems would no longer be among us.
* There are some people (unqualified in these professions) who are found helpful for specific purposes, such as Alan Carr. He has helped thousands of people to stop smoking.
? Why are there such differences in people's needs and wants? Should everybody want the same things?

3. Why not? (Dangers and abuses of psychological therapy)

- Therapy has been accused of many abuses. So has every other profession.
- There are bad doctors, bad lawyers, bad teachers, bad preachers and bad accountants. In any profession there are rules, ethics, guidelines and professional practices and procedures that the professionals must follow or be educated, disciplined or expelled.
- Sometimes the rules are unfair, old-fashioned or too rigid and even bent by the complainant. Often the person complaining has a good case and the right and just verdict is passed.
- There are also good guys in every profession. Usually most of the professionals are doing their best under the circumstances.
- The worst abuses of trust in the professional relationship in psychoanalysis and psychotherapy are probably physical violence or sexual exploitation.
- It is always unethical for a psychoanalyst or psychologist to have sexual intimacy with a client, patient or trainee.
- It is based on a lot of experience that sexuality and a professional relationship don't work well together in the long run as far the client is concerned.
- Neither do surgeons now usually operate on their close friends or family for the same reasons – although famous people like Freud, Jung, Klein and Perls all did therapy or analysis on their lovers or children in the past.
- It is important to seek someone professional whose natural interests are independent of your welfare.

- That is the primary difference between a psychotherapist and a friend. Much as the analyst may care about you as a person, it is a paid professional relationship and the analyst's sexual satisfactions should come from elsewhere.
- If a therapist suggests or gives in to any suggestion of sexual intimacy, please seek help from another professional as soon as possible. It is an emergency and a sign that the therapeutic relationship is seriously endangered.
- It is a sad fact that many of the people most seriously in need of the best help in our society rarely get it.

! If you are worried about any behaviour, requests or actions of your psychoanalyst, immediately consult an independent practitioner.
* Many people do have very loving and sometimes sexual feelings or dreams about their therapists. This is a frequent and normal exercise of affectionate feelings and fantasies. The job of therapy is to talk about it and explore it to the benefit of the patient's other relationships in their outside life – not to do it in therapy.
? For many people, their first experience of being listened to, given space to cry or be angry and understood comes from the experience of being in counselling. Why is this so? Why can't people do it for each other – or can they ?

4. What else? (Alternatives to therapy)

- Therapy is a good and effective way to help them reach their goals for many people. But, it is not the only way. There are many alternatives to therapy which may need to be explored first or at the same time.
- Sometimes medical conditions cause mental problems and emotional disturbances. All people should consult their general practitioners also about psychological problems, to ensure that there is not a physical reason for their distress which can be comparatively easily handled – for example, through medication for an hormonal imbalance or dietary adjustment.
- Anxiety, insomnia, impotence and depression are such cases. They are quite frequently associated with drinking too much coffee or alcohol or as a side-effect of other medication or lifestyles that can be adjusted without expensive time-consuming psychotherapy.
- There is some evidence that some behaviour disorders of children are associated with preservatives or nutritional deficiencies or imbalances. Investigate alternative resources in your country from your family doctor, recommended nutritionist or institute of complementary medicine.
- Sometimes people simply need more education in order to solve their problems themselves. Institutions for adult education, sex education clinics, assertiveness training classes, communication skills

workshops, parent effectiveness courses, and many other such resources exist in your community.

- Check out your doctor, community nurse, local library or social services, health food or magazine shop where you could get more information on any topic under the sun which may be bothering you. Professionals can be very hindering or very helpful. Keep going until you find the helpful ones for you.
- Life itself is a great teacher. Notice the lessons life brings and try to learn them. Many people have found that crises and catastrophes have in the end brought them endurance, understanding and deeper fulfilment than they would ever have thought possible. Read or visit the wisdom teachers. Stay discriminating.
- Sometimes people should stop considering others for all their lives and take care for themselves first for a change. Go to a retreat, have a massage, put an ad in for a friend or a lover, buy or make something extravagant and beautiful.
- Sometimes people get well by starting to take care of others. Visit an old people's home, give to a charity, do something about injustice where you see it, act on behalf of a political ideal. Check out which one is your habitual pattern and try the other one for a while.

! Therapy is not a panacea. It is not the answer to all of human ills. It is not an inoculation against life's ups and downs. It does not magic answers. It does sometimes help some people in some ways.

* There are many alternatives to therapy – explore them.

? Why do people let themselves first 'be abused' and then complain about it? How does this happen? What can be done to prevent it?

5. Who? (Different professional disciplines involved)

- There are many different professional disciplines involved in the provision of psychotherapy, psychoanalysis or counselling psychology.
- The major divisions are between counsellors, psychotherapists and psychologists.
- In terms of what they actually do with clients there is probably not a great deal of difference between them. However, their training, range of competence, education, personal experience and supervision requirements may differ considerably.
- In most countries there are different registers and different requirements for training and practice for each of these. Sometimes these registers are law (as in the US and Austria), some are voluntary (as in the UK).
- Do find out your local or national situation. Your doctor should know. Any professional must be able and willing to tell you where

and how they are registered, show you their professional code of ethics and licensing board certification as well as give you full information about their conditions of work.

- There are many disputes about the differences between these professions. On the one hand some practitioners say there are no differences at all, on the other hand some practitioners say that the differences are both significant and important.
- Counselling or clinical psychologists have a university degree in psychology (or equivalent) with special training, supervision and personal experience of counselling psychology.
- Psychotherapists or psychoanalysts may or may not be graduates from any of the other professions. They usually will have had a special training, supervision and personal experience of the psychotherapy or psychoanalysis they offer to clients or patients. (Psychotherapists may or may not have had special training in psychotherapy or psychoanalysis.)
- Psychoanalysis is only one of the forms of psychotherapy which is derived from Freud, Klein or Jung. It is usually means a form of such treatment which involve the patient in sessions of 50 minutes three to five times a week.
- Counsellors usually do not have a medical or psychological degree, but they have a specialised training in one form of counselling or another. This may range from Rogerian counselling to bereavement or employee counselling.
- Some professionals may have training and experience as counsellors, psychologists and psychotherapists. That is, they may have training and qualifications in all three relevant disciplines.
- These professionals may be more flexible with a wider range of skills, understanding and competencies than someone who is trained only in one discipline. This does not necessarily mean that they may be the best for you.
- Your family doctor, university counselling service or local hospital should be able to give you the information on professional registers of such professionals in your area.
- The field is still young and quite confusing to the client who wants to use it or the person who wants to qualify in it.

! Watch out for people who advertise or sell their services as counsellors, psychotherapists, psychoanalysts or anything which sounds similar and who do not belong to some national or international organisation with a code of practice and ethics and a professional body looking after standards.
* Do try to read, ask questions and to understand the field as much as possible, but do not be disheartened if you get confused. Most of the professionals are not that clear either.
? Perhaps the differences between these disciplines have to do with money (psychologists generally can charge more than counsellors),

education (psychologists and psychotherapists are often graduates) or status (who gets to play 'Mine's better than yours'). What do you think?

6. How? (Different approaches involved)

- If you went to a doctor with a broken leg and he or she offered you 450 kinds of treatment and asked you to take responsibility for choosing the right one, what would you think?
- This is the current situation in psychotherapy. There are at least 450 different kinds of psychotherapeutic treatment. What are the differences?
- The major differentation between different approaches to therapy is the theory on which they are based – that is, the teachings of the founder teacher of the school or approach in which the practitioner trained.
- There are many ways of discussing such differences. Many people find it most useful to think of dividing all these 450 schools roughly into 3 major traditions.
- Using these three major traditions – which all started around the beginning of this century – can be helpful in locating the original sources of any clinician or counsellor who is practising today.
- It's a bit like getting to know the grandparents. It does not contain all the information you need, but at least it's some indication.
- All approaches have by now influenced each other. Pure forms of any approach are exceptionally rare, unusual and probably questionable.
- One grandfather is Freud. From him came all psychoanalytic approaches including those of Jung, Klein, Bowlby and Winnicott.
- Psychoanalysis generally stresses the past, the unconscious, the transference of feelings onto the therapist from childhood, interpretation of the unconscious, sexual and aggressive drives. These procedures are usually long-term – an average psychoanalysis now is said to be 11 years at 5 times per week.
- Another grandparent is Pavlov. From him came all behavioural and cognitive behavioural approaches including constructivist, rational-emotive and desensitisation techniques including Skinner, Ellis, and even NLP.
- Cognitive behavioural approaches generally stress the present, the influence of learning and thinking, therapist and client working together for change, the provision of techniques, teaching of skills and specific help – often short-term – weeks or months.
- The other grandfather is Moreno. From him came all the humanistic and existential approaches including Gestalt and transactional analysis. Existential psychotherapists come from a philosophical tradition, but also belong in this group, as well as perhaps the transpersonal approaches such as psychosynthesis.

- Humanistic and existential approaches tend to stress the past and future as well as the present, the choice and responsibility of the client, the capacity for genuine relationship, the creative, healing and transformative forces in the psyche as well as the regressive or destructive forces.
- But – in each one of these there may be hundreds of practitioners who are all different anyway and who may take different aspects of their own training alone or together with elements from either or both of the other main approaches.
- The trend nowadays is towards integrative psychotherapy or integrative approaches to counselling or psychotherapy, which draw on many traditions and do not adhere to only one 'truth'.
- In the US, most psychologists say they are integrative; and it is likely in the next few years to become more established in the UK (Dryden, 1984). As these professions develop I hope that there will be a rich representation of both specialist and integrative approaches to the field from which clients can choose whether they are seen in hospitals or in private practice.
- Practitioners throughout the world nowadays tend to integrate both within and between approaches. Research has also shown that the more experienced clinicians become, the less there are observable differences between their actual practices – whatever their theoretical orientation!
- How is a prospective client to choose between them? It may be easier than it first appears.
- Research studies show that certain client characteristics, including motivation for change and the willingness to take responsibility for their part in the process is also very likely to result in a successful outcome. (Successful outcome here is judged by both client and therapist.)
- Research also shows that theoretical differences between 'schools or approaches' is far less important in terms of successful outcome of counselling or psychotherapy, than the quality of the relationship between counsellor and client.

! There are probably some exceptions and disagreements and qualifications to much of what I have written here. Please check out lengthier and more formal discussions in the books included in the Further Reading list.

* The therapeutic relationship does appear to be more important than theoretical orientation in all instances – except for drug treatment for psychosis and in cognitive behavioural therapy for acute phobias, compulsions and some kinds of depression.

? Why did psychoanalysis break into three different streams and then into many more schools? Why are there more than five different approaches to Jungian analysis which can be located within very different traditions – often at loggerheads with each other?

7. Which kind? (Different modalities available)

- Therapy comes in many different forms. There is short-term or brief therapy as well as long-term therapy.
- Short-term therapy is sometimes called brief focal therapy or it may have another name. It tends to refer to therapies or counselling which are planned to take from 2 sessions to 6 months and can vary enormously.
- Short-term therapy is not necessarily less effective than long-term therapy. It may be worthwhile to try it first before investing years of time and money in long-term work.
- The biggest criticism of short-term therapy is that it may only provide symptom relief without dealing with ~he underlying causes.
- Sometimes people want just relief from their symptoms, their pain, their distress. If it can be achieved without disruption to their lives or great expense, it may be worth doing as a short-term experiment.
- Sometimes the search for underlying causes is more the interest of the therapist than to the benefit of the client. There are many instances where the causes are inherited tendencies, obscure or simply not applicable.
- Many people who have had terrible childhoods grow up to have happy fulfilling adult lives of love and achievement.
- Some people who have had childhoods full of privilege, love and attention grow up to be mentally ill, suffering from addictions and racked with misery and despair.
- Even psychologists may find it hard to explain how this happens, but we know it does. There are no simple cause–effect explanations.
- Then there is couples' or marital therapy if both partners in a love relationship want to work together to save or improve their partnership. It is generally not a good idea for the individual therapist of either to be the couples' therapist. The couples' therapist should not have a special private relationship with either.
- Family therapy is particularly good for families where there are difficulties or one or more of the children are in trouble, sick or very unhappy. Family therapy can be very confusing, but it is often very effective. Normally all members of the family need to attend sessions and a number of different professionals are involved in order to ensure adequate supervision and the best quality work.
- Occasionally a parent and child pair may arrange to work with a therapist, for example, to help a mother form a good bond with a baby or infant or an adoptive parent to understand or respond better to a child. It is advisable to seek out someone with specific training and experience in this field.
- Child therapy, play therapy or therapy with children or adolescents on their own is usually somewhat different from individual or group

therapy with adults. Play material, arts, puppets, toys, sand and musical instruments may form an important part of the work. It is vital that the parents or teachers respect the child's right to privacy and confidentiality.

- There are also short-term counselling or special therapy services specially designed for particular problems such as gambling, families of drug addicts, bereavement, HIV, violence in the family, women who are married to bisexual or cross-dressing men, people with eating disorders, children who have been sexually abused or sent to boarding school and so on and so forth.
- For almost any kind of problem, there may be a service or counselling form that is formulated for it. Your general practitioner (or local librarian) should be able to tell you where to start the search if your newspaper does not.
- Group therapy can be used instead of or in addition to individual therapy. It is a very powerful and effective form of therapy and has many safeguards against abuse. This is partly because there are a number of other people in the group forming a kind of 'laboratory' of life where people can learn, experiment with relationships and benefit from the experiences of the other group members in addition to the expertise of the group leader.
- Many people report benefit from group therapy. It is also usually cheaper than individual therapy. It may even be more effective, but this is not proven. Ensure your therapist is appropriately qualified, supervised and open to questions of his or her conduct in the group.
- Sometimes therapy intensives or marathons can be useful. These are shorter or longer events where participants may or may not be in a place of residence with the group leader(s) for a couple of days or more.

! Be wary of any therapy which – against your will – drastically interferes with your basic life patterns such as prohibiting you from going to the toilet, changing your eating habits, demands sexual behaviours, signing over or lending large sums of money and other dubious signs. These are the indications that you may be getting involved with a cult of some kind – no matter if it has a scientific sounding name. Check them out.

* Of course many people may change many of their habits during and after therapy if they choose. This frequently affects their families, their relationships and even their work. Not all apparently negative consequences of going into therapy are destructive. They may just be temporary upheavals and disturbances until the person balances again – hopefully at a more effective and better level.

? Many spouses resent their partners being in therapy and get quite jealous of the therapist if they are not also in therapy or counselling for themselves or with their partner. Why should this be so?

8. Which one? (How do I choose?)

- Research does not show that any one form of therapy is better than another, with two exceptions: drug therapy for acute psychosis, and cognitive behavioural therapy for some specific kinds of phobias (irrational fears) and depression-inducing obsessive thoughts.
- However, this research is also contested (like almost everything else in this field).
- What appears just about unarguable and widely accepted on all sides is that the quality of the relationship between client and therapist is the most important factor in determining the success of psychotherapy, psychological counselling or psychoanalysis.
- Notwithstanding all the libraries of books written about different theories and different approaches, it seems as if theoretical orientation is not very important in the effectiveness of psychotherapy.
- The relationship and the client's motivation for change are more important.
- Research has shown that very experienced clinicians in different approaches resemble each other more than beginners and experienced people in any one approach. This means that the more experienced professionals in this field become, the more what they actually do in the consulting room becomes similar to each other rather than different.
- Thorough investigation reveals that the relationship is differently emphasised or given different terminology in the different approaches, but that some possibilities are always present.
- I have identified five kinds of therapeutic relationship. Not all therapists recognise or use all five. I think they are all potentially present in any healing encounter.
- It is important to remember these are not stages but states in psychotherapy or psychoanalysis, often subtly 'overlapping', in and between which a client construes his or her unique experiences. The five kinds of relationship are as follows:
    - The *working alliance* is the part of client–psychotherapist relationship that enables the client and therapist to work together even when the patient or client may not feel like it. You may not want to go to the session or be frightened of telling the therapist that you admire them or that you are angry with them.
    - The *transferential/countertransferential relationship* is the experience of transferring (carrying over) or projecting (pushing out) unconscious wishes and fears on to the therapist. Countertransference refers to the feelings, attitudes and behaviours of the therapist in the consulting room toward the patient.
    - The *reparative/developmentally needed relationship* is when the therapist intentionally provides a corrective, reparative, or replenishing experience where the original parenting was

deficient, abusive or overprotective. In its simplest form it may mean that the therapist listens and understands your feelings in a way that no-one ever has done before.

- The *person-to-person relationship* is the real relationship or core relationship. It shows the humanity of the therapist and deals with the genuine presence of the therapist as person equally human with the client.

- The *transpersonal relationship* is the timeless facet of the psychotherapeutic relationship, which is impossible to describe, but refers to the spiritual or inexplicable aspects of the healing relationship. Everyone puts in here what they want to. Not all practitioners want to work with such ideas. At the very least it makes allowance for all those things which our science does not know or understand yet.

• The ancient physicians used to say : 'I administer the medicine, but it is Nature (or God or Physis) which cures'. Many modern doctors of the body or the soul would agree with them.

! Be cautious of any therapist, analyst, psychologist or counsellor who will not explain the theoretical basis of their work. All theories carry values about what is good, normal, healthy and so on. These values will affect the way you are treated. It is vital to get clarification on such issues before getting involved in long-term work. This is particularly important for anyone belonging to any minority group in a culture.

* It may be difficult to decide whether very positive or very negative feelings about your therapist are useful or destructive. You must be able to discuss these with your therapist. If such feelings persist, seek a second opinion from an independent psychologist – telling your therapist that you will be doing so.

? Therapists usually explain that they take their clients for supervision – and so they should. Why should clients not be able to take their part of the therapy for supervision or consultation?

9. First aid (Frequent problems and emergencies)

• 'Whenever I criticise my therapist he (or she) just throws it back at me and makes it my problem.' This is impossibly difficult to judge unless we know a lot more about the situation. Keep trying. If that does not work the therapist may be right or you may need to seek a second independent opinion.

• 'I want to leave therapy, but my therapist says I would be making a mistake if I leave now.' Sometimes people feel like stopping therapy when they're just about to be really successful or make a major break-through. Sometimes people feel like stopping just before or after a vacation break. Sometimes they've just 'had enough'.

- It is best when your feeling that it is time to leave coincides with the opinion of the therapist. Always investigate both sets of motivations about leaving or staying on.
- It is not necessary to be sick or mad or unhappy to be in therapy. Many people stay on well after they have been 'cured' because they say 'I enjoy being in a healthy space with supportive and challenging people where I can grow and develop' or 'I was in an unhappy negative family for 18 years, surely I can allow myself a couple more in this my new family even though I am not sick anymore.'
- There is often a very human tendency to diminish or 'make bad' a partner, job or therapy that we are leaving behind. If we can make them bad, the parting may not feel so sad or so hard. Be aware of this tendency, anticipate it before you leave therapy and try to transform it into gratitude and joyful remembrance if that is true for you.
- 'I don't think this person is the right therapist for me'. This is not uncommon or unusual. Talk through with the therapist what the worries, concerns or dissatisfactions are rather than keeping them secret. Give both of you the chance to resolve it or give yourself a date by which time you will make a decision to leave.
- Try not to do anything rash (giving all your money away, starting an affair, etc.) while you are in therapy without discussing it with your therapist first.
- If he or she is to give you their best professional service, you need to tell them as much about yourself as honestly as you can in order to get the best from them. Otherwise it may be a case of 'garbage in, garbage out'.
- Ensure that your therapist has made provision by giving you a locum or helpline number, for example, in cases of emergencies such as illness or a death (in your family or theirs) or when he or she will be away or unavailable.
- Most therapists charge patients for sessions they miss. Ensure right at the beginning that you understand all the conditions of working together – including the policy about cancelling of sessions from either side.
- Occasionally you may come across your therapist in other, perhaps unexpected, settings such as a shopping mall, conference or concert. They may acknowledge you warmly or not. Do talk about it when next you see them.
- Try to avoid gossiping about your therapist or discussing your counselling in detail with other people. It can be quite a problem to keep this boundary, but probably very helpful to you in the long run. Other people close to us can get too involved in this very personal voyage of discovery.
- This does not mean that you should not seek a second opinion in a case where you are very doubtful. You should. Seek independent advice when you are in doubt for any length of time.

! Do not destroy the goodness you have made or taken from your therapy as result of what may happen to you after you leave. It is yours. Treasure or transform it.

* There are almost always rough, difficult and/or boring patches in any psychoanalysis or therapy, the same as in life. The working alliance is the mutual commitment of therapist and patient to 'hang in there' while they work it out. Honour the working alliance.

? Why can't people just simply do their own psychoanalysis (as Freud tried to do)? Do we really need someone else who is paid to be in this therapeutic relationship?

10. Where to train or to find out more

* There are now hundreds of opportunities and advertisements for training courses in counselling, psychology and psychotherapy. It is important to be selective since they do not all give access to all the major registers or have equal academic or career advantages.

* Remember that much international research evidence fails to show differences between schools on the basis of theory. Of course, as with almost everything else in this field, this is debatable.

* However, the professional choices prospective trainees make can have far- and long-reaching effects. Take time to consider whether and how the differences between practising as a counsellor, psychologist, psychotherapist, psychoanalyst or another variety of helping professional will affect you in terms of choices, fees, employment opportunities and freedom to practice.

* Seek advice from someone who understands all aspects of this complex field and who has experience and training in different modalities and different theoretical schools before you make a major commitment. For example, why do an MSc when you could do a PhD in the same time?

* Here follows a selection of good comprehensive sources. Each contains many more points of information or resource. If what you need is not here, ask your general practitioner or librarian.

! Watch out for titles which may be misleading, for example, The New York Institute of Something-or-other may consist of one man and his wife. An organisation may have a title such as The Hebridean Society of Psychotherapy implying that they are a national or very wide association of psychotherapists. This may not be intentional, but this may also not be the case. Do not be misled by titles and names you do not understand. Ask. If it is not possible to find out, stay away.

* There are now very many articles, books and programmes about therapy and related fields and almost everybody has their own opinions. Read, listen, observe your own experience and make up your own mind – improving it from time to time!

? Why, since we've now had 'a hundred years of psychotherapy', is 'the world getting worse'?

Further reading

Aveline, M. and Dryden, W. (eds) (1988) Group Therapy in Britain. Buckingham: Open University Press.

Brown S.D. and Lent, R.W. (eds) (1992) Handbook of Counselling Psychology. New York: Wiley

Clarkson, P. (1995) The Therapeutic Relationship. London: Whurr.

Dryden W. (ed.) (1984) Individual Therapy in Britain London: Harper & Row.

Dryden W. (ed.) (1990) Individual Therapy: A Handbook. Milton Keynes: Open University Press.

Hillman, J. and Ventura, M. (1992) We've Had a Hundred Years of Psychotherapy and the World's Getting Worse. San Francisco: Harper & Row.

Huxley, L. (1994) You are not the Target, San Francisco, CA: Metamorphous Press.

Masson, J.M. (1989) Against Psychotherapy. London: Collins.

Norcross, J. C. and Goldfried, M. R. (1992) Handbook of Psychotherapy Integration. New York: Basic Books.

Roet, B. (1989) A Safer Place to Cry. London: Macdonald Optima.

Roth, A. and Fonagy, P. (1996) What Works for Whom? A Critical Review of Psychotherapy Research. New York: Guilford Press.

Appendix 2
Dysfunction in Training Organisations

CHRIS ROBERTSON

When we are trying to understand the nature of abuse, we can look in two ways: either to the past for a historical perspective such as the repetition of childhood abuse, or systemically to the wider circle in which the abuse occurs, seeing it as a symptom of the dysfunction of that wider circle. James Hillman has recently suggested that the language of psychopathology needs to be extroverted towards the social and cultural systems. In many ways this is not such a different message from that of Ronnie Laing's challenges to our 'sick society' or Annie Schaffer's notice of an addicted one.

Abuse by an individual practitioner may reflect unresolved issues within her or his past, and it may also be a symptom of the abusive nature of the training in which they participated. The fact that training organisations occupy such a pivotal and powerful position is sometimes missed by those investigating therapeutic abuse. We tend to hold the individual practitioner as ultimately responsible, when they may also be the victims of dysfunctional patterns arising from their training.

It seems to me that we can integrate both systemic and historical perspectives by looking at training organisations as mini-cultures in which therapists develop. Whatever the explicit skills, awareness and practices the students learn, they inevitably pick up many implicit ones. Unfortunately, it is often the worst habits that students imitate and then unconsciously perpetuate in their own work. Where they have been the victims of abusive trainers or training systems, students may unconsciously act out this abuse with their clients. Just as dysfunctional families tend to produce abusive parents for the next generation, dysfunctional training organisations tend to produce abusive therapists. Having an explicit code of ethics will not of itself prevent unconscious acting out by those who are carrying the pathology of their training 'parents'.

Students are often susceptible to picking up the attitudes from the training's mini-culture. By the time they graduate, students have allowed this culture to pervade them, and so it is all the more pernicious. Like a fish in water, the graduate counsellor or therapist may be the last to recognise the difficulties.

One aim of this appendix is to stress the inevitability of such abusive phenomena in training organisations, and the impossibility of inoculation against it. The 'it can't happen here' attitude makes any organisation particularly susceptible to abusive patterns. As with individual abuse, organisational abuse is frequently denied, and those bringing the possibility out into the open may be attacked for exposing the shadow side of the organisation. This is not intended as a cynical or negative approach but, rather than being controlled by the fear of accreditational or media exposure, we can create an atmosphere in which we can recognise abuse with compassion and therefore contribute to its acknowledgement.

Paradoxically, through accepting the reality of abuse in organisations, trainers can learn the humbling and salutary lessons within their organisations rather than passing on their group pathology to the graduates. This learning could include how to pay attention to the symptoms of abuse; what training structures can do to facilitate their recognition; how to provide a place for the painful working through of the experience; and helping potential students to know what to watch out for in a training.

In the chart that follows I have used cult phenomena as a mirror for organisational dysfunction. Cult organisations may seem to be too extreme an example to act as a mirror for the subtle levels of abuse that are perpetrated in training, yet pathology shows itself more clearly in extreme forms. Having seen the characteristics that lead to abuse within cults, we may more readily recognise the symptoms within our counselling and psychotherapy training organisations. I hope that the reader will recognise from the chart that elements of the cult phenomena, rather than the trappings of a full-blown cult, are prevalent in all organisations. It is the extent of the phenomena that is significant in whether or not the organisation is dysfunctional.

Research on cults seem to agree that there are four key characteristics to any group forming itself into a 'cult'. These are:

1. A closed system
2. Group conformity
3. Idealisation of the leader(s)
4. Scapegoating

I have added four other characteristics which, although less generally found, have a strong psychological dimension. These are:

5. Charismatic mission
6. Denial of shadow
7. Group narcissism
8. Secrets

As you examine the chart you may recognise characteristics within your own training organisation and you may have reactions to these recognitions. What is healthy to a degree may, when mixed with other characteristics, become a fanatical dogma that leads to disempowerment and abuse. While the chart analyses and separates different ingredients of what make an organisation dysfunctional, it should be remembered that it is the systemic whole that makes the organisation what it is.

I am aware that there are many aspects of this chart that might need further elucidation and that I have not suggested what sort of training structures might be put in place to recognise, contain and potentially transform group pathology. Yet I hope that I have provided something to chew on, and that it will help you come to your own conclusions about abuse in training.

Cult characteristics	Training organisation symptoms
A closed system	
A protective cocoon to shelter the family	*As training expands graduates become trainers.*
Enmeshment and incest	It is kept in the 'family'. Junior staff gain
Outside world filtered out	vicarious power through allegiance with
Outside influences e.g. from family are discouraged	founders/directors. Further training for staff is in-house, outside influence is minimised and the 'group-think' built. Outside trainers are devalued or brought in on the periphery so that they do not create dissonance or confusion for students.
	No boundaries between trainers and therapists.
	Therapists are graduates of the training and participate in the training and assessment of students. The students do not have a 'safe' space outside of the organisation to 'think' or voice disquiet/dissatisfaction.

(contd)

Cult characteristics	Training organisation symptoms

Group conformity

Ideology at variance with cultural norm	*Screening off of the 'wrong sort of person'*
Security provided through belonging	*through initial selection procedure*
to distinct group	*Group norms governed by implicit rules.*
Fear of disapproval of leader	Mysteriousness of process disempowers
Punitive measures	newcomers until they 'get it' or have been
Belief in the 'truth' of what is being	'got'. The trainers' skill is a manipulation.
taught without checking	Deviants humiliated in the group or
	assessed as unsuitable.
	Authority to give or withhold professional
	recognition gives trainers great power;
	moving the goalposts.
	Subjective assessment by trainers creates
	dangers of negative and positive counter-
	transference, e.g. favourites. Arbitrary
	judgements mean students cannot self-
	assess, and lose confidence in their own
	experience. They become alienated and
	dependent.

Idealisation

Charismatic leadership offers the	*Powerfully transforming experiences lead*
promise of fulfilling needs	*newcomers to idealise trainers.*
Sexual acting out	*Therapeutic work evokes the inner child*
High expectations can trap leader into	*and leads to projection and transference*
inflated role of supplying unmet	*on to trainers.*
dependency	If trainers do not acknowledge this uncon-
Leader denies their own limitation and	scious reality, it gets played out through
becomes inflated; no humility	their unconscious fantasies of power and
	healing – the charlatan.
	Students cannot afford the risk of negative
	parental projection with their professional
	investment at stake, so splitting off
	negative feelings or denying them.
	Founders/directors may not have been
	thoroughly trained themselves and avoid
	testing from outside authority.

Scapegoating

Coheres group around the exclusion	*Dissenters who are not silenced are*
of what is 'bad'	*expelled, carrying the split-off feelings,*
Fear in the group of being labelled 'bad'	*the shit, with them.*
	Resistance to group norms is labelled
	pathological, defensive and unprofes-
	sional, and student is expected to 'work
	through' their deviance. Individual group

(contd)

Cult characteristics	Training organisation symptoms
	members who do not 'shape up' are picked on by the trainer and group forces may be used to break down defences. This lack of respect often rationalised as necessary therapeutically.

Charismatic mission

The vision of the leader has a transpersonal perspective that is inspirational. It connects with the hopes and dreams of the followers. It offers a promise for which sacrifices have to be made. *The dream of a paradise restored* – a strong pull for those who feel lost	*Mission of the organisation often identified with charismatic persona of founders/directors.* The cost of carrying these projections may lead founders/ directors into denying their own human needs and thereby creating an atmosphere that is anti-feminine and not nourishing, but which focuses on striving. How can you put your own selfish needs first when the planet, society, new project, or accreditation meetings call? Exploitation of junior staff to work for nothing or of students to do menial community' tasks not connected to their training, e.g. cooking and washing for organisation is rationalized as part of further training. *The promise may pull on the students' unmet needs of their inner child – the 'orphan' hopes to have found home – but this may be a regressive move.*

Denial of shadow

Prevalent in spiritual groups seeking salvation Light-good/dark-bad split Abusive behaviour of leader rationalised as spiritually necessary for follower	*Shadow issues not addressed in training course yet they operate in organisation unrecognised.* Like Sparrow Hawk In Ursula LeGuin's *Earthsea Trilogy*, our shadow may enter in through the door of the training institute unnoticed in terms of our need for power. *Success can lead to arrogance and self-importance. The inferior, wounded side of trainers gets hidden as they attempt to live up to expectations of their new status.* Double-talk is prevalent, e.g. talking about vulnerability while being invulnerable.

(contd)

Cult characteristics	Training organisation symptoms

Group narcissism

Followers had narcissistic parents and, in seeking to be special, repeat pattern of deprivation and abuse	*Organisation fears testing itself outside and becomes more and more self-referring and self-absorbed.*
Failure to challenge superego rules and develop autonomy leads to regressive fantasies	The organisation creates a false-self with which to face the world that is blown up with inflated fantasies and fuelled by the importance staff and students give to their own activities.
The leader becomes God through a collapse of levels	Trainers and students mirror each others' narcissistic needs and protect each other from painful disconfirmation. The false-self becomes impervious to external criticism as a way of defending against the hollowness inside.
	Lack of differentiation within the organisation leads to an inflated organisational ego which subsumes the 'soul'.
	Founders/directors are often the focus of projected fantasies of omnipotence which they may accept as realistic confirmations.

Secrets

They help bind the group together – they are sworn to secrecy	*Secrets give power to those who know them and mark them off as the 'in' group within a hierarchy, excluding others.*
Family secrets are picked up unconsciously and acted out by the children. Family myths are created around these secrets and constellate in potentially destructive rules of behaviour	*Secrets give a rational base for paranoid defences against the loss of the secret to 'unbelievers'.*
	The secret can take on mystical properties of the organisational life-blood which if revealed through an act of betrayal would mean the death of the organisation. In fact it may shatter the false self of the organisation.

Index

abandonment of client by therapist, 98
academic issues, see training of therapists
accidental disclosure of information, 6
accidental receipt of information, 6
accuracy in publications, 220
Achilles, 223
administrative/ancillary staff, 122
   code of ethics and grievance procedure, 124
   collegial relationship, 125
   confidentiality, 122
   conversations
      about counselling and training, 124
      about people, 123–124
   emergencies, 125
   handling complaints, 124–125
   security of information
      spoken, 123
      written, 122–123
Allen, Woody, 268
American Psychological Association (APA)
   code of ethics, 145, 254
   copyright, 200
   ethical dilemmas, 3, 6, 13–16
ancillary staff, see administrative/ ancillary staff
Anderson, R., 258, 262, 272, 275, 277
Anderson, W.T., 71, 96
animism, 21
anomie v. invasion, 35–36

apartheid, xv, 105
Apollo, 223
appointments books, 123
Arendt, Hannah, 147
Asclepiades, 224
Asclepius, 223
assertiveness, 125
audit, 111
avowed v. enacted values, 54

Ball, S.J., 260
Barber, P., 259
Barfield, O., 264
Barkham, M., 226
Barrett, M., 272
Bauman, Z., xiii, xx, 20, 130–131
Becker, H.S., 273
Beitman, B.D., 229
Benson, Lord, 242
Bergson, H., 238, 239
Berman, J.S., 188
Berne, E., 237, 238
Bersoff, D.N., 222
betrayal v. reductionism, 31–33
Better Regulation Task Force, 244
bias, and judicial review, 245–246
bibles v. illiteracy, 36–38
bibliographies, 213
Bond, Tim, 114, 146, 255
Bor, R., 264
boundaries of therapeutic relationship, 89–90, 161
Bowlby, John, 228
brainstorming, 211

311

Braud, W., 258, 272, 277
British Association for Counselling
    (BAC)
  code of ethics, 113, 114, 124
  collegial working relationships,
    141, 142
    libel, slander and defamation,
    151–152
  complaints, 113
  death of a therapist, 168, 171
  plagiarism, 205, 206
  supervision, 154, 158, 161, 173,
    177–182
British Association for Psychoanalytic
    and Psychodynamic Supervision
    (BAPPS), 154
British Confederation of
    Psychotherapists (BCP)
  collegial working relationships,
    141
  organisation of professions, 187
  training and organisational
    contexts, 2, 183
British Psychological Society (BPS)
  collegial working relationships,
    132, 141, 142
    libel, slander and defamation,
    150–151
  ethical dilemmas, 1–2, 3, 6, 13–16
  integrative relational research 272
  judicial review, 260
  organisation of professions,
    186–187
  plagiarism, 206
  presidential addresses, 1
  regulation of therapists, 16
  supervision, 177–182
  training and organisational
    contexts, 183
Brown, L.S., xviii, 257–258, 281–282
Brown, M.T., 174
Bruner, E.M., 271, 274
Bulger, James, 73
bystanding, 57, 61, 260
  definitions, 62, 73
  motivations for, 62
  neutrality myth, 57, 63–71
  power of, 63
  rationalisations for, 62–63
  v. responsible involvement, 73–74

Canadian Psychological Association, 1

case studies
  asking the client's permission, 107,
    112, 212
    caveats, 112
    examples, 108–109
    issues, 109–110
    suggested practice, 111
  dual relationships, 86
  publishing, 211–212
changing therapists, 92–93
charging contracts, 9
charismatic mission, 309
child abuse, 5–6
Chiron, 223
Christ, Jesus, 223
Clandinin, D.J., 259, 264–265, 267
Clarkson, P.
  integrative relational research, 265
  judicial review, 247
  physis, 240
  relationship, therapeutic, 29–30,
    118–119
closed system, 307
clubs v. professions, 246–247, 248
codes of ethics, xvi, 1–2
  administrative/ancillary staff, 122,
    123, 124
  collegial working relationships,
    126–127, 135, 136, 138–139,
    141–146
    libel, slander and defamation,
    150–152
  death of therapist, 168, 171
  dual relationships, 75
  integrative relational research,
    257–258
  v. oaths, 17–18
  plagiarism, 205–207
  for publications, 219–221
  spirit of the law, 113–114
    communication implies value
    judgement, 115
    conflicting demands, 114–115
    prioritising the therapeutic
    relationship, 120–121
    protection of counsellor,
    119–120
    relationship, basic assumption,
    117–119
    value-free counselling, 115–117
  supervision, 164
coercion v. defensiveness, 28–31

colleagues' conduct
   ethical dilemmas, 8–9, 13–14,
      128–138
   supervision, 166
collegial working relationships
   administrative/ancillary staff, 125
   libel, slander and defamation,
      150–152
   research findings, 126–137
   self-regulation, 137–148
   writing, 208–209
Colley, A., 1, 255
Collis, W., 245
collusion, 141, 142
competence issues
   ethical dilemmas, 9, 12, 13–14,
      131–132, 144
   publication, 220–221
   supervision, 182
   training, 183–185
complaints and grievances
   administrative/ancillary staff,
      124–125
   collegial working relationships,
      129, 137, 138–141, 144–145
   ineffectiveness, 187–188
   integrative relational research, 257
   thought experiments and imagi-
      nary dilemmas, 250–252
   see also self-regulation
confidentiality
   administrative/ancillary staff,
      122–124, 125
   case studies, asking client's permis-
      sion, 111
   collegial working relationships,
      132
   ethical dilemmas, 5–7, 13, 14, 15
   prospective clients, information
      for, 90–92, 95
   tape-recording training sessions, 95
   writing, 219
conflicts, professional, 9
Connelly, F.M., 259, 264–265, 267
consent, see informed consent
contracts, charging, 9
conversations
   about counselling and training,
      124
   about people, 123–124
copyright, 199–201
Copyright Act 1988, 201

Cornell, W., 76
Corney, R., 188
Cottone, R.R., xx
countertransference
   case studies, 109–110
   collegial working relationships,
      135
   dual relationships, 83
   integrative relational research, 266,
      269–271, 279
   supervision, 155, 160, 161, 163,
      179
   therapeutic relationship, 25, 31–33
   values, 54
   victim's vengeance, 102
Craddock Jones, Ann, 207
Crone, T., 152, 200, 201
cult organisations, 306–310
cultural differences
   ethical dilemmas, 12–13
   supervision, 174–177
   training and organisational
      contexts, 185–186
   values, 55
   see also ethnicity issues

Dalton, Clare, 232
Daniel, 223
Data Protection Act, 123
death in therapist's family, 166
death of therapist
   case studies, 112
   discussion issues, 171–172
   ethics, 171
   organisational management of, 186
   plagiarism, 202–203
   practicalities, 170–171
   psychotherapeutic executor's role,
      168–170
decision-making hierarchy, 41–43,
      45–47
   sample dilemmas, 43–45
defamation, 137, 150–152
defensiveness v. coercion, 28–31
defensive psychotherapy, xviii, 56, 86,
      179–180
   emergence, 98–100
delayed (recovered) memory,
      101–102, 182
Demeter, 223
Denzin, N.K., 263, 267, 272–274, 275
dependency v. deprivation, 33–35

Deurzen-Smith, E. van, 203
developmentally needed relationship, 26
    dependency v. deprivation, 33–35
    integrative relational research, 266, 271–273, 280
diakonia, 272
Diamond, N., 127
dilemmas, ethical, 1–2
    psychotherapists v. psychologists, 13–16
    research study, 2–13
disabilities, counsellors with, 114, 175
discretionary ethical principles, xvii
Dominicans, 224
Dostoevsky, Fedor, 68, 229
Douglas, J.D., 273
Douglass, B.G., 273
Dryden, Windy, 225, 258–259
dual relationships, 75–76
    clients in training, 79–82
    clients not in training, 82–86
    ethical dilemmas, 7–8, 13–14, 133
    prospective clients, information for, 89–95
    recommendations, 86–87
    supervision, 181
    ubiquity, 76–79, 118–119
Durlak, J.A., 188

education, see training of therapists
Eiser, J.R., 268
Eliot, T.S., 199
Elkin, I., 226
Elliot, R., 231
Ellis, M.V., 175–176
emergencies, 93, 125
emotional discourse domain, 194
enacted v. avowed values, 54
entanglement theory, 27
equal opportunities for publication, 220
Erickson, Milton, 25
Eros, 237–238
ethnicity issues
    conflicting demands, 114
    relationship, therapeutic, 30
    supervision, 158–159, 164–165
    see also cultural differences
European Association for Psychotherapy, 154

European Federation of Professional Psychologists Associations (EFPPA), 1
executor, psychotherapeutic
    plagiarism, 202–203
    role, 168–171
exorcism, 223–224
Eysenck, H.J., 188, 226

facilitators, collegial working relationships, 145
fairness issues, case studies, 110
family therapy, 30
Farrell, B.A., 56, 230
fear in supervision, 179–181
Feltham, C., 188
feminist ways of research, 274
Ferenczi, 77
Feyerabend, P., 278
Feynman, Richard, 279
Fiedler, F.E., 22
financial issues
    charging contracts, 9
    prospective clients, information for, 94
    supervision, 181
    training, 188–189
Fine, M., 259, 276
Fletcher, J., 54
Fonagy, P., 226
Foster Report, 244
Foucault, Michel, 230, 275, 276
Fox, M., 56
Frank, J.B., 261, 262, 278
Frank, J.D., 69, 222, 261, 262, 278
Freud, Sigmund, 224–225
    bystanding, 66
    dual relationships, 77
    physis, 237
    relationship, therapeutic, 25
    transference, 279
    values, 49, 54, 115
Friedson, E., 126–127
friendship, 188
    and supervision, 159–160
Fry, Marianne, x–xii, 261
full hearing, judicial review, 245
fundamental ethical principles, xvii

Galen, 224
Galileo Galilei, 37

Garcia Lorca, F., 277
Gawthop, J.C., 146
Gee, H., 25, 259
Gelso, C.J., 269–270
General Medical Council (GMC),
    186–187
general practitioners (GPs), 6
Genovese, Kitty, 73
Gergen, K.J., 263
Gergen, M.M., 263, 265, 268, 273
Gestalt Psychotherapy Training
    Institute (GPTI), 151, 168, 171
Goodman, Paul, 66
Goodwin, Brian, 24, 239, 240, 278
Goulding, Mary M., xxi, 25
Goulding, R.L., 25
government regulation of
    psychotherapy, 244, 249
Greek mythology, 223
grievances, see complaints and griev-
    ances
group conformity, j308
group therapy, 90–91, 92, 94
Guba, E.G., 264
Guggenbühl-Craig, A., 61, 160

Haley, J., 30
Hariman, R., 206
Hartle, Jim, 266
Haskins, Lord, 244
Hattie, J.A., 188
Hauke, C., 26
Havel, V., 257
Hawthorne studies, 270
Hecate, 223
Heidegger, M., 189
Heine, R.W., 22
Hekman, S.J., 1, 256, 274
Helman, C.G., 230
Heraclitus, 209, 240
Hercules, 223
Hermes, 223
heuristics, 254, 255, 273
hierarchy of decision-making, 41–43,
    45–47
    sample dilemmas, 43–45
Hillman, James, 20, 56, 63, 305
Hinshelwood, R., 26, 265
Hippocrates, 32, 224
Hippocratic oath, 21, 117
Hoffman, Lord, 246

honesty in publication, 220
Howarth, 29

idealisation, 308
illness of therapist, 112
inappropriate disclosure, 9
incompetence, see competence issues
infantilisation, 67–68
informed consent
    confidentiality issues, 6
    integrative relational research, 268
    for publication, 220
    values, 55, 116
    working alliance, 29
Institute for Transactional Analysis
    (ITA), 151, 168, 171
Institute of Management Consultants
    xix
institutional issues, 182–183
    collegial working relationships,
        134–135
    complaints procedures, ineffective,
        187–188
    cultural and difference issues,
        185–186
    death of psychotherapist, 186
    dysfunctions, 305–310
    ethical dilemmas, 196–197
    financial concerns, 181, 188–189
    organisation of professions,
        186–187
    supervision, 164–165
integrative psychotherapy, 225
    relational research, 253–262,
        281–282
        five kinds of relationship,
            264–280
        method, 262–264
interpreters, 6
invasion v. anomie, 35–36
Irish Psychological Society, 1
isolation v. over-intimacy, 35–36

Jager, B., 253
Jason, 223
judicial review of self-regulation,
    242–246, 249, 260
    club v. profession, 246–247
    UKCP, 139, 187, 246, 247–249,
        260–261
Jung, Carl, xiv, 233, 237

Kant, Immanuel, 1
Kaplan, J., 260
Keter, Vincent, 248
Kidder, L.H., 276
Kiesler, D.J., 259
Kitching, Andrew, 202–203
Kitzinger, C., 78
Klein, Melanie
    dual relationships, 76, 84
    rescuers attacked by victims, 104
    values, 54
Kleinman, A., 230
Knapp, S., 176
Koestler, A., 37
Koocher, G.P., 258
Korman, M., 13
Kottler, J.A., 82, 84
Kvale, S., 66, 71, 266

Ladany, N., 175–176
Laing, Ronnie, 305
Landrum Brown, J., 174
lateral violence, 105
Leahey, T.H., 64
leave stage, judicial review, 245
legal issues, supervision, 164
Leith, W., 103–104
Lerman, H., 258
libel, 137, 150–152
Lincoln, Y.S., 263, 272–274, 275
Lindsay, G., 1, 255
Little, M., 32
Lloyd, A.P., 66, 78
Lofland, J., 276
Lofland, L., 276
Lunt, I., 141, 243–244, 249
Lyotard, J-F., 230–231

Macdonald, K., 247
MacIntyre, A., 48
Mahrer, Alvin R., 98, 207, 259
Malcolm, J., 77
Mangold, R., 254
manipulation charge against
    psychotherapy, 66
Marsella, A.J., 12
Martin, E.A., 152
Marzillier, J., 139
Maslow, A.H., 278
Masson, J.M., 56, 66

Maturana, H.R., 195, 266
May, R., 25
McCarthy, John, 24
McLennan, J., 188
McLeod, J., 261, 267, 272
media, 6
mediation, collegial working relation-
    ships, 145, 146
Merleau-Ponty, M., 35, 193, 276
meta-methodology, 228
Metanoia Psychotherapy Training
    Institute, 168, 200, 201–202
Milan School, 30
Milgram experiments, 62, 191, 270
Miller, A., 103
Miller, H., 70, 217
mind control, 98
Moiso, C., 25
Moodley, R., 262
moral rights, 201–202
Moreno, J.L., 225
    social engagement, 66, 115
    values, 50, 54
Morrow-Bradley, C., 231
Mothersole, Geoff, 248
Moustakas, C., 254, 255, 273, 276
Murray, G., 238, 239, 240

Nadirshaw, Z., 185
narcissism
    and bystanding, 67
    group, 310
Nebuchadnezzar, 223
Neufeldt, S.A., 176
neutrality and bystanding, 57, 63–71
Newton, R.R., 263
nominative discourse domain,
    193–194
normative discourse domain, 192
Norton, N.C., 188

oaths, 17–18
    Hippocratic, 21, 117
    psychotherapy and counselling,
        18–19
Obholzer, 242
O'Donohue, W., 254
Old Testament, 223
Olivier, G., 56
Oppenheimer, Robert, 268

organisational issues, see institutional
        issues
organisation of profession, 186–187
over-intimacy v. isolation, 35–36

Palmer Barnes, F., 136, 140, 142, 143,
        146, 187
Paracelsus, 29
Pavlov, Ivan, 49, 224–225
pecuniary bias, and judicial review,
        246
Pedersen, P.B., 12
permission for case study, 107, 112
        caveats, 112
        examples, 108–109
        issues, 109–110
        suggested practice, 111
Persephone, 223
person-to-person relationship, 26
        integrative relational research, 266,
                273–276, 280
        invasion v. anomie, 35–36
philosophy, 146, 229
physiological discourse domain, 194
physis, 237–241
        writing, 209
Pilgrim, D., 258
Pinel, Philippe, 63, 224
plagiarism, 202–204, 205–206
Plato, 21–22
political exploitation of clients, 81
Polkinghorne, D.E., 225
Polster, E., 25
Polster, M., 25
Polyani, M., 262
Pope, K.S., 133, 139, 176
Popper, K., 135
Porter, N., 258
prerogative units, 244–245
Prevention of Professional Abuse
        Network (POPAN), 75, 139, 187,
        243, 257
Prioleau, L., 23
prioritising the therapeutic relation-
        ship, 120–121
privacy, therapist's invaded by client,
        104
professional conduct guidelines for
        prospective clients, 92–94
professional conflicts, 9
professionalisation rhetoric, 69–70

professionalism and case studies, 110
professions v. clubs, 246–247, 248
prospective clients, information for,
        89, 94, 289–304
        confidentiality, 90–91
                and outside relationships, 91–92
        creating space for growth and
                change, 92
        practical details, 94
        professional conduct guidelines,
                92–94
        protection of boundaries, 89–90
        tape-recording sessions, example
                letter for, 95
Psychologist Act, 16
Psychotherapists and Counsellors for
        Social Responsibility, 66
public opinion, 99

qualified privilege, 152

race, see ethnicity issues
racism, 164–165
rational discourse domain, 192
re-accreditation, 111
reactive countertransference, 109
Reason, P., 266
recovered memory, 101–102, 182
reductionism v. betrayal, 31–33
references, text, 213–214, 220
referrals, 9
reflection, 135
regulation of psychotherapists, 16
        see also self-regulation
relationships, ethical, 20–24
        basic assumption, 117–119
        five therapeutic relationships,
                24–38
        physis, 239–240
religion
        psychology as, 64
        transpersonal relationship, 36–38
reparative/developmentally needed
        relationship, 26
        dependency v. deprivation, 33–35
        integrative relational research, 266,
                271–273, 280
reputation, professional, 132, 144,
        150–152
rescuers attacked by victims, 103–104
research, integrative relational,

253–262, 281–282
five kinds of relationship, 264–280
method, 262–264
research relationship
objective aspects, 267–269, 279
projective aspect, 269–271, 279
reparative aspect, 271–273, 280
subjective aspect, 273–276, 280
transformative aspect, 276–279,
280
Rield, Rupert, 96
Rilke, Rainer Maria, 288
risk behaviour, 6
Roth, A., 226
Rowan, J., 266, 276–277
Rudestam, K.E., 263
Rumi, J., 277
Russell, R., 227
Ryle, Gilbert, 232

Salmon, 260
Samaritans, 93
Samuels, Andrew, xxi, 56, 66, 68, 115,
158
Sarason, S.B., 259
scapegoating, 308–309
Schaffer, Annie, 305
Schindler's List, 63
scholarship, 204–205
schoolism, 222–224, 232–233
contemporary situation, 225–227
first three 20th century 'schools' ,
224–225
privileging of theory, 227–229
reasons/rationalisations for,
229–232
Sechehaye, M., 77–78
secrets, 310
security
of spoken information, 123
of written information, 122–123
self-doubt, 135
self-regulation, 242–244, 249
collegial duty as principle of,
137–148
government, 244
judicial review, 139, 187, 244–249
seven domains of discourse, 191–195
supervision, training and organisations, 195–198
Severin, F.T., xvi, 67
sexual issues

abuse by clients, 5–6
abuse of clients by therapist, 97
ethical dilemmas, 9–11, 13–15
group therapy, 92
prospective clients, information
for, 92, 93
relationships with clients
bystanding, 65
ethical dilemmas, 7, 9–10, 11,
132, 139, 144
relationships with students, 132,
139, 144
values, 117
victim's vengeance, 104
shadow denial, 309
Shapiro, D.A., 226
Shapiro, M.K., 50
Shelef, L.O., 262
Shotter, J., 228
Silverman, D., 230
Simmer, S., 204–205, 213, 215
Simons, H.W., 69, 113
Skynner, R., 182
Slade, Peter, 65, 141, 243, 249
slander, 137, 150–152
Smith, J.A., 257, 263, 268
Smith, M.L., 69
Smuts, J.C., xv
social relationships between clients, 8
society and supervision, 158–159
social relationships with clients, 7–8
socioeconomic issues, 30
solitary confinement, 24
Solzhenitsyn, A., xxvi
spirituality, 36–38
spoken information, 123–124
Steedman, P.H., 253
Steiner, C., 66
Stern, Itzhak, 63
Stewart, I., 232
Stone, A.S., 145
Stone, M.H., 77
Styles, Joseph, 276
suggestion boxes, 124
suicidal patients, xviii
supervision, 173–174
appreciation of ethical complexities, 179
case studies, asking permission for,
110, 111
competency issues, 182
confidentiality issues, 91–92

conflicts, 114, 159–162
culture, 174–177
ethical dilemmas, 11–12, 178–179,
    195–198
fear, 179–181
financial concerns, individual and
    organisational, 181
map, 155–159
organisational contexts, 164–165
recovered memory, 182
requirements, 114
responsibilities of supervisor,
    162–164
    professional, 165–166
theory and practice, 154–155
Szapocznik, J., 13
Szasz, T., xviii, 142, 188

Tantam, D., 228
tape-recording sessions
    defensive therapy, 100, 179–180
    prospective clients, information
        for, 91–92
Tarasoff case, 97
Taylor, H., xvi
teachers, protection of, 120
temptation, 118
termination of therapy, 168–169
    financial concerns, 181
    see also death of therapist
Thanatos, 237–238
theoretical approach to therapy,
    22–23, 227–229
    see also schoolism
theoretical discourse domain,
    192–193
Thompson, A., 136, 137–138, 140,
    143, 145
time management, 207–208
touching
    appropriate, 86, 100
    inappropriate, 93
        see also sexual issues
    in supervision, 157
    truth, perspectives on, 98
training of therapists, 2, 182–183
    case studies, asking permission for,
        111
    conflicting demands, 114
    cultural and difference issues,
        185–186
    dual relationships, 79–82

dysfunction, 305–310
ethical dilemmas, 11–12, 13–14,
    195–198
incompetence, 183–185
organisation of professions,
    186–187
supervision, 161–163
tape-recording of sessions, 95
validity, 188–189
transference
    case studies, 109, 110
    dual relationships, 83
    Freud on, 279
    integrative relational research, 266,
        269–271, 279
    supervision, 160, 161, 163
    theory, xx, 25
    therapeutic relationship, 25
    truth, perspectives on, 98
    values, 55
    victim's vengeance, 102–103,
        119–120
transpersonal discourse domain, 195
transpersonal relationship, 26
    bibles v. illiteracy, 36–38
    integrative relational research, 266,
        276–279, 280
Traynor, Barbara, 202–203
triangulation, 263
truth, perspectives on, 96–98

Uhleman, M.R., 146
Ulichny, P., 259
United Kingdom Council for
    Psychotherapy (UKCP)
    bystanding, 65
    codes of ethics, 114, 119
    collegial working relationships,
        127–137, 141
    libel, slander and defamation,
        151
    complaints, 113, 257
    ethical dilemmas, 2–16
    organisational context, 183
    organisation of professions, 187
    plagiarism, 206
    self-regulation, 243, 244
    judicial review, 139, 187, 246,
        247–249, 260–261
    supervision, 177–182
    training, 2, 183
    truth, perspectives on, 98

values, 51
unprofessionalism, 9

values, 48–49
  avowed, 54
  and communication, 115
  discovering your own, 59–60
  enacted, 54
  heritages, 49–50
  imposition of, 55–57
  integrative relational research, 274
  prospective clients, information
      for, 93
  psychology as value-free science,
      50–52
  ubiquity, 52–53, 115–118
VandeCreek, L., 176
Varela, F.J., 266
Ventural, M., 20, 56, 63
Vetere, A., 2
Vetter, V.A., 176
victim's vengeance, 119–120
  defensive psychotherapy,
      emergence, 98–100
  displaced, 104–105
  reasons for, 101–102
  reality consequences, 102–103
  on rescuers, 103–104
  transference aspects, 102
  truth, perspectives, 96–98
Voster, John, xx
voyeurism, 108

Walden, B., 69–70
Watkins, C.E., 230

Watkins, Edward, 176
Watkins, J.G., 98
Watson, John, 64
Watts, M., 264
Weigert, A., 69, 113
Weldon, Fay, 63, 98
Wertz, F.J., 275
Whyte, C.R., 65
wills, 169–170
Witmer, 224
Wittgenstein, L., 204, 233, 240–241,
      279
Wolman, B.B., 273
working alliance, 25
  coercion v. defensiveness, 28–31
  integrative relational research, 266,
      267–269, 279
writing, 199, 217
  codes of ethics, 205–207, 219–221
  copyright, 199–201
  dual relationships, 85–86
  mistaken assumptions, 207–208
  moral rights, 201–202
  plagiarism, 202–204
  process, 209–217
  reasons for, 208–209
  scholarship, 204–205
written information, security of
  administrative/ancillary staff,
      122–123
  death of therapist, 169, 170
Wundt, Wilhelm, Max, 224

Ziegler, A., xx

Printed and bound by CPI Group (UK) Ltd, Croydon, CR0 4YY

09/06/2025

14685982-0002